SPONTANEOUS HEALING

SPONTANEOUS HEALING

*How to Discover and Enhance
Your Body's Natural Ability to
Maintain and Heal Itself*

ANDREW WEIL, M.D.

Fawcett Columbine   NEW YORK

A Fawcett Columbine Book
Published by Ballantine Books

Copyright © 1995 by Andrew Weil, M.D.

All rights reserved under International and Pan-American Copyright Conventions. Published in the United States by Ballantine Books, a division of Random House, Inc., New York, and simultaneously in Canada by Random House of Canada Limited, Toronto.

This edition published by arrangement with Alfred A. Knopf, Inc.

Library of Congress Catalog Card Number: 96-96016

ISBN: 0-449-91064-4

Cover photo by Curt Richter

Manufactured in the United States of America

First Ballantine Books Edition: May 1996

20   19   18   17   16   15   14   13   12

For Diana

CONTENTS

II. OPTIMIZING THE HEALING SYSTEM

III. IF YOU GET SICK

SPONTANEOUS
HEALING

INTRODUCTION

A MAN WHOSE lungs are filled with cancer is sent home to die, having been told that medicine can do nothing for him. Six months later he reappears in his doctor's office, tumor free. A young woman—diabetic, a heavy smoker—lies unconscious in a coronary care unit following a bad heart attack. Her doctor anguishes over the fact that her cardiac function is rapidly declining and he is powerless to save her. But the next morning she is awake and talking, clearly on the way to recovery. A neurosurgeon tells grieving parents that their son, who is in a coma following a motorcycle accident and severe head injury, will never regain consciousness. The son is now fine.

Most doctors I know have one or two stories of this sort, stories of spontaneous healing. You will uncover many more of them if you seek them out, yet few medical researchers do. To most doctors, the stories are just stories, not taken seriously, not studied, not looked to as sources of information about the body's potential to repair itself.

Meanwhile, modern medicine has become so expensive that it is straining the economies of many developed nations and putting itself beyond the reach of much of the world's population. In many countries politicians argue about how to pay for health care, unaware that a philosophical debate about the very nature of health care has been ongoing throughout history. Doctors believe that health requires outside intervention of one sort or another, while proponents of natural hygiene maintain that health results from living in harmony with natural law. In ancient Greece, doctors worked under the patronage of

Asklepios, the god of medicine, but healers served Asklepios's daughter, the radiant Hygeia, goddess of health. Medical writer and philosopher René Dubos has written:

> For the worshippers of Hygeia, health is the natural order of things, a positive attribute to which men are entitled if they govern their lives wisely. According to them, the most important function of medicine is to discover and teach the natural laws which will ensure a man a healthy mind in a healthy body. More skeptical, or wiser in the ways of the world, the followers of Asklepios believe that the chief role of the physician is to treat disease, to restore health by correcting any imperfections caused by accidents of birth or life.

Political debates about how to cover the costs of medical care mostly take place among followers of Asklepios. There has been no argument about the nature of medicine or people's expectations of it, only about who is going to pay for its services, which have become inordinately expensive because of doctors' reliance on technology. I am a dedicated follower of Hygeia and want to interject that viewpoint into any discussions of the future of medicine.

Let me give an example of how these different philosophies lead to very different courses of action. In the West, a major focus of scientific medicine has been the identification of external agents of disease and the development of weapons against them. An outstanding success in the middle of this century was the discovery of antibiotics and, with that, great victories against infectious diseases caused by bacteria. This success was a major factor in winning hearts and minds over to the Asklepian side, convincing most people that medical intervention with the products of technology was worth it, no matter the cost. In the East, especially in China, medicine has had a quite different focus. It has explored ways of increasing internal resistance to disease so that, no matter what harmful influences you are exposed to, you can remain healthy—a Hygeian strategy. In their explorations Chinese doctors have discovered many natural substances that have such tonic effects on the body. Although the Western approach has served us well for a number of years, its long-term usefulness may not be nearly so great as the Eastern one.

Weapons are dangerous. They may backfire, causing injury to the user, and they may also stimulate greater aggression on the part of the enemy. In fact, infectious-disease specialists throughout the world are now wringing their hands over the possibility of untreatable plagues of resistant organisms. Just today I received a copy of *Clinical Research News for Arizona Physicians,* a publication of the university medical center where I teach, that featured an article on "Resistance to Antimicrobial Agents: The New Plague?" It reads in part:

> While antimicrobial agents have been considered the "wonder drugs" of the 20th century, clinicians and researchers are now acutely aware that microbial resistance to drugs has become a major clinical problem. . . . A variety of solutions have been proposed. The pharmaceutical industry is attempting to develop new agents that are less susceptible to current resistance mechanisms. Unfortunately, the organisms appear to rapidly develop new resistance mechanisms. . . . In the inpatient setting, strict adherence to infection control procedures is essential. Health care workers need to understand that antimicrobial resistance is an accelerating problem *in all practice settings* that can directly compromise patient outcomes.

The phrase "can directly compromise patient outcomes" is euphemistic. It means patients will die of infections that doctors formerly could treat with antibiotics. In fact, antibiotics are rapidly losing their power, and some infectious-disease specialists are beginning to think about what we will do when we can no longer rely on them. We might have to revert to methods used in hospitals in the 1920s and 1930s before there were antibiotics: strict quarantine and disinfection, surgical drainage, and so forth. What a reversal that will be for technological medicine!

Meanwhile, resistance does not develop to the tonics of Chinese medicine, because they are not acting *against* germs (and do not therefore influence their evolution) but rather are acting *with* the body's defenses. They increase activity and efficiency of cells of the immune system, helping patients resist all kinds of infections, not just those caused by bacteria. Antibiotics are only effective against bacteria; they are of no use in diseases caused by viruses. Western medicine's powerlessness against viral infections is clearly visible in its ineffectiveness against AIDS. Chinese herbal therapy for people infected with HIV looks much more promising. It is nontoxic, in great contrast to the Western antiviral drugs in current use, and may enable many of those with HIV infection to have relatively long, symptom-free lives, even though the virus remains in their bodies.

The Eastern concept of strengthening internal defenses is Hygeian, because it assumes that the body has a natural ability to resist and deal with agents of disease. If that assumption were more prominent in Western medicine, we would not now have an economic crisis in health care, because methods that take advantage of the body's natural healing abilities are far cheaper than the intensive interventions of technological medicine, as well as safer and more effective over time.

Asklepians are most interested in treatment, while Hygeians are interested in healing. Treatment originates outside; healing comes from within. The word "healing" means "making whole"—that is, restoring integrity and balance. I have long been interested in stories about healing, and I assume you are too. Perhaps you know someone who experienced a spontaneous remission of cancer, in which widespread malignant disease disappeared, to the amazement of doctors in charge of the case. Maybe the disappearance was temporary or maybe it was permanent. What happened? Or perhaps you know someone who was healed by prayer or by religious fervor.

I have titled this book *Spontaneous Healing* because I want to call attention to the innate, intrinsic nature of the healing process. *Even when treatments are applied with successful outcomes, those outcomes represent activation of intrinsic healing mechanisms, which, under other circumstances, might operate without any outside stimulus.* The main theme of this book is very simple: The body can heal itself. It can do so because it has a healing system. If you are in good health, you will want to know about this system, because it is what keeps you in good health and because you can enhance that condition. If you or people you love are sick, you will want to know about this system, because it is the best hope for recovery.

Part One builds a case for the existence of a healing system and presents evidence for its operation, including its interactions with the mind. At every level of biological organization, from DNA up, mechanisms of self-diagnosis, self-repair, and regeneration exist in us, always ready to become active when the need arises. Medicine that takes advantage of these innate mechanisms of healing is more effective than medicine that simply suppresses symptoms. This section includes stories of people I have known who have recovered from illness, often in spite of the predictions of doctors who saw no possibility of recovery or insisted that improvement could occur only with a great deal of Asklepian effort. As I have made it known that I am interested in cases of this sort, I have found more and more of them, and I believe that anyone who looks will find others. Spontaneous healing is a common occurrence, not a rare event. We may marvel at stories of spontaneous remissions of cancer but pay little attention to more commonplace activities of the healing system, such as the repair of wounds. In fact, it is the ordinary, day-to-day workings of the healing system that are most extraordinary.

Part Two of the book tells you how to optimize your healing system. You will find here specific information on modifying lifestyle to increase your healing potentials, including facts about food, environmental toxins, exercise, stress reduction, vitamins, supplements, and tonic herbs that can help you maintain your well-being. I will also suggest an eight-week program for gradually changing lifestyle in a manner that will enhance your natural healing power.

Part Three gives advice on managing illness. It analyzes the strengths and weaknesses of conventional and alternative treatments and identifies a number of strategies used by successful patients. I give suggestions here for using natural methods to ameliorate common kinds of illnesses and also include a chapter on "Cancer as a Special Case," because that disease poses a unique challenge to the healing system, and the selection of treatments for it requires careful analysis of each individual's condition. An afterword, "Prescriptions for Society," considers how existing medical institutions would have to change to accommodate Hygeian philosophy.

Until now few doctors and scientists have looked for examples of healing; therefore, it is not surprising that the phenomenon of spontaneous healing seems obscure and the concept of an internal healing system odd. I contend that the more we embrace that concept, the more we will experience healing in our lives, and the less reason we will have to use medical interventions that are unnecessary, sometimes damaging, and consume so much money. Healing-oriented medicine would serve us much better than the present system, since it would be safer and surer as well as cheaper. I have written this book in an effort to help bring it into existence.

PART ONE

THE HEALING
SYSTEM

1

PROLOGUE IN
THE RAIN FOREST

LET ME TAKE YOU with me to a faraway place I visited more than twenty years ago: the sandy bank of a wide river on a sultry afternoon in 1972. The river was a tributary of the Río Caquetá in the northwest Amazon, near the common border of Colombia and Ecuador, and I was lost. I was searching for a shaman, a Kofán Indian named Pedro, who lived in a remote hut somewhere in the huge, dense forest, but the trail that was supposed to take me there left me at an uncrossable river with no sign of how to proceed. It was getting late in the day.

Two days before, after a long, hard drive, I left my Land-Rover at the end of a dirt road and took a motorboat to a tiny frontier settlement, where I spent a restless night. The next day, I found some Indians who took me by canoe to the beginning of a trail they said would eventually bring me to the clearing where Pedro lived. "Half a day's walk," they told me, but I knew that half a day's walk for an Indian might be more for me. I had a backpack with essentials, but not much food, since I expected to be staying with the shaman. After several hours in dark forest, the trail forked. No one had said anything about a fork. I listened for the whisper of intuition and decided to go to the right. After another hour I came upon a clearing with several huts and five Kofán men painting each other's faces.

I was terribly hot and thirsty and asked in Spanish for water. The men ignored me. I asked again. They said they had no water. "No water?!" I exclaimed. "How can that be?" They shrugged and continued to apply their makeup. I asked for the shaman. "Not here," said one of the Indians. "Where can I find him?" There was an offhanded indication of a trail beyond the huts. "Is it far?" I asked. Another shrug.

This was a new experience for me. In the hinterlands of Colombia I had always found Indians to be exceedingly hospitable. It was the inhabitants of the rough frontier towns, the mestizo fortune hunters, who were unfriendly and intimidating. Once I passed through them to Indian territory, I always felt safe, assured that the native people would take in a stranger, help him find his destination, and certainly give water to a thirsty traveler.

The five Kofán men were young, handsome, and, obviously, vain. They wore simple cotton tunics, had long, glossy, black hair, and were intently devoted to their cosmetic art. After one would apply new markings to forehead or cheek, the recipient would spend long minutes evaluating the additions in a broken piece of mirrored glass, grunting approval or requesting further embellishment. This was clearly going to take all afternoon. My presence held not the slightest interest for them, and after half an hour of being ignored, I put on my pack and continued down the trail, until, several hours later, it disappeared in a dense thicket at the edge of the big river, leaving me stranded.

It was strikingly beautiful there, although I was inclined to view the river and forest more as obstacles than as sources of sensory pleasure. Big, billowy cumulus clouds floated above the canopy of trees. The river was swift and clear. There was not a sign of human presence, no sounds except those of insects and birds. Were it not for the sandflies, small biting pests that are out in great numbers from dawn to dusk, I would not have minded camping there. I had a hammock and mosquito net in my pack and could have spent the night if necessary, but I felt anxious at the prospect of being lost, and discouraged by the fruitlessness of my quest.

This shaman, so difficult to reach, was said to be a powerful healer. In a year I spent wandering in South America, most of the shamans I met were disappointing. Some were drunks. Some were clearly out for fame and fortune. One, when he learned I was a doctor from Harvard, was interested only in persuading me to obtain for him a certificate from that institution testifying to his powers so that he could one-up his rivals. I had plenty of adventures during these travels, but in the end, none of them had taught me how to be a better doctor.

Pedro was my last hope. He was unknown to the outside world. I would be the first gringo to visit him, and I had high hopes that he would teach me the secrets of healing I had so long been searching for.

But now I was lost, and the brilliant Amazon sun was taking on the rich golden tones of the end of afternoon. Night would come quickly here, meaning surprising chilliness along the river and no chance of reaching a habitation. I'm not a smoker, but I lit up three cigarettes at once, Pielrojas ("Redskins"), the local cheap brand, with a picture of a North American Indian on the pack. I puffed on them and blew smoke all around me, hoping for the usual temporary relief tobacco smoke brings from biting sandflies.

When in doubt, eat. I broke into my meager stores and found a packet of cocoa mix and some dried fruit. I set up a little butane stove, boiled some river water, and soon was sipping the hot liquid, which never tasted better—a bit of comfort and familiarity in this, for me, strange environment.

I was in this remote part of South America because I was searching for something I believed to be exotic and extraordinary, something worlds away from my ordinary experience. I was looking for insight into the source of healing power, and the interconnectedness of magic, religion, and medicine. I wanted to understand how the mind interacts with the body. Above all, I hoped to learn practical secrets of helping people to get well. I had spent eight years in a prestigious institution of higher learning, four studying botany and four studying medicine, but I had found no clear answers to my questions. My botanical studies awakened a desire to see the rain forest, meet native practitioners, and help rescue fast-disappearing knowledge of medicinal plants. My medical training made me want to flee from the world of invasive, technological treatment toward a romantic ideal of natural healing.

Three years before, in 1969, when I finished my basic clinical training, I made a conscious decision not to practice the kind of medicine I had just learned. I did so for two reasons, one emotional and one logical. The first was simply a gut feeling that if I were sick, I would not want to be treated the way I had been taught to treat others, unless there were no alternative. That made me uncomfortable about treating others. The logical reason was that most of the treatments I had learned in four years at Harvard Medical School and one of internship did not get to the root of disease processes and promote healing but rather suppressed those processes or merely counteracted the visible symptoms of disease. I had learned almost nothing about health and its maintenance, about how to prevent illness—a great omission, because I have always believed that the primary function of doctors should be to teach people how *not* to get sick in the first place. The word "doctor" comes from the Latin word for "teacher." Teaching prevention should be primary; treatment of existing disease, secondary.

I am uneasy about the suppressive nature of conventional medicine. If you look at the names of the most popular categories of drugs in use today, you will find that most of them begin with the prefix "anti." We use antispasmodics and antihypertensives, antianxiety agents and antidepressants, antihistamines, antiarrhythmics, antitussives, antipyretics, and anti-inflammatories, as well as beta blockers and H_2-receptor antagonists. This is truly antimedicine—medicine that is, in essence, counteractive and suppressive.

What is wrong with that? you may ask. If a fever is in the danger zone, or an allergic reaction is out of control, of course those symptoms should be counteracted. I have no objection to use of these treatments *on a short-term basis for the management of very severe conditions*. But I came to realize, early in my hospital days, that if you rely on such measures as the main strategy for treating illness, you create two kinds of problems. First, you expose patients to risk, because, by their nature, pharmaceutical weapons are strong and toxic. Their desired effects are too often offset by side effects, by toxicity. Adverse reactions to the counteractive drugs of conventional medicine are a great black mark against the system, and I saw more than enough of them in my clinical training to know that there has to be a better way. Botanical medicine appealed to me because it offered the possibility of finding safe, natural alternatives to the drugs I had been taught to use.

The second problem, less visible but more worrisome, is the chance that over time suppressive treatments may actually strengthen disease processes instead of resolving them. This possibility did not occur to me until I read the writings of a great medical heretic, Samuel Hahnemann (1755–1843), the German prodigy and renegade physician who developed homeopathy, one of the major schools of alternative medicine. Homeopathy relies on very small doses of highly diluted remedies to catalyze healing responses. I am not a homeopath. I disagree strongly with the many homeopaths who oppose immunization and find the whole system puzzling as well as incompatible with current scientific models of physics and chemistry. Nonetheless, I have experienced and observed homeopathic cures and admire the system for its use of treatments that cannot harm. What is more, I find some of Hahnemann's ideas useful.

One of his most important teachings concerns the danger of suppressing visible symptoms of illness. Hahnemann used the example of an itching, red rash on the skin. Better to have disease on the surface of the body, he taught, because from the surface it can exit outward. Suppressive measures may drive a disease process inward toward more vital organs. The itching rash may disappear, but worse trouble may appear down the road, trouble that may resist the strongest suppressive treatments.

Hahnemann had this insight long before the discovery of corticosteroids, the very powerful anti-inflammatory hormones that conventional doctors now dispense without much thought for the harm they can do. Topical steroids are very effective suppressants of skin rashes and are now even sold over the counter in the United States. Again and again I see patients who become dependent on them. As long as they use the steroid creams and ointments, their rashes are held in check, but as soon as the treatment is stopped, the symptoms reappear more severely than before. The disease process is not resolved but merely held at bay, gathering power for renewed expression as soon as the outside, counteractive force is removed.

When steroids are given systemically, their suppressive power and toxicity is even greater. Patients who take drugs like prednisone for months or years to control rheumatoid arthritis, asthma, and other autoimmune and allergic disorders commonly suffer terrible toxicity (weight gain, depression, ulcers, cataracts, weakened bones, acne), but cannot stop taking the drugs because their symptoms will return in full force. What happens to the energies of such suppressed diseases? Where do they go?

My experience with patients confirms Hahnemann's warning. Recently I saw a woman in her mid-thirties who, two years before, had developed symptoms of a serious autoimmune disease: scleroderma. The disease began with episodes of painful blanching of the hands on exposure to cold. This is Raynaud's phenomenon, a sign of neurovascular instability that can exist by itself or herald deeper disturbances of nervous and circulatory function. In this case it was followed by joint pain and swelling of the fingers. Then the skin of her fingers and hands began to thicken and harden, the classic, visible manifestation of scleroderma (the word means "hard skin"). The hands of patients with advanced scleroderma are often cold, purplish, shiny, hard, and immobile, but this external change, while disfiguring, is not the worst effect of this disease. When scleroderma involves internal organs of the digestive and cardiorespiratory systems, it can kill.

Doctors quickly diagnosed the problem and started the patient on high doses of prednisone and other immunosuppressive drugs. She responded dramatically. Within a few months, her skin returned to normal, all joint pain disappeared, and her physician pronounced her to be "in complete remission." Unhappily, a year later she developed shortness of breath. X-rays revealed pulmonary fibrosis, a progressive disease in which normal lung tissue is replaced by abnormal fibrous tissue. She was told that this condition was not related to the previous scleroderma; but, in fact, pulmonary fibrosis is a well-known, albeit uncommon, manifestation of the same process, only in a much more vital area of the body and much more resistant to treatment. Her hands were warm, pink, and soft. There was no visible sign of disease on the surface of her body. Inside, however, she was being crippled by a disease in her lungs that now resisted all the counteractive power of conventional medicine.

By the time I completed my medical internship, I had seen enough variations on this theme to convince me that I did not want to practice conventional medicine or take any further training in it. I did not know what else to practice, however, and that uncertainty led me to undertake my present quest. But after two difficult years of searching, I had learned little about healing. Shortly before coming to Kofán territory I had concluded that I must not have made a sufficient effort to explore new terrain. The healers and shamans I had located were already discovered, too well known, too easy to find. What I was looking for must be still farther away, I thought, still harder to reach, more obscurely hidden in the Amazon forest.

And so there I was, cocoa finished, day coming to an end, lost.

I did eventually find Pedro the shaman, and I remember our meeting very well, even though it happened long ago, because it was a major turning point in my life. Of course, at the time I had no idea of its real significance, regarding it as just another in a long series of frustrations. In fact, it was the first step of a new path, one that would take me back to a place where I would discover what I had known all along but had been unable to recognize.

Having packed up my equipment and shouldered my pack, I noticed a sandbar a short distance upriver. I thought that from its vantage point, I might get a better view of the area and be able to make an educated guess as to the direction of Pedro's hut. I waded to the sandbar, and as I scanned the shore I spied what looked like a bit of trail farther upstream. It was. I got to it by walking just at the water's edge and, once on it, felt my anxieties melt away, even as the sun got low in the west. After forty-five minutes I came to a clearing where a small river entered the big one. At the junction, elevated on stilts, was a lone, thatched hut of ample size. I ran up to it just as the sky was blazing with the colors of a tropical sunset, and climbed a rude staircase up to a deck overlooking the confluence of the rivers.

There was no shaman in sight. The only inhabitant was a young Indian girl, who spoke Spanish hesitantly and looked at me as I might regard an extraterrestrial. She told me that Pedro was gone. He had left ten days ago and should have been back the day before. I asked if I could stay. She did not object, so I took off my pack and strung my hammock between two poles at the edge of the deck.

For the next four days and nights, I stayed mostly in my hammock, Pielroja cigarettes blazing in my fingers, watching the long, hot days pass into clear, starry nights. Occasionally I would brave the sandflies to go for an afternoon swim in the river. I tried, unsuccessfully, to engage the young woman of the house in conversation. And I sought refuge from the world of heat, humidity, blinding sun, and dense forest in a collection of Jack London's tales of the Far North that I had brought with me for just such a circumstance. It was an inspired choice, the perfect literary escape into a world with igloos, ice fields, and numbing cold. But sadly, it came to an end, so I reread it and reread it again.

There was one other diversion. Pedro had killed a jaguar shortly before he left. The jaguar had a young cub that was now in a cage in the house. It was appealingly cute and kittenish and wanted interaction. On one occasion I had it out of the cage and was playing with it on the floor until its play became too rough for me. I wanted it to stop, but my attempts to push the cub away and calm it down stimulated the wild-animal circuit in its brain. Suddenly it was no longer a cute kitten but a vicious hellcat. The Indian girl came at it with a broom and together we managed to get it back in its cage. I came away with nasty scratches and two good bites on my arms.

Then, one afternoon, Pedro appeared and greeted me matter-of-factly. He was a vigorous, solemn man in his early forties. I liked him at once, but he told me soon into our conversation that there would not be any point in my staying, because he had stopped practicing his profession. Instead of working as a healer, he had become a political activist and was trying to organize his fellow Kofán to fight a great threat to their way of life, the presence in their forest of "La Texas." This was the local name for Texaco, which had come to the northwest Amazon to exploit its rich reserves of oil. I had once stayed briefly in a frontier town that served as Texaco's base and was appalled by what I saw and heard: it was a center of noise, mud, fumes, thieves, whores, and roughnecks that was spreading devastation from its margins. But the town was hundreds of miles from this peaceful region, and I could not imagine how it impacted on Pedro's life.

He told me that the noise of Texaco's helicopters had driven game from the forest and that, at the same time, fish were disappearing from the rivers. Hunting and fishing had declined drastically in the past two years, which he blamed entirely on the oil explorations. All of his efforts were now going to collecting signatures on a petition demanding reparations from Texaco. He was sorry I had come such a long way for nothing. I was, too. At least, I now understood why Kofán men would not be hospitable to a gringo walking through their forest.

The next morning I left. Eventually I got back to my Land-Rover and left Kofán territory for good.

I was to spend another year wandering in Colombia, Ecuador, and Peru, but I never again made such an arduous journey in search of an exotic, magical healer. Instead I studied medicinal plants in Ecuador and Peru, learned about the cultivation and use of coca leaf, worked with a Colombian filmmaker to document the use of drug plants by shamans, and looked for unusual fruits, spices, and dyes. Although I did not admit it to myself consciously, on some level I realized that what I was searching for was not to be found in the wilds of Amazonia or any other exotic location. I remained as committed as ever to finding answers to my questions: What is the source of healing? What is the relationship between treatments and cures? How can doctors and patients access healing more of the time? What my search for Pedro taught me was that I was looking for answers in the wrong way, that I did not have to turn from my own land and culture, my formal education, and my own self to find the source of healing. But I did have to spend those years wandering in order to figure that out.

Almost a quarter of a century has passed since I left Pedro's hut at the junction of the two rivers. In that time the destruction of the rain forest caused by the removal of oil has reached levels that Pedro and his people could never have imagined. Road building, oil spills, the dumping of toxic chemicals into rivers, and a cynical disregard for native cultures by both national governments and foreign businesses have damaged vast areas of Colombia and Ecuador irreparably. Simply put, the Kofán people have been put out of business. They are finished, terminated, and any knowledge held by their wise elders and traditional healers is soon to be lost forever. Other tribes now face the same threat. Whether they can avoid the fate of the Kofán is uncertain.

The years have been much kinder to me. I found what I was looking for and more, found it much closer to home in ways both unexpected and satisfying.

THE FACES OF HEALING: KRISTIN

KRISTIN KILLOPS SHOULD not be alive today. Certainly she should not have children. Not only did her doctors send her home to die; they were quite clear that the treatments she received had destroyed her reproductive capacity.

Kristin's story begins with the appearance of unexplainable bruises on her body in 1974. She was nineteen and living with friends on the island of Maui in Hawaii. A doctor suggested she take iron supplements, but after two weeks without improvement, she underwent blood tests that yielded alarming results. All her blood counts were very low: red cells, white cells, and platelets. Platelets are the elements in blood responsible for clotting, and their low level was the cause of the bruising that attracted Kristin's attention. She was scheduled for a bone-marrow biopsy to determine why she lacked blood cells, and this result was even more ominous. Her marrow had almost no cells in it, only two percent of the normal number. The diagnosis was aplastic anemia—a medical calamity, because it represents loss of one of the body's most vital tissues, the source of all the formed elements of the blood. Kristin was evacuated to a Southern California hospital for full-scale technological intervention in an attempt to save her life.

The word "aplastic" means "without form"—a good description of a process that wipes out the normal components of bone marrow, leading to "empty marrow syndrome," in which there are empty spaces and fat where blood-forming cells should be. Bone marrow produces the red cells that carry oxygen, the various white cells that are central to the body's defenses, and the platelets. Normally, there is continuous production of all these elements, each one arising from its own ancestral cell line, maturing in stages, and finally migrating from the marrow cavity of large bones into the bloodstream. The ancestral cells themselves have a common ancestor called the stem cell, a "primitive," embryonic cell, native to the marrow, with the potential to differentiate into all other forms. Presumably, aplastic anemia results from failure of this stem cell, as a result of injury or suppression of some kind.

In Kristin's case, failure of bone marrow had no identifiable cause, but there was suspicion of a toxic exposure. Six other people on Maui developed marrow and blood abnormalities at the same time; all of them were dead within months. Such a cluster of cases suggests an environmental cause. Agricultural chemicals are used immoderately and carelessly in Hawaii, especially on the ubiquitous sugar cane and pineapple fields. Might these unfortunate people have had some genetic susceptibility to a pesticide or herbicide that entered their systems? We will never know.

Kristin arrived in Santa Barbara, California, desperately ill. Imagine the plight of someone with almost no functioning marrow. Severe depletion of red cells can damp down metabolism and stress the heart, which has to work harder to compensate for the low oxygen content of the blood. Deficiency of white cells knocks out resistance to infection. The hospital had to keep Kristin in a protective "reverse isolation" environment to minimize her contact with germs, as well as maintain her on antibiotics and give her daily washes with disinfectants. Absence of platelets creates the risk of abnormal bleeding, internally and externally.

Treatment of aplastic anemia requires drastic measures. Doctors often give high doses of steroids and other immunosuppressive drugs, which work in some cases but not others. Such treatment seems irrational, given the fact that the immune system is already crippled by the disappearance of its armies of white cells; but it is possible that some form of autoimmunity mediates the damage to the marrow, and steroids would suppress that. Maybe exposure to certain chemicals or viruses sets off an autoimmune reaction in which the immune system attacks marrow stem cells; the reaction then becomes self-perpetuating, independent of the triggering event.

Kristin's doctors began steroid treatment but thought she was too critically ill to survive. Instead they sent her to UCLA Medical Center in Los Angeles for a bone-marrow transplant. This operation may be the best hope for people with aplastic anemia, especially young people, who often respond well; but it is a major procedure, with uncertain results, limited by the availability of a suitable donor: preferably an identical twin or a sibling who is antigenically compatible. Luckily, Kristin had both a brother and a sister who matched and were willing to donate marrow, but she wanted to avoid the ordeal of a transplant. "I did many things to try to avoid it," she says, "including visualizations, meditation on healing, and taking a lot of vitamins and supplements. Then I found a healer to work on me, but it was just too late. The doctors gave me a firm deadline, and the healer did not have enough time to help me." Kristin received two bone-marrow transplants, but here she was not so lucky; her body rejected both of them. That was the medical profession's best shot. There was nothing else to offer her but general support and comfort. Her doctors had no hope.

Not so, Kristin. She was determined to find other sorts of treatments, and her inclination was to experiment with psychic healing and visualization. The hospital psychologist had referred her to a researcher at UCLA who studied psychic healing. Through him she found a healer who used hypnotherapy as well as the laying on of hands. While still hospitalized Kristin had two sessions a week with him for two weeks. At the end of that time, tests showed a modest increase in bone marrow, which her doctors told her was unheard of. But although her blood counts rose dramatically, they did not get high enough for her to escape isolation rooms, and she required transfusions. Finally, the doctors said they could do nothing more. After discussions with the patient and her mother, they discharged her from the hospital. Her mother understood that her daughter was being released so she could die at home.

Kristin persevered in her search for healers. She saw another who came five days a week to do the laying on of hands. After two weeks, results were again miraculous: blood counts rose and bordered on low normal. She hung on. Then she contracted serum hepatitis from the transfusions and became very ill, with a fever that remained over 100 degrees for a month.

She heard of a woman who could prescribe healing diets by psychic intuition. The diet prescribed for her was not easy to follow: no sugars or starches of any kind, two eggs and an extra yolk each day with steamed vegetables, vegetable broth and salad without oil, a little steamed fish or chicken, and one glass a day of pomegranate or grape juice, diluted fifty percent with water. Kristin followed this regimen for nine months. "It was the hardest thing I've ever done," she said. She lost weight. "But it pulled me through. Within a few days, there was dramatic improvement in the symptoms of the hepatitis."

In all, Kristin spent half a year in the hospital. One year from the onset of her illness, she knew she was going to live, although the road back to health remained slow and difficult. "They told me I would never have children, due to the drug they had given me to suppress rejection of the marrow transplants," she remembers. "Because of the risk of uncontrollable bleeding, they couldn't let me have periods, so they also gave me high doses of female hormones. In addition I got prednisone to try to control reactions to the transfusions and male hormones to try to stimulate my bone marrow. I didn't have a period for a year, and one psychic healer who put her hand over my pelvis said she sensed 'total blackness' there. But then I went on a fast for a week, and my period started! It's been completely regular ever since."

Twenty years later, Kristin is a healthy, vital woman, and the mother of four natural, healthy children. Her recovery was so unusual from the medical point of view that one of her doctors presented her case at an international conference on aplastic anemia. Kristin writes: "I am not just alive but quite healthy and strong. I've always thrived on physical activity and found as I got better that I could become as strong as I wanted to be. Daily bicycling, regular running, and ocean swimming helped get me over the final hurdle to excellent health.

"Today I am happy and busy raising my four children. I am a licensed naturopathic doctor but have not practiced since becoming a mother. I teach yoga and am writing and illustrating a children's book. Our family is very active—we ski, and windsurf, and I run regularly. Unless I mention my medical history, others do not suspect it; in fact those I do tell are quite surprised to learn that I was ever seriously ill."

What reserves of healing power did Kristin draw on to reactivate her bone marrow, neutralize whatever was the original cause of the disease, and undo the toxic effects of invasive treatment? I am fascinated by her unwavering confidence through her ordeal. "I always believed there was a way to live," she told me. "I just had to find it in time. That belief and the search fueled my undying optimism and made me an active participant in the healing process."

And what would she tell others facing grave medical crises?

"There may be different ways to healing for different people," she says, "but there is always a way. Keep searching!"

2

RIGHT IN MY
OWN BACKYARD

⸱

WHEN I FINISHED my South American travels in 1973, I began a
long process of settling down in the vicinity of Tucson, Arizona,
where I live to this day. I felt a strong affinity with the natural environment of the desert and made good connections with people and
places in the area. One of those connections was with Sandy Newmark, a graduate student in anthropology at the University of Arizona, who became one of my neighbors in Esperero Canyon in the
foothills of the Catalina Mountains. Sandy subsequently left anthropology to be a farmer in the White Mountains of central Arizona;
then he returned to Tucson to enroll in medical school. Today he is
my family's pediatrician.

Sandy and his wife, Linda, now a clinical psychologist, have a
daughter, Sophia, who is developmentally retarded. When Sophia
was a baby, many of the Newmarks' friends offered suggestions for
treatment. One was to take the baby to an unusual osteopathic physician named Robert Fulford, who had a good record of working with
children suffering from all sorts of problems. Sandy and Linda were
so impressed with him that they took Sophia for a number of his gentle sessions of "cranial therapy," and Sandy, then in his first year of
medical school at the University of Arizona, worked with Dr. Fulford
for a time. He kept telling me I should meet him, but I was not interested, partially due to my ignorance about osteopaths. With the usual
prejudices of medical doctors, I considered them second-rate M.D.'s
who dabbled in the kind of manipulation of the body more frequently done by chiropractors. I was also probably still attached to

the romantic notion of finding a healer/teacher in some far-off, very different culture—this despite my repeated experience of coming back emptyhanded from trips to remote places. It took many people telling me many times that I had to meet Dr. Fulford before I finally paid him a visit.

Bob Fulford was then in his late seventies. He had come to Tucson from Cincinnati in retirement from an overwhelming practice. One night, after spending a year recovering from exhaustion, he received a desperate call from a friend whose baby was severely ill with pneumonia. The baby was in the hospital, not responding to antibiotics. Dr. Fulford went to the hospital, gave hands-on treatment, and the next morning the baby was out of danger. Within hours people began calling him with requests for treatment, and he found himself drawn inexorably out of retirement and back into the practice of his own special form of osteopathic medicine.

I was struck by the simplicity of Dr. Fulford's office: a waiting room with a nurse-receptionist and two treatment rooms. Except for a diploma from the Kansas City College of Osteopathy on the wall, there were no distinguishing features and none of the equipment normally associated with a medical office. Dr. Fulford appeared kind and grandfatherly. He was tall, strong, and relaxed, with large, wonderful hands. He spoke quietly and sparingly. I told him I had heard much about his effectiveness and wanted to experience his treatments for myself.

"Well, what's wrong with you?" he asked.

"Not much," I told him. "My neck's been bothering me a little; sometimes it gets pretty stiff and sore."

"Well, let's see what we can do about it," he said.

He asked me to stand, put his hands on my shoulders, and observed my breathing. Then he moved my head in different directions. "Just get up here on the table," he directed. I lay on my back and watched him wheel over a stand with a curious instrument on a long power cord. The instrument was his "percussion hammer," a modified dentist's-drill motor with a thick, round metal disk that vibrated up and down. Dr. Fulford sat on a stool next to the table, adjusted the vibration rate, and put the disk in contact with my right shoulder. I could feel the vibrations through the whole right side of my body, pleasant and relaxing but hardly major therapy. After several minutes, Dr. Fulford's hand gave a little jerk and he muttered, "There she goes." With that he removed the percussion hammer and placed it in a new spot on my right hip. He continued this routine for twenty minutes, while I drifted in and out of daydreams; then he turned off the machine, moved his stool to the end of the table, and put his hands on the sides of my head, his fingers around my ears.

For the next few minutes, he cradled my head, applying the gentlest of pressure, now here, now there. It was one of the least dramatic forms of body work I had ever felt, so much so that I doubted it could accomplish anything. At the same time it felt reassuring to be held by such experienced, confident hands.

When this phase of the treatment was over, Dr. Fulford checked the mobility of my limbs, then asked me to sit up. He finished with a few, more familiar manipulations to crack my spine.

"There, that should do it," he said.

"What did you find?" I asked.

"Not much," he replied. "A few little restrictions in the shoulder that were probably causing your neck to get sore. Your cranial impulses are very good."

I had no idea what cranial impulses were, but I was glad to hear mine were good. As for "restrictions in the shoulder" and how they might cause a stiff neck, I was equally in the dark. But no further explanation was offered, and Dr. Fulford indicated that our time was up. He told me I was welcome to come back anytime and watch him work.

I was pleasantly surprised to learn that the charge for this session was only thirty-five dollars, clearly a bargain, if only for the relaxation it provided. Still, I failed to see how this minimal intervention could account for all the stories I had heard about Dr. Fulford's clinical successes. I resolved to come back and watch him treat others.

The next day I was surprised to find that I was fatigued and sore. I called Dr. Fulford to ask if this could be a result of his work. "Oh, yes," he said, "that's perfectly normal; you might feel it for a couple of days." And so I did. After that I felt fine, and my neck did, indeed, bother me less, but I did not notice any other change.

About a month later, I began spending a few hours a week in the doctor's little office on Grant Road, watching the old man work with patients. His office was always full, often with parents and children, representing a cross-section of the diverse groups that populate southern Arizona, including Hispanics and Asians, city folk and country folk. All came with high expectations and gratitude just for the chance to see this man. At the least, Dr. Fulford was a wonderful role model of the old-fashioned, caring family doctor who made people feel better just by the warmth of his presence and his own personal example of good health.

Observing him, I was surprised by the brevity of his histories and physical examinations. He asked very few questions when a new patient walked in the door—"What's the problem? . . . How long has it been bothering you? . . . Did you ever take any bad falls in childhood? . . . Do you know anything about the circumstances of your birth?" and maybe a few more. Then he stood people up, checked the patients' limbs and breathing, rotated their heads, and asked them to lie on the table. He administered to most people the same kinds of treatments I received: a slow going-over with the percussion hammer, held to various parts of the body until some sort of release occurred (when his hand holding the instrument would jerk suddenly), then slow, imperceptible hands-on manipulation of the head, and finally a few adjustments of the back. He rarely volunteered explanations of what he thought was wrong or what he aimed to do; but if people asked, he would do so in a few words. Most people did not ask; they just seemed to entrust themselves or their children to the doctor and let him work in silence. Everyone relaxed in Dr. Fulford's hands, even restless, fussy children, who would calm down almost as soon as he touched them.

Often, at the end of the session, he gave people strange daily exercises to perform, exercises that I had never seen before. One he recommended frequently went like this: Stand with your feet apart at shoulder width and extend the arms to the side fully with the left palm facing up and the right palm facing down. Breathe deeply and regularly, holding this position until the strain in the upper arms and shoulders becomes unbearable. Then, as slowly as you can, raise the arms above the head, keeping them fully extended, until the hands touch. Then lower the arms and relax. What was that supposed to do? I asked him. "It opens the chest and allows the breath to expand," was the answer. Another Fulford exercise was to sit on the edge of a chair with feet flat on the floor and shoulder width apart, then bend forward and, with the arms inside the legs, grasp the bottoms of the feet with the hands. Hold this position for a few minutes, and it gently stretches the lower vertebrae, allowing for greater motion of the spine. Sometimes when patients came back, Dr. Fulford, on examining them, would say, "You haven't been doing your exercise," or "Good, you've been doing your exercise," and the patients would confirm that this was so.

He often told patients not to come back. "When do you want to see me again?" they might ask as they got off the table. "I don't need to see you again," Dr. Fulford would say. "You're fixed." "But don't I need any follow-up?" they might persist. Dr. Fulford smiled and shook his head. "I took the shock out of your system," he would say. "Now just let old Mother Nature do her job." If there was any disappointment among Dr. Fulford's patients, it had to do with their not having to see him again, since the experience of his treatment was so satisfying.

Gradually, I began to realize that I was seeing something quite extraordinary. This old man of strong hands and few words was, in fact, fixing people who came to him with a wide range of disorders, often in one session of therapy that, on the surface, seemed minimal. I heard tale after tale of longstanding problems resolved after one or two visits to Dr. Fulford, problems that had not responded to conventional medicine. And these were not just aches, pains, and other musculoskeletal ailments but also hormonal and digestive disturbances, sleep disorders, asthma, ear infections, and more. How could such undramatic treatment give such dramatic results?

I began to ask Dr. Fulford about the why and wherefore of his methods. What was the theory behind them? Just what was he doing? The answers I received sounded like nothing I had learned at Harvard Medical School.

Bob Fulford was a pure, old-time osteopath in the tradition of the man who founded the system, Andrew Taylor Still (1828–1917) of Kirksville, Missouri. A. T. Still, "the Old Doctor" to his contemporaries, was a renegade physician who disowned the toxic drugs of his colleagues in favor of a drugless system of therapy based on manipulation of bones. His idea was to adjust the body mechanically in order to allow the circulatory and nervous systems to function smoothly, bringing natural healing power to any ailing part. The new profession that he founded in 1874 was very successful in its early years, but by the middle of the twentieth century it was eclipsed by the spectacular rise of modern scientific medicine, also known as allopathic medicine. In response, osteopaths abandoned Still's teachings and began to behave increasingly like M.D.'s. Today the M.D. and D.O. degrees are equivalent; most osteopaths rely on drugs and surgery, and few use manipulation as a primary modality of treatment.

Nevertheless, there has always existed within the osteopathic profession a minor tradition of healers who use no drugs and continue to refine A. T. Still's insights into the nature of the human body and its potential to heal itself. One of those was William Sutherland, who in 1939 announced to his colleagues his discovery of an aspect of human physiology he called the primary respiratory mechanism, and a technique for modifying it that became known as cranial therapy, or craniosacral therapy. Sutherland worked on his theory for many years to ensure its correctness before going public. Nonetheless it met with great resistance, and only a small percentage of osteopaths accepted it. One of those was the young Robert Fulford, then just beginning his general practice in Cincinnati.

Sutherland's insight was that the central nervous system and its associated structures were in constant rhythmic motion, and that this motion was an essential feature—perhaps the most essential feature—of human life and health. He identified five components of the mechanism:

- Motion at the cranial sutures, the joints linking the twenty-six bones of the skull
- Expansion and contraction of the hemispheres of the brain
- Motion of the membranes covering the brain and spinal cord
- A fluid wave within the cerebrospinal fluid that bathes the brain and spinal cord
- Involuntary, subtle motion of the sacrum (tailbone).

Sutherland thought the rhythmic expansion and contraction of this system resembled breathing, but since it was occurring in the most vital, most essential organs, he called it "primary respiration" to indicate its importance in the hierarchy of body functions and distinguish it from "secondary respiration," the familiar motions of the chest, lungs, and diaphragm associated with the exchange of air. He postulated that an intact, freely moving primary respiratory mechanism was necessary to full health; any restrictions in it could lead to disease, since the central nervous system regulated all other organs.

One of the main heresies in Sutherland's formulation was the notion that the cranial bones move. Generations of anatomists had taught that the joints of the skull are fixed and immobile. Not only

M.D.'s but also most D.O.'s refused to consider the idea of cranial motion. Dr. Fulford was not one of them, and he started training himself to feel those motions by putting his hands on people's heads.

It is only in recent years that researchers at Michigan State University's College of Osteopathic Medicine have confirmed Sutherland's theory with X-ray films of living skulls that show cranial motion. Those motions can be measured by sensitive instruments. Bob Fulford would argue that the most sensitive instruments are the hands of a practiced physician. He trained himself to feel a human hair under seventeen sheets of paper, and he says that anyone can develop similar touch sensitivity with enough practice.

Under Dr. Fulford's guidance I began feeling heads myself to see if I could detect cranial impulses. At first I felt mainly my own pulse, but as I practiced I began to feel the subtle breathlike motion that Dr. Fulford considers the most vital expression of life. At least I felt it in people who had well-running primary respiratory mechanisms. Once he asked me to feel the head of a woman who, he said, had no detectable cranial impulses. She had been in several bad accidents, one twenty years before, and now suffered extreme fatigue, insomnia, migraine headaches, weak vision, poor digestion, and increased susceptibility to infection. Her head felt like a bag of cement, a dead weight, the rhythm of life not present. After several sessions of treatment, her cranial motions began to return, and as they did, her health began to improve.

"What causes impairment of this system?" I asked Dr. Fulford.

"Trauma," was the answer. "Three kinds of trauma. The first is birth trauma. If the first breath of life is not perfectly full, the cranial rhythms are restricted from the start. That first breath is so important. In my lifetime I've seen problems of this sort increase steadily, which, I think, is a black mark against our obstetrical practices. The second common reason is physical trauma, especially in early life. Any fall or blow that knocks the wind out of you, that causes the breath cycle to be interrupted, even for a moment, can cause permanent, lifelong restriction in the primary respiratory mechanism. It's possible to feel and identify and undo those restrictions with your hands. That's what I call taking the shock out of the body. And a third reason, maybe less common, is major psychological trauma—again, especially in early life. I estimate that ninety-five percent of people have restrictions of one degree or another in this function."

Around the time Dr. Fulford was teaching these new concepts to me, I was helping a friend through a medical crisis. Kim Cliffton was a thirty-four-year-old marine biologist who spent most of the year on the Pacific beaches of southern Mexico, trying to save an endangered species of sea turtle that was being hunted to extinction. He directed a World Wildlife Fund project that kept him in the field leading a rough, adventurous life except for the summer months, when the turtles headed out to sea. Then he would come up to Tucson, looking bedraggled, to tell his stories and gather his strength. For several years he had suffered from intestinal problems: episodes of severe diarrhea in Mexico, inability to digest many foods, and abdominal pain. He would routinely take courses of antibiotics and antiparasitic drugs, but year by year the episodes became more frequent and more intense. Now he came to me having lost twenty pounds, saying that he had not had a formed bowel movement in months, that his stool frequently contained blood and mucus, that he had constant abdominal pain and increasing debility. He did not think he would be able to continue his turtle work.

Kim wanted prescriptions to knock out what he thought were more parasites in his gut, but the picture he presented was not one of infection. Instead, he seemed to me to have chronic inflammatory bowel disease, possibly ulcerative colitis, and I urged him to see a highly recommended gastroenterologist at the University of Arizona Health Sciences Center. Kim was the son of a pulmonary surgeon in New York, and he had great faith in conventional medicine. That faith was tested, however, when, after a long and expensive series of tests, culminating in a biopsy of the colon, the gastroenterologist could not identify the nature of the problem, except to say that Kim's colon was severely and chronically inflamed. Ulcerative colitis was definitely a possibility. "I think we should go in and take out more tissue," the gastroenterologist told me. "Then maybe we'll find out what the hell he's got." This did not sound encouraging, and since Kim was paying for it out of his own pocket, I suggested looking for another approach. Then it occurred to me to send Kim to Dr. Fulford.

Kim had a long history of playing contact sports, including boxing—he had been a heavyweight in the army—and had suffered many traumatic injuries. I noticed that he always breathed through his mouth. In addition to the intestinal problems he complained of episodes of bad back and neck pain. It seemed to me that Dr. Fulford might be able to make sense of this whole picture, but I foresaw two problems. The first was that Dr. Fulford was now only seeing patients under thirty, a limit he imposed because his practice was again getting out of hand as his reputation grew. "I'm almost eighty," he said to me one day, "and I can't work myself to exhaustion anymore. My energies go further with younger folks; their healing responses are stronger." He had invented the percussion hammer to make things easier on himself, too. What it accomplished could be done by hand, he said, but with much more effort.

A second problem was that Kim, having grown up with conventional medicine and lacking any experience with alternative practitioners, might be reluctant to trust himself to one. I did my best to explain to both Dr. Fulford and Kim why they should see each other, and I succeeded, except that Kim couldn't see how an osteopath was going to help his colon. "Just tell him all your symptoms," I urged him, "all the intestinal symptoms as well as the pains in your back and neck."

I was unable to be in the office that day and waited expectantly to see Kim when he came home. "He's a quack," were Kim's first words. "I mean, he's a nice old man, but he doesn't do anything."

"What did he tell you?" I asked.

"He said I was in critical condition, that my cranial motions were completely shut down because of old injuries, and that the cranial nerve controlling the digestive system was not functioning as a result. Also that the same injuries make me breathe through my mouth, and that doesn't nourish my brain as breathing should."

"Did he say he was able to help you?"

"He said he took care of most of it and that I should come back in three weeks. But he seemed so feeble, and he's got all these nervous tics; I felt sorry for him. At least it didn't cost much."

"What do you mean by 'nervous tics'?" I asked.

"You know, when he has that vibrator on you, every few minutes his hand flies up in the air and his whole body jerks."

"Really?"

"Yes, it's kind of sad."

I called Dr. Fulford for his view of the session. "Mr. Cliffton came in not a moment too soon," he told me. "His whole primary respiratory mechanism was shut down. I think he would really have gone downhill fast."

"Were you able to help him?"

"Oh, yes, I got major releases from many parts of his body, undid a lot of the trauma, and got the impulses flowing again. Once the vagus nerve kicks in, he'll be all right. He should just take it easy now and let old Mother Nature do her job."

Six hours after the treatment, Kim's diarrhea stopped for the first time in eight months, never to return. Over the next three months he regained all of his lost weight and energy. The back and neck pain disappeared, and he stopped breathing through his mouth.

"He saved my life," Kim told me later. "I'm convinced that man saved my life." He has since become a passionate convert to alternative medicine in general, and osteopathy in particular. This cure was so impressive that I tried to arrange a conference to discuss the case with Dr. Fulford, Kim, myself, and the university gastroenterologist. That doctor said he was interested but failed to show. When I asked him why, he told me, "Look, I'm not going to argue with success, but I can't believe that osteopathic treatment had anything to do with the outcome."

Shortly afterward I had another opportunity to witness Dr. Fulford's skill with the human body, this time firsthand. I was working in my garden with a friend. In a freak accident that I could never reconstruct, he stood up as I bent down, and his shoulder hit me hard in the right side of my face, just forward of my ear. There was a sharp pain, and I could neither open nor close my mouth fully. It felt as if my jaw were partially dislocated, and I couldn't get it to go back, no matter what I did. I called Dr. Fulford and told him what had happened. "Get on down here," he said. I drove myself to his office and walked in, still in pain and still unable to make my jaw work. He made time in his lineup of patients and told me to get on the table.

As soon as he put his hands on my head, he named the bone in my skull that was out of place. Then he began the gentlest of manipulations. After a few minutes, he said, "There, it's back." I felt nothing happen and no change in the discomfort. He said I could get up. "It still hurts," I said, disappointed.

"Oh, the muscles will be sore for a little while," he replied. "Well, I've got to get busy."

I left, unconvinced that I had been helped, contemplating a visit to the emergency room of the university hospital. But ten minutes later, as I was sitting at a stop light, I suddenly realized that the pain was not there, and that I could open and close my mouth normally. Incredible! Thank you, Dr. Fulford! Then I thought: What would you have done if you didn't know about him? Probably, I would have visited an emergency room, undergone X-rays, and been sent home with painkillers, muscle relaxants, and the expectation of a large bill. Possibly I would have remained unhealed for weeks or months.

Now I was truly inspired to learn everything I could from Dr. Fulford. I also became increasingly frustrated in trying to explain my excitement to colleagues. Most doctors were no more interested in my stories than the gastroenterologist had been. It was especially annoying to try to talk with pediatricians about the Fulford approach to ear infections in children.

Recurrent infection of the middle ear—otitis media—is the bread and butter of pediatricians; so common is it that an ever-growing number of people in our society accept it as a normal part of growing up. The conventional treatments are antibiotics and decongestants and sometimes surgical placement of tubes through the eardrums to equalize pressure. Commonly the drug treatments end episodes of infection sooner or later, only for new episodes to recur at frequent intervals.

Bob Fulford was outstandingly successful at permanently ending this cycle in young children, often with just one session of treatment in which he concentrated on freeing up the sacrum. "I just beat the heck out of their tailbones" was the way he put it, because he found that the sacral end of the craniosacral system was often the one that was locked up in children, probably from trauma suffered during birth. Here is how he explained the situation:

"When the sacrum is restricted, the whole primary respiratory mechanism is impaired. Along with this goes a pattern of restricted breathing, and it is the force of the breath—the rhythmic pressure changes in the chest—that pumps the lymphatic circulation. With inadequate lymphatic circulation there is poor fluid drainage from the head and neck. Stagnant fluid builds up in the middle ear, providing an ideal breeding ground for bacteria. You can wipe out the bacteria all you want with antibiotics, but if you don't correct the underlying problem of fluid stagnation, they're just going to come back." Certainly that is the usual experience of kids, parents, and pediatricians; the bacteria just come back.

I saw case after case go through Dr. Fulford's office in which this simple treatment cured otitis media permanently. Often I could see a change in breathing as soon as the child got off the table: greater, more symmetrical expansion of the chest, deeper breaths. Yet I could not get one pediatrician from the Tucson medical community to come to Dr. Fulford's office and watch. Instead of being interested in my accounts of his treatment, the medical men seemed threatened. Finally, one practitioner, an Englishwoman, agreed to watch. She even sent a patient, with such good result that she consented to help me make a documentary film of Dr. Fulford with the biomedical communications department of the University of Arizona.

The more I watched Bob Fulford work, the more I was impressed by his own health and vigor. At eighty he was an inspiration for successful aging. Once I asked him for his personal secret of good health. "I'll show you," he said, and with that took a deep, slow breath that went on so long that I stared in disbelief. His chest expanded enormously. Then he exhaled as spaciously. "The more air you can breathe in and out, the more nourishment you can give to the central nervous system," he said afterward. "Good breathing is the key."

The medicine I saw Bob Fulford practice was the kind of medicine I had longed for during my years of clinical training and my years of wandering. It was nonviolent medicine that did not suppress disease but rather encouraged the body's own healing potential to express itself. Dr. Fulford was the first practitioner I met who adhered religiously to the two most famous admonitions of Hippocrates: "First, Do No Harm" (*Primum non nocere*) and "Honor the Healing Power of Nature" (the *vis medicatrix naturae*).

I learned so much by simply watching him work, being worked on by him, and having informal discussions with him. His answers to my questions were always brief and in ordinary language, unsophisticated by the standards of academic medicine but bright with wisdom and full of useful practical information. Here are some ideas I took away from my time with him that I have found most useful in my own work as a physician:

• *The body wants to be healthy*. Health is the condition of perfect balance, when all systems run smoothly and energy circulates freely. This is the natural condition, the one in which least effort is expended; therefore, when the body is out of balance, it wants to get back to it. Treatment can and should take advantage of this tendency to return to the condition of health.

• *Healing is a natural power.* When Dr. Fulford told patients to relax and "let old Mother Nature do her job," he was expressing in a folksy way his great faith in the *vis medicatrix naturae* of Hippocrates, a concept missing from conventional medicine. Never in my years at Harvard Medical School did anyone mention it to me and my classmates, nor do medical school professors talk about it to students today. That seems to me to be the greatest single philosophical defect of modern medicine, a defect that has immense practical significance, since it underlies our inability to find cost-effective solutions to common health problems.

My friend Linda Newmark said that Dr. Fulford told her the best thing she could do for her husband, Sandy, while he was in medical school, was to take him out in nature for regular walks. He explained to her, "He'll need that to balance all the other stuff they're putting into his head."

• *The body is a whole, and all of its parts are connected.* Dr. Fulford had a brilliant, intuitive understanding of the body as a unified functioning system. When a patient came in complaining of pain in the knee, he did not automatically conclude that the problem was in the knee and proceed to work there. He knew that the knee is the compensating joint for both the ankle and the hip. If there is a restriction in an ankle, as a result of an old injury, the ankle will not be able to respond as it should to gravity and motion and will transmit a distorted force up the leg. The knee will compensate for the distortion in order to keep the pelvis in its normal position, and the strain of the compensating effort might be experienced as knee pain. If the knee is locked for any reason, the distortion from the ankle can reach the hip, causing lower back pain. How many knee and back operations were performed, Dr. Fulford wondered, for problems that actually originated in locked-up ankles? I saw him cure cases of chronic knee and back pain by unlocking ankles with his percussion hammer.

Bob Fulford thought the restrictions he talked about occurred in the fascia, the tough connective tissue that covers muscles and separates spaces inside the body. Anatomists teach that fascia exists as separate sheets, but Fulford worked on the premise that all of the fascia throughout the body is one big, convoluted piece. If a restriction occurs anywhere in it, it distorts the fabric of the whole; hence local changes can have global effects.

Similarly, when Kim Cliffton came with his complaints of back and neck pain, mouth breathing, and chronic bowel disease, Dr. Fulford looked at this whole picture of disturbed physiology and identified a common root in an old traumatic injury of the head. The gastroenterologist, who looked only at Kim's colon, could make no sense of the problem and had no treatments to offer except drugs to suppress the inflammatory process in the colon.

• *There is no separation of mind and body.* Just as Dr. Fulford believed that psychological trauma could interfere with the respiratory motions of the central nervous system, so also did he presume that physical interventions, by their effect on the nervous system, could improve psychological function. He regularly raised IQs of learning-disabled children by his cranial therapy; in fact, he was so successful at this that a state hospital for developmentally retarded children in Louisiana had him come for a few weeks every year to work on its patients.

• *The beliefs of practitioners strongly influence the healing powers of patients.* Dr. Fulford believed that the patients he treated could get better. He had a simple, genuine, and very beautiful faith in their potential for healing, which he communicated in many ways, both verbal and nonverbal. That was one reason so many people gravitated to him. He was also careful to select those cases he thought he could help. If you had a broken bone, he would tell you, "There's nothing I can do for a broken bone. Let nature heal it, then come to me, and I'll take the shock of the injury out of your system." Neither would he treat problems requiring surgery or other forms of emergency care.

As he got older, and the demands on him increased steadily, he kept lowering the age limit of patients he accepted. Soon it was twenty-five, then twenty. Ideally, he would have liked to restrict his practice to infants, "because their healing potential is so great, and the restrictions have not had time to become fixed in body structures." He also thought all newborns should have prophylactic treatment, because "so many illnesses in later life are long-term consequences of traumatic birth, and for the first twenty-four hours of life, the bones are just like jelly; it takes no effort to put them back the way they should be."

Dr. Fulford did not succeed with everyone, but he had a higher percentage of successful outcomes than any other practitioner I have met.

Eventually, the workload became overwhelming, and Bob Fulford, to the great dismay of his patients and followers, announced that he was going into permanent retirement and moving back to southern Ohio. He did so; but, as I write this, he is still, at the age of ninety, actively teaching cranial therapy. He travels around the country lecturing, instructing students in technique, and inspiring new generations of physicians to become true doctors.

Discovering Dr. Fulford in my own backyard after chasing all over the world was a powerful lesson: I did not have to look Out There for what I wanted. Neither do most people have to look Out There for healing. Of course, it is worth searching for the best treatment, since treatment comes from outside. But healing comes from within, its source in our very nature as living organisms.

THE FACES OF HEALING:
HARVEY AND PHYLLIS

IN THE SUMMER of 1992, when he was fifty years old and six months into a happy second marriage, Harvey Sandler developed a disturbing set of symptoms. His vision became blurred, he would wake up in the middle of the night drenched in sweat, he began to urinate frequently, and he became impotent. The last change was the most disturbing, because he and Phyllis, his new wife, had enjoyed a passionate sexual relationship for some time. "It got more and more difficult for me to perform," Harvey remembers, "so I just stopped coming to bed." He chalked it all up to stress and did not visit a doctor.

Phyllis says, "I didn't want to pressure him, but after a while it got me down." Harvey's job as a money manager gave him some stress; but in Phyllis's words, "Really, our lives were pretty good." After several months, Harvey sought help from a psychiatrist specializing in sexual dysfunction. She suggested blood tests, one of which, for a pituitary hormone, was abnormal. Then an eye doctor ordered an MRI scan of the brain, and this test revealed a tumor directly behind Harvey's eyes. In this location it was pressing on the hypothalamus, a vital center that controls the pituitary gland, and through it, many involuntary functions of the body. It was also affecting the optic nerves.

From its location and appearance, Harvey's doctors thought the tumor was benign—either a glioma or a craniopharyngioma. The former is a solid tumor arising from cells that support neurons. The latter arises from embryonic cells left over from fetal development and tends to be cystic, containing fluid-filled sacs in addition to tissue; it usually appears in people younger than Harvey, but may grow slowly for a long time before it reaches a size that affects brain function.

The brain is one part of the body where the distinction between benign and malignant tumors is not as immediately important as it usually is. The problem here was a space-occupying lesion, exerting pressure on vital centers in a confined area. It would have to be removed or shrunk.

Harvey and Phyllis made the rounds of neurosurgeons in New York. Most were "very alarmist" about the tumor and prospects for removing it without causing permanent brain damage. "Finally we found one neurosurgeon who told us what we wanted to hear," Phyllis says. "He told us the operation would be 'a piece of cake,' and he could have Harvey in and out of the hospital in two days. We decided to go with him."

The operation took place in November 1992. When exposed, the tumor turned out to be the size of a small egg, situated between the optic nerve and the hypothalamus. The surgeon, unable to remove the tumor because of its location, drained fluid from it to reduce the pressure it was causing and took a sample of the tissue, which identified it as a craniopharyngioma. He then sent Harvey for thirty radiation treatments to shrink the tumor, ending just around Christmas.

To everyone's dismay, the patient got worse as treatment progressed. His vision deteriorated to the point of near blindness, leaving him unable to read anything or see what was on a television screen. To prevent brain swelling, doctors had prescribed Decadron, a strong steroid; it caused Harvey to gain forty pounds and changed his personality. "He was angry, aggressive, and nasty and slept most of the time," Phyllis says. Harvey says only, "I don't remember any of it." He began to lose his memory and his mind. He would get lost in his apartment, describe events that never happened. "I didn't know who this person was," Phyllis recalls. According to the doctors, none of this should have happened, and they had no explanation for the deterioration. "Nobody would take responsibility for it, either," Phyllis says. "The surgeon said, 'I'm only the carpenter here; my job is done'; the endocrinologist told us to see the neurologist, and the neurologist told us to see the endocrinologist. I got really scared."

About this time, a counselor named Deborah, who is skilled at working with seriously ill people, took Phyllis away for a weekend break, arranging for Harvey's son to come in and care for him. Deborah's brother was a distinguished neurosurgeon in Philadelphia, and he was called in for another opinion. After reviewing the case, this doctor told his sister: "Harvey Sandler will never make an independent decision again in his life. He will never recover. You should try to prepare Phyllis to accept his condition; it will be lucky if he stays the same and doesn't deteriorate further."

Phyllis became hysterical when Deborah reported this conversation, and as Deborah recalls: "Phyllis screamed, 'There's no way he's not coming back!' I said, 'Okay, I'm with you,' but in my heart I didn't believe it."

Phyllis returned home feeling she could not afford to waste time. "I called all the smartest and best-connected people I knew," she says, "always asking for help. I told them I had to find the one doctor in the world who had done more of these procedures than any other. Well, I got sent on one wild-goose chase after another. I talked to doctor after doctor. Finally, I found one who seemed right, but he specialized in aneurysms, not tumors. Then the eye doctor called me and said, 'Time is of the essence. What vision he has left is going.' I dragged my poor husband from doctor to doctor, even though he was exhausted and never wanted to go out. Usually, I had to dress him and half-carry him, and usually he fell asleep in the doctors' offices; once he wandered out of an office and got lost. Finally, I found a neurosurgeon who was willing to operate, one who had done a lot of these procedures and wasn't put off by such a high-risk case."

The second operation to remove the tumor took place in mid-February 1993. Harvey did not wake up for a long time after the surgery. Then he almost died from fluid filling his lungs. On the fourth day after the operation he lapsed into a coma, and the doctors again were at a loss.

It was Phyllis who saved the day. She wondered whether Harvey's coma might be the result of withdrawing him from Decadron too quickly. The drug is used short-term to prevent brain swelling after surgery, but this team of doctors did not know that Harvey had been maintained on very high doses of Decadron since the previous operation. When Phyllis pointed that out to them, they tried giving Harvey some Decadron intravenously. The next morning he was sitting up and talking. He stayed in intensive care for two weeks, in a regular hospital room for another two weeks, then began a long and steady recovery.

"It took him a whole year to catch up," Phyllis says, "and he remained amnesic for the three months prior to the second operation. Slowly he got stronger physically and recovered some of his memory. He had to develop a whole new way of thinking and approaching life. He had to learn what had happened to him, then to be frightened about it, then to be reborn."

Deborah remembers Harvey's frustration during this period. "Everyone expected him to be transformed by the experience," she recalls, "but it seemed that everyone *but* him got transformed. Harvey had had it all. He was rich, successful, good-looking, enjoying life immensely. His friends were deeply affected by what happened. Almost overnight, he turned into one of life's unfortunates: brain-damaged, overweight, angry and abusive, disoriented, with a good chance of dying or being a vegetable. People said, 'If this can happen to him, it could happen to me.' It really got people thinking about their vulnerability and motivated them to clean up their acts. Now, after the second operation, the more Harvey heard about the effect he had had on others, the more he resented the fact that nothing magical had happened to him."

Phyllis spent time every day trying to help Harvey learn to walk again. He would fight with her a lot and remembers her asking him constantly, "So what's different now? How is your life changed as a result of all this?" All he could think to say was, "I just want to get back on the tennis court."

About a year after the second operation, the magic happened. In Harvey's words: "I started thinking. I had always let Phyllis do the thinking for me, and I had always shied away from power and responsibility. Now it seemed the tumor and the surgery had reawakened parts of me that had been asleep and at the same time lessened other parts of me. My ability to perform sexually came back six weeks after the operation, but my sexuality in general was diminished. I think it had been too dominant before. On the other hand, thinking and emotion increased. In general, I felt more balanced. To make a very long story short, I've assumed responsibility for my life. I'm a more responsible human being now, and I'm using my power appropriately. This illness is one of the biggest gifts I've ever had.

"On a practical level, my vision is better than it was before, and my memory is excellent. I'm working and playing and living much more the life I want to live. I've changed my work so that I can stay at home and don't have to go in to an office. I play tennis every morning."

I also talked to Phyllis about her perspective on the saga. She said, "Throughout the darkest days I remember thinking, 'There are going to be gifts coming from this, and I'm going after every one of them.' We were very isolated during that period; I didn't let many people into our lives. If I had believed the doctors all knew more than me, I would have accepted their pessimistic outlook and not kept pursuing the possibility of a cure. It's hard to believe they don't know it all. The surgeon who finally took us on told me he couldn't guarantee that Harvey would live or have any vision or even recover consciousness. He is as surprised and thrilled at the extent of the recovery as anyone else. A year after the operation, we invited him and his wife to come for dinner and celebrate with us.

"Really, Harvey has been reborn. He was given a chance to redesign himself, and he's come out a more generous person, someone who is more sensitive to people and wants to be the best person he can be. I've been reborn in the process too. Our adventure has inspired both of us to keep trying to heal the parts of ourselves that are not yet healed. We are still processing it and appreciating it."

Phyllis wanted me to know that this was not the first dramatic healing she had witnessed. "Seven years ago I developed excruciating sciatic pain. I had it for two and a half years and went to more than twenty doctors but could get no relief with any of the treatments they prescribed. Then my first grandchild was born, and I really wanted to be with the baby. I knew I had to make myself better if I was going to be able to enjoy being a grandmother. I listened to tapes, visualized, got acupuncture, ate healthy food, and took vitamins. In just four weeks I was pain free, a hundred percent. I think the most important thing I did was to visualize more blood going to my back. That and telling myself, 'I really want to be healed.' "

3

TESTIMONIALS

AS A PHYSICIAN with botanical training and a long-standing interest in medicinal plants, I work as an advisor to several groups promoting research on herbal medicine, one of which is the American Botanical Council in Austin, Texas. Recently, the director of the council, Mark Blumenthal, asked me to comment on a letter he received from a woman in Chicago, extolling the health benefits of ginkgo. She was taking pills containing an extract of the leaves of a tree, *Ginkgo biloba,* native to China and now widely planted in cities throughout the world, because it is resistant to air pollution. The tree has attractive, fan-shaped leaves, used for centuries in traditional Chinese medicine, and the female trees provide edible nuts. Only in recent years has a concentrated, standardized extract of ginkgo leaves become available in the West. This product has become very popular in Germany as a treatment for circulatory disorders and now is available in all health food stores in this country. The medical profession here remains mostly ignorant of it.

Let me quote at length from the letter:

An 84-year-old friend of mine (I am 60) called to ask me if I knew anything about Ginkgo biloba. I said no, but I would do some research on it. My research led me to two books. . . . Then I did a little research elsewhere, coming up with a few things.

My own reaction to Ginkgo was so astounding that I became a walking advertisement for it. I started noticing activity on the third day I started taking it (one pill a day in the beginning). In a few days there was more activity. During the second week I began taking three a day, one with each meal. I believe it was the third week that I lost my depression and began feeling like the world was a wonderful place in which to live.

I began having more energy. In a six-week period I noticed more and more changes. . . . One of the most outstanding was when the Ginkgo reached my equilibrium. I had been walking with a cane because my gait was so unsteady. Suddenly, while walking in a store, I noticed that I wasn't using my cane, and I had a longer stride, a steady stride. Not minutes later I ran into someone I knew and excitedly told her what had just happened to me. I was *swinging my cane instead of using it to steady myself.* I was so excited that I made a spontaneous rapid turn-around (something I hadn't done in years!). (I know people must have thought I was crazy!) I was all smiles—as was the person I met!

I lost the pain in my legs and feet. I was regaining normal breathing action. Now, a year later, I have lost my night blindness (and have gotten my ophthalmologist interested in Ginkgo). My vision is better, and my hearing has improved immensely. (My TV is now on low sound rather than loud.)

I called and wrote to people I knew. People needed to know what was happening to me. Those who saw me after I was on Ginkgo were amazed.

A beautician had a lot of pain in her wrists from working with her hands so much. After listening to me she began taking Ginkgo and claims she not only has eliminated her pain but also sleeps much better. A woman in her late 40s could rarely get out of her house, and when she did, she needed to have a wheelable can of oxygen with her and be using it all the while she was out. Now she uses the oxygen very little—and is able to go many places. This shocks a lot of people who know her and her background.

I have TMJ (temporo-mandibular joint) problems—or I should say *I did have them.* Suddenly I no longer suffer from the pain! It had to be Ginkgo! It just *had to be!* I figure as long as I am on Ginkgo I'm not going to be bothered by it. Even the clicking sound is gone!

I have a 94-year-old mother in a nursing home and this year she changed doctors. . . . The new doctor was agreeable to Mom taking Ginkgo if I would pay for it. I certainly was willing to do that.

The last Wednesday of January 1994 this doctor okayed the Ginkgo. He allowed her only one pill a day. I wasn't concerned about that since I had seen the 84-year-old woman who originally talked to me about Ginkgo do amazingly well with only one pill a day!

Mom started with Ginkgo the very next day. From Thursday to Sunday she changed amazingly! She was no longer depressed. She was happy. She was filled with life. Her voice volume had changed from a weak, soft voice (you could hear illness in its tone) to a strong, solid voice. I could feel electricity in that room between us! I was so happy to see her changes and she was thrilled to feel so much better! She also had a very miraculous improvement in her hearing! This placed her life in an entirely new category! Previously she walked in her own little world—not being able to hear others speak unless they yelled loudly (and few bothered to do that), and not being able to think clearly (short-term memory loss, confusion, anxiety, etc.). . . .

Suddenly she was hearing! For the first time she wanted to know how to fix her hearing aid! And one day she started talking to the people at her dining room table—something she had never done before! . . . It was obvious that her short-term memory loss was improving. . . . Her hemorrhoids also have improved. I expect a lot more things to improve. . . .

IT IS SO WONDERFUL TO BE ABLE TO FEEL LIFE AS IT SHOULD BE FELT—BE WILLING TO BREATHE AND ENJOY LIFE AS IT SHOULD BE ENJOYED! A PERSON JUST DOESN'T WANT TO STOP!

A man I know took one Ginkgo a day for approximately six months. He suffered from ringing in the ears. At six months he lost the ringing. He quit the Ginkgo. The ringing returned.

I believe it is necessary to continue taking Ginkgo if you intend to retain any of the benefits it offers. For those who suffer greatly it certainly is worth the cost! Far too many people feel that life isn't worth living. I wish I could reach them all and tell them the wonders of Ginkgo!

This letter is a classic example of a testimonial to a health product. As such it would likely be dismissed by most medical scientists, who tend to drop all testimonials into wastebaskets labeled Anecdotal Evidence. In medical usage, "anecdotal evidence" means "of no scientific value or importance." I take a different view of this material, and I am interested in why so many doctors have a hard time with it.

I suppose the simplest answer is that doctors and scientists do not like to be made to look like fools, and they sense danger in endorsing products or techniques whose claimed effects may turn out to be false or unprovable by controlled experiments. But it is equally foolish to ignore testimonial evidence, because it may suggest directions for experimental inquiry as well as provide clues to the nature of healing.

Many scientists reject testimonials out of hand on the assumption that the information is false, that people are either deluded or have simply made up the stories for one reason or another. The essence of good science is open-minded inquiry, so would it not make sense to try, at least, to verify the stories? My experience, overwhelmingly, is that whenever I have met and interviewed persons who have written testimonial letters to me, I have found no reason to disbelieve them, although I may not agree with their interpretations of their experiences. For example, I believe the writer of the letter quoted here experienced the positive changes she reports in her own health and the health of relatives and friends. I am not sure I agree with her statement that "it had to be Ginkgo! It just *had to be!*"

Science is the orderly gathering of knowledge by methodical inquiry and experiment, but where do you get ideas to inquire about or experiment with except through your experience of the world around you? Experimenting blindly, without starting from reasonable hypotheses suggested by experience, often wastes time, money, and effort. I became interested in Dr. Fulford and through him in cranial osteopathic theory and practice as a result of paying attention to testimonials about his work. Testimonials have led me to discoveries of other useful practices as well.

Some years ago I got a letter from a man in California describing remarkable experiences with a preparation of an herb called bloodroot, which he said miraculously dissolved moles and other growths on the skin, including, in at least one case he had witnessed, a malignant melanoma. He urged me to order the product from an old man in Utah who prepared it, and to experiment with it. I did order it (it was quite inexpensive), and shortly afterward a container of oily, blood-red paste arrived in the mail with no instructions. I went to my bookshelf to read about the plant.

Bloodroot is a small woodland herb, *Sanguinaria canadensis,* native to the North Central United States and Canada. Its taproot exudes a bloody juice, which probably inspired Native Americans to experiment with the plant as a medicine. Bloodroot was one of the most popular herbal remedies among Plains Indians and the European settlers who came later, used internally for sore throats and respiratory ailments and externally for growths on the surface of the body. The plant fell into disfavor in modern times with the demonstration that it was toxic: taken internally, it interferes with cell division and may promote mutations and cancer. The Food and Drug Administration has it on a list of most dangerous herbs. But I was able to find a number of references to its peculiar ability to dissolve abnormal growths on the skin without harming normal tissue, even to dissolving some breast cancers that had eroded through the skin, in the days before current cancer treatments were available. As a topical application, it seemed safe.

Since I had no immediate use for the paste, I put it in my refrigerator and forgot about it. I only remembered it six months later, when I had to make a decision about veterinary treatment for my dog, Coca, a female Rhodesian ridgeback, six years old and in good health except for a growth that had developed on her right side, near the shoulder. It had started as a black skin tag but had steadily enlarged until it was now the size of a marble and looked like a little black cauliflower. My vet told me it should come off. "These things can turn into melanomas," he said. Taking it off would mean putting the dog under general anesthesia, which I did not want to do, since general anesthesia is a risky procedure, more so in dogs than humans. I did nothing, and the tumor kept growing.

Then I remembered the container in my refrigerator. Here was a perfect opportunity to test the power of bloodroot. I smeared a thin coating of the paste over the growth, and repeated the application every morning for three days. On the fourth day, when I called Coca over for the treatment, I was alarmed to see blood running down her side. The tumor had turned grayish and seemed to be separating from the skin, leaving a gaping wound underneath. I stopped applying bloodroot, cleaned the area with hydrogen peroxide, and resolved to keep an eye on the area. Two days later, the whole tumor, then whitish gray, fell off, leaving a raw, circular area that quickly healed over. The end result was a perfectly circular, slightly depressed area of skin, with no trace of tumor. The bloodroot had removed it more neatly than one could have done with a scalpel. Later, hair grew over the spot, concealing it completely. I could not have asked for a better outcome, especially as the dog had showed no signs of discomfort.

So much for my animal trial; I was ready to go on to humans. Shortly afterward a friend came to visit who showed me a mole he was worried about on his chest. His name is John Fago, a photographer, who had lost a leg to bone cancer some years before. He had been an avid downhill skier before the operation and now was an avid and very skillful one-legged skier. Statistically, John's chances of being cured of his cancer were excellent, and he was careful to follow a lifestyle that increased them even more. Still, he was understandably nervous about strange growths. This one was a pigmented mole that had been enlarging. When I told John about the bloodroot cure of my dog, he did not hesitate. "Let's do it," he said.

Unlike my dog, John had no coat of fur, so it was easier to watch the process. On the second day of applying the paste, the skin around the base of the mole became inflamed, an obvious immune reaction, and John said it was quite sore. On the third day, the mole turned pale and began to swell. On the fourth day, it fell off, leaving a perfectly circular wound that healed quickly. Later I asked John to describe his experience to a group of medical students. He did so, with the result that I began getting requests for nonsurgical removal of moles. Over the years, I have given out bloodroot paste and instructions on how to use it to a number of medical students, and the outcomes have been consistent and satisfactory. The most recent was a young woman with a large mole at the collar line at the base of the neck. A dermatologist wanted to take it off, but his description of the size of the incision he would have to make put her off, and she knew that healing would be difficult because of the location. She asked me if I knew any alternative to surgery. Bloodroot solved her problem. "It got pretty scary-looking on the third day," she told me afterward, "but I remembered your description of what would happen, and I tried not to worry. Now the mole is gone completely, and I think it's a much better job than the dermatologist could have done. I'm amazed."

So here is an example of a discovery made by paying attention to a testimonial. I would hope it would inspire scientific inquiry into the mechanism by which bloodroot is able to stimulate rejection of abnormal tissue and into possible applications of it for treatment of growths other than moles.

Talking about herbal cures with doctors is particularly difficult because they have no training in medical botany and because the subject is highly polarized, with some authorities claiming that the use of plants in medicine is not only unscientific, being based on purely anecdotal evidence, but also dangerous. This is an uninformed position. Not only do many pharmaceutical drugs in current favor come from plants; there is quite an active effort today to study traditional plant remedies by the methods of modern science. In general, herbal medicines are safer than pharmaceutical drugs simply because their active constituents are diluted by inert material and modified by secondary components. On the other hand, manufacturers of herbal products often make unsubstantiated claims for them in order to sell their wares in a competitive and largely unregulated market.

Take *Ginkgo biloba*. Dozens of scientific articles about its chemistry and pharmacology, based on both animal and human experiments, have appeared in good, peer-reviewed journals, although the journals are not ones read by American physicians. (I cannot think of one physician I know who reads *Planta Medica,* a German journal and one of the best.) If you will review the hefty technical literature on ginkgo, you will find experimental evidence that it increases blood flow throughout the body, especially in the head. It has been shown to be an effective and nontoxic treatment for disorders of hearing and equilibrium due to impaired circulation to the ear and for deficits of memory and mental function due to impaired blood supply to the brain. Its lack of toxicity is in great contrast to pharmaceutical drugs used to treat these conditions.

The known actions of ginkgo extract are consistent with some of the favorable results reported in the testimonial letter from the woman in Chicago, but the effects she says she has experienced go beyond those known actions. Besides, the dose she was using is low. The effective dose range is two tablets of the standardized material taken three times a day. Even with that, patients are advised to be patient; the beneficial effects of ginkgo usually do not appear before six to eight weeks of continuous usage. So even if we accept the stories as true, there is a question about the assignment of cause and effect. Did ginkgo cause the beneficial changes?

This question raises a thorny issue that leads even more doctors to throw testimonials into wastebaskets. It is well known that belief in medicines can cause favorable outcomes even if the medicines are ineffective. This is the placebo response, which most doctors dislike because it muddies their experiments and seems inherently unscientific from the point of view of the biomedical model. I regard the placebo response as a pure example of healing elicited by the mind; far from being a nuisance, it is, potentially, the greatest therapeutic ally doctors can find in their efforts to mitigate disease. I believe further that the art of medicine is in the selection of treatments and their presentation to patients in ways that increase their effectiveness through the activation of placebo responses. The best way to do this as a physician is to use treatments that you yourself genuinely believe in, because your belief in what you do catalyzes the beliefs of your patients.

Unfortunately, this view of placebo medicine is very much out of fashion today. Most doctors want nothing to do with placebos, favoring instead "real" treatments that work through identifiable biochemical mechanisms. They also like treatments that produce very specific effects ("magic bullets"). If a drug begins to work in too many different conditions, most doctors lose interest in it, because they think lack of specificity means lack of an underlying mechanism. In other words the drug could be—perish the thought!—merely a placebo.

I might mention that this way of thinking is unique to Western medicine. In traditional Chinese medicine, drugs, which are mostly herbal, are classified into three categories, called superior, middle, and inferior. Inferior drugs are those with specific effects in specific conditions, the magic bullets that are Western medicine's highest therapeutic ideal. Middle drugs have broader powers because they strengthen body functions. Superior drugs are the tonics and panaceas, those that work for everything. Ginseng is an example; its Latin name, *Panax*, comes from the same root as *panacea*, meaning "all heal." In the Chinese conception, superior drugs work by stimulating the defensive functions of the body, making it more resistant to assaults of all kinds. These drugs are not toxic, not weapons against specific diseases; but by increasing resistance, of course they work for everything.

This short digression into medical philosophy and the differences between Western and Eastern medicine is meant simply to point out the many reasons why most scientifically minded doctors in this country would ignore testimonials such as the one above. In short: they tend to disbelieve the stories without attempting to verify them, possibly out of fear that someone is trying to put something over on them; they are unwilling to endorse (or even consider) types of treatments falling outside their area of experience, such as herbal remedies; and they are reluctant to put cause-and-effect interpretations on anecdotes of this sort because they fear the reported benefits, even if true, may turn out to be "nothing more" than placebo responses.

Over the years that I have been writing and speaking in public I have received hundreds and hundreds of testimonials. For every testimonial letter that has come to me I have heard dozens more stories that were not written down. In these accounts patients have sung the praises of an astonishing variety of therapies: herbs (familiar and unfamiliar), particular foods and dietary regimens, vitamins and supplements, drugs (prescription, over-the-counter, and illegal), acupuncture, yoga, biofeedback, homeopathy, chiropractic, surgery, prayer, massage, psychotherapy, love, marriage, divorce, exercise, sunlight, fasting, and on and on. I collect this material, save it, and take it seriously. In its totality and range and abundance it makes one powerful point: *People can get better.* More than that, they can get better from all sorts of conditions of disease, even very severe ones of long duration.

Like my colleagues, I also question the simple cause-and-effect interpretations placed on these reports and hesitate to endorse products and practitioners; but unlike most of them, I do not throw out the reports. Testimonials are important pieces of evidence. They are not necessarily testimony to the power or value of particular healers and products. Rather, *they are testimony to the human capacity for healing.* The evidence is incontrovertible that the body is capable of healing itself. By ignoring that, many doctors cut themselves off from a tremendous source of optimism about health and healing.

THE FACES OF HEALING: AL

OF THE PEOPLE I have interviewed for their personal accounts of healing, Alan Kapuler is one of the most unusual and delightful. A molecular biologist turned New Age gardener, he combines a formidable intellect and wide-ranging knowledge of life processes with a deep sensitivity to and reverence for the natural world. Al is the co-founder and director of Peace Seeds in Corvallis, Oregon, a family business specializing in the preservation, propagation, and distribution of heirloom and other unusual varieties of flowers and vegetables. He is also research director of Seeds of Change, a national organic seed company. Al works hard, loves his plants, collects and packs thousands of packets of seeds by hand, and is committed to nonviolence as a general principle.

Al Kapuler was graduated summa cum laude in biology from Yale University in 1962 at the age of nineteen. He considered going to medical school and remembers that in an admissions interview for New York University, he was asked why he wanted to be a doctor. "I want to cure cancer," he replied. Instead he studied cancer at Rockefeller University for six years, eventually earning a Ph.D. in life sciences. Much of his research experience was devoted to developing new chemotherapy agents and understanding their mechanisms of action on DNA.

Soon after completing his studies, Al dropped out of what he now calls the "whole materialistic system." He moved to the country, became a most-of-the-time vegetarian, and started farming. Since then, he has lived simply and worked the soil. In 1987 he settled with his wife and young children in Corvallis, where he set up Peace Seeds as a for-profit endeavor. "I was really working compulsively at that point," he recalls, "doing twenty-five thousand packets of seeds, growing and cleaning hundreds of seed crops, trying to solve the problem of 'right livelihood,' and all this with only part-time help; I was under a lot of stress."

You would think that given his biomedical background, he would have been alarmed by the appearance of swollen lymph nodes in his groin in June 1989, but the nodes were painless, and Al thought they would go away. They didn't. He tried putting hot and cold compresses on them with no success and just continued with his exhausting work. "I had no idea what they were," he told me. The enlarged nodes were on both sides, the size of quarters. Eventually he sought the advice of a physician friend he had known since graduate school. The friend recommended a CT scan of the whole body; it revealed between twenty-five and thirty abnormal nodes from the neck to the groin, two of which were biopsied and sent off for diagnosis. The result was mixed cell lymphoma, cancer of the lymphatic system. "They told me I had a seven-year life expectancy, that it would probably be two to three years before it got bad, and that I had to start chemotherapy."

Al's mother-in-law, an advocate of natural foods, sent him a book on healing cancer with a macrobiotic diet. He read it along with other books on dietary approaches to cancer. The books on macrobiotics made the most sense to him. "They used less pseudoscience than the others. They just said that certain patterns of eating cause cancer, and here's what you can do to reverse it. I thought I ate a pretty healthy diet, but, in fact, we consumed a lot of sugar in the form of honey and fruit juice, and I smoked tobacco. I also drank coffee—two cappuccinos a day with honey. From the macrobiotic point of view, all this is terrible. I realized I had to cut out everything unhealthy from my life." In November 1989 he went on a strict macrobiotic diet: brown rice, miso soup, beans, cooked vegetables, and sea vegetables, or in his words, "your basic Oriental monastic diet." The diet allowed no fruits or salads, no oils, no bread, no dietary supplements, and, of course, no meat or milk products, no sugar, and no alcohol.

"Did you ever consider doing chemotherapy?" I asked.

"Are you kidding? I'm a molecular biologist. I know what that crap does to people. And I knew that poisoning myself made no sense. Besides, I remembered telling that medical school interviewer years before that I wanted to cure cancer. I thought to myself, 'Ha! Now I've got a chance to do it.'

"Actually, I've come to love brown rice and vegetables, and on this program, I could have as much of those as I wanted. I had to chew my food very well. The diet agreed with me. I've been macrobiotic ever since, becoming more or less strict as changes in my health dictate."

For the first eleven months of this regimen, Al saw no change in his lymph nodes: no new ones developed, but there was no improvement. During this time he went to an oncologist in Eugene, Oregon, who did blood work every two months to look at the numbers of abnormal lymphocytes in Al's circulation. The numbers would fluctuate, and the oncologist pressured Al to start chemo. "He told me he'd just give me a 'light dose.' But I'd look around his office, and everyone was eating candy all the time. There were candy boxes on the counter where patients met the receptionists and receiving nurses. The secretaries and nurses and patients were all into it, and then you'd see the patients going into the chemo room. I told him, 'Never mind; the diet will take care of me.' "

In September 1990, just around the time of his forty-eighth birthday, Al noticed that the nodes in his groin seemed to be shrinking. By the end of October they were gone, and his groin was completely back to normal. His blood work returned to normal too, and the oncologist was amazed. Al recalls, "And another well-known oncologist told me I was the only patient he knew with a confirmed diagnosis of cancer who got into complete remission as a result of diet therapy alone."

There was no sign of abnormality in Al's lymphatic system until the beginning of 1993, when he was again under unusually heavy stress as a result of his work. His income had dropped, he was trying to work with another organization, and he felt he was at a crossroads in his career, with the future direction uncertain. In response to this stress, he abandoned his strict diet and began to eat sweets. Shortly afterward he developed a gum infection on the right side of his mouth. This was followed by an infection in his left ear. As the ear infection drained, the lymph nodes in the left side of his neck swelled. They were tender, suggesting reaction to infection rather than any malignant process; but when the infection resolved, the lymph nodes remained enlarged. Al now had six abnormal nodes in his neck. He also developed a rash on three fingers of his right hand; it would come in cycles, beginning with itching and developing into weeping pustules that would eventually become crusted and disappear. Having his hands in the soil made it worse. Al decided he had to take further action.

"My diet had become looser in the previous couple of years when I was feeling completely well. I decided I would go back on the strict regime. Also, I saw a documentary film that a friend of mine had made about the Hoxsey cancer therapy, and another friend, an acupuncturist, told me he had seen a patient cured by this method. I decided to go to Mexico, to a clinic in Tijuana that offers it."

The Hoxsey treatment is a tonic, composed of seven herbs and potassium iodide, and a diet. The diet, which prohibits pork, tomatoes, and vinegar, among other things, was much less restrictive than Al's macrobiotic regimen, which he continued. The idea of an herbal tonic appealed to Al's sympathies with plants, especially since many of the plants in the Hoxsey formula have anticancer properties.

"I went to Tijuana in the spring of 1993, and I must say I got better treatment at that clinic than anything I've seen from the medical profession in this country. The staff were very humane, very caring. You've got to remember that my father was a doctor, and I've had a lot of conventional treatment in my life. I had polio as a kid—in the 1949 epidemic—and was out of school for six months. Then I had chronic tonsillitis and was on endless cycles of antibiotics for years. So I'm very familiar with that kind of medicine, and I liked the kindness and patience of the doctors in Tijuana much better. They were so impressed with my diet that they told me I'd respond very quickly to the herbal therapy."

Al returned home with a supply of the Hoxsey formula and took a small amount of it after each meal. Within two months the nodes in his neck were down, and he has had no problems since. "Actually, I think I'm in better health now than I was five years ago," he says. "I've got incredible energy now." Having visited with him recently, I can confirm this. Al gives every appearance of being in excellent health.

"What have you learned from all this?" I asked him.

"Oh, so much, so much," he replied. "First of all, the cancer was a great gift, truly one of the best things that's ever happened to me. As a result of it, I understand so much more about how the body works. I've become really sensitive to the effects of food on my system, for instance. If I eat the wrong food, I know it within a half hour by how I feel. Also, I discovered something very interesting about the process of healing from cancer. It's not a simple one-step thing. I think there was a relationship between that rash on my fingers and the nodes in my neck. Something was being discharged through the skin, as if the internal aspects of the disease were moving to the surface and then out of the body. No conventional doctor would see that relationship, but I'm sure of it. Now I have nothing on my skin; it's completely clear.

"Most of all, I've learned that you are your own physician and have to heal yourself. The trick is to get your ego out of the way, get your concepts out of the way, and just let the body heal itself. It knows how to do it."

4

MEDICAL PESSIMISM

IT IS DIFFICULT for me to write about the failings of my profession, but these failings have negative consequences for all of us. Simply put: too many doctors are deeply pessimistic about the possibility of people getting better, and they communicate their pessimism to patients and families. Many of the patients who come to see me have been told by doctors, in one way or another, that they will not get better, that they will have to learn to live with their problems or expect to die from them, that medicine has nothing more to offer them.

I see patients from all over the country as well as from other countries, the vast majority of them refugees from conventional medicine. About ten percent of them are well—they have no immediate problems and want preventive lifestyle counseling. I wish more people would come to me before they get sick, because I have a great deal of information about how to reduce risks of heart disease, cancer, stroke, and other diseases that kill and disable us prematurely. I also know of ways to protect and enhance the body's healing system, which are set forth in the second part of this book. My advice concerns diet, patterns of activity and rest, and ways of handling stress, along with intelligent use of vitamins, supplements, herbs, and practices that take advantage of mind/body interactions.

Of the remaining ninety percent of my patients, about half have routine complaints: allergies, headaches, insomnia, anxiety, sinus trouble, arthritis, back pain, and so forth. To these people I offer genuine alternatives to conventional medicine. From my extensive travels and studies of many different therapeutic systems, I have assembled a large collection of methods and remedies that I find to be safer, more effective, and certainly more cost-effective than the drugs and surgeries offered by mainstream medical practitioners. For the management of common, everyday ailments, conventional methods are best described as therapeutic overkill—heavy artillery that should be used only as a last resort, after simpler and safer methods have failed. The problem is that doctors are not trained in the use of simple methods that take advantage of the body's own healing potential.

The last group of patients are those with serious illnesses, where the probability of healing is less. I see many people with cancer, many with chronic degenerative diseases. Often, these people tell me they regard me as their last hope, since they have exhausted all other possibilities for medical help. In such cases I act as an advisor, helping patients weigh their options and make intelligent choices about how to use conventional medicine selectively and how to combine it with alternatives. For example, many of the cancer patients decide to undergo surgery and chemotherapy or radiation therapy, but they want to know what else they can do to prevent recurrences. Typically, their oncologists tell them they do not need to do anything else once they have been treated. The patients know better. They want to learn about anticancer foods and supplements, ways of using the mind to boost immune defenses, and so forth. My job is to make that information available.

Whether they are relatively healthy or relatively sick, the patients who come to my office are highly motivated to take responsibility for their own health. Motivated patients are a pleasure to work with. They are seeking information, which they will act on once they obtain it. Such patients tend to be intelligent and well educated, attributes consistent with the findings of surveys here and abroad of people who go to alternative practitioners. Finally, many of them have suffered physically, emotionally, or financially as a result of encounters with conventional medicine. Here are the complaints I hear most commonly:

"Doctors don't take time to listen to you or answer your questions."

"All they do is give you drugs; I don't want to take more drugs."

"They said there was nothing more they could do for me."

"They told me it would only get worse."

"They told me I would just have to live with it."

"They said I'd be dead in six months."

The last four statements are particularly disturbing, because they reflect deep pessimism about the human potential for healing. At its most extreme, this attitude constitutes a kind of medical "hexing" that I find unconscionable. Anthropologists and psychologists have studied medical hexing in shamanistic cultures, where, on occasion, a shaman or witch doctor will curse someone (usually at the behest of the person's enemy), and the victim of the curse then withdraws from society, friends, and family, stops eating, and weakens. The medical literature contains reports of chronic illness and death resulting from this process, with some speculation about physiological mechanisms that might account for it, such as derangement of the involuntary nervous system. So-called voodoo death is the ultimate example of a negative placebo response. Although it is easy to identify this hexing phenomenon in exotic cultures, we rarely perceive that something very similar goes on every day in our own culture, in hospitals, clinics, and doctors' offices.

Two years ago a man in his mid-thirties came to me for a second opinion about his illness. After several months of worsening episodes of diarrhea and abdominal pain, his family doctor referred him to a gastroenterologist, who diagnosed the problem as ulcerative colitis and started the patient on a standard suppressive drug but gave him no information about modifying his lifestyle. The man disliked the side effects of the drug and did not think it controlled the symptoms very well. He also suspected that his problem had something to do with stress. He complained about the drug treatment and persisted in questioning the gastroenterologist about other possible strategies, without success. "Do you know what that doctor said to me on my last visit? He said, 'Listen, I've got nothing else to offer you, and, anyway, the chances are you'll eventually develop colon cancer.' "

People with ulcerative colitis are statistically more likely than others to get colon cancer, it is true, probably because chronic inflammation and destruction of the lining of the colon leads to increased cell division and with increased cell division comes increased risk of malignant transformation; but the probability of colon cancer in any individual with ulcerative colitis is low, especially if the disease is controlled and, as in this case, mild. Besides, even cases of not-so-mild ulcerative colitis can respond dramatically to changes in lifestyle and outlook. I remember a woman in her mid-forties who had suffered for years with a severe form of the disease, managed imperfectly with high doses of prednisone and other suppressive drugs, who was told that surgical removal of the entire colon was her only option. She went on a macrobiotic diet, and the disease promptly disappeared. Fifteen years later, when she consulted me about an unrelated problem, it had still not returned.

How did the gastroenterologist's words of doom affect my patient? "I didn't sleep for three nights," he reported. "All I could think was, 'I'm going to get cancer of the colon,' and, frankly, the idea still haunts me." I gave him a program to follow, including referral to a hypnotherapist to help undo the medical hex and teach him how to use his mind to improve his condition. Had it been feasible, I would have put him in touch with the woman whose colitis had disappeared. That was the second opinion he really needed.

Here is another instructive story: Five years ago a fifty-three-year-old man from Canada came to see me. Actually, it was his wife who came to see me. He stayed in his car in the driveway, because, his wife said, he was terrified of doctors and couldn't bring himself to see another one. I took the history from her, then went out and persuaded him to come in. He had had several years of urinary disturbances, which he had ignored. When he did finally go to a urologist, the problem turned out to be prostate cancer that had already escaped the gland and gone to the bones of the pelvis, making for a poor prognosis. He went to a university hospital, where the only treatment offered him was female hormones to antagonize the growth of the tumor.

The main impression I had of this man was of someone in the grip of fear. He had seized on visualization therapy as his best and only hope and told me that he spent two hours a day in fierce concentration, trying to visualize his immune cells gobbling up the cancer cells. But he had made no effort to change his lifestyle in a manner that might have improved his general health and immunity; he continued to smoke cigarettes at the rate of two packs a day, for example. When

I asked about the smoking, he said: "Three months ago, I was at University Hospital, in the office of the chief urologist. He explained the hormone therapy to me and said that it was not worth doing any other treatment. I asked him, 'Should I stop smoking?' and he said, 'At this point, why bother?' "

Were I to ask that urologist about his reply—assuming he even remembered making it—he would probably say that he was doing the patient a favor by sparing him further trouble. What the patient heard, however, was "You are going to die soon." A high priest of technological medicine, enthroned in his temple, had uttered the equivalent of a shamanistic curse, for doctors in our culture are invested with the very same power others project onto shamans and priests. Those words were the source of the patient's terror, a terror that paralyzed him and prevented him from making constructive efforts for his own survival and well-being. Yes, metastatic prostate cancer has a poor prognosis, but this patient was still in relatively good general health, and it is not hard to find examples of people with metastatic prostate cancer who remain relatively healthy for years. Why prejudice the outcome?

There is a difference worth noting between the hex in this case and in the previous one. Here the urologist revealed his pessimism in an unthinking way, without any intent to upset the patient. The gastroenterologist who predicted colon cancer for the man with early ulcerative colitis may have been annoyed by a patient who questioned his treatment and repeatedly demanded information he was not able to provide. My experience is that thoughtless medical hexing is much more common than intentional hexing, though it is no less harmful.

Some of the stories I hear are so outrageous that all I can do is laugh; when I can get patients to laugh as well, I feel that the curses are dispelled. A woman from Helsinki in her late forties came to see me one February. She had early multiple sclerosis that had caused muscle weakness in one leg. I was more alarmed by her emotional state. She was depressed and wooden throughout the telling of the story, which she related as if it had all happened to someone else. It did not take much to make her feel better; traveling from Helsinki to Tucson in February was salutary in itself. Since she was able to stay for a while, I put her in touch with several therapists who worked with her on matters of body, mind, and lifestyle. After a month, she had brightened considerably and had adopted a more hopeful outlook.

"You wouldn't believe what those doctors did to me in Finland," she confided. I asked for details. "It took them a long time to make the diagnosis, many tests. Then finally, the head neurologist took me into his office and told me I had multiple sclerosis. He let that sink in; then he went out of the room and returned with a wheelchair. This he told me to sit in. I said, 'Why should I sit in your wheelchair?' He said I was to buy a wheelchair and sit in it for an hour a day to 'practice' for when I would be totally disabled. Can you imagine?" She related this tale with a healthy laugh that I strongly encouraged. Wheelchair practice, indeed!

I could go on and on recounting stories of medical hexing, intentional or unintentional, funny or—more often—sad, but I believe I have made my point. I have more uplifting subjects to write about. I cannot help feeling embarrassed by my profession when I hear the myriad ways in which doctors convey their pessimism to patients. I would like to change this pattern and am working to require instruction in medical school about the power of words and the need for physicians to use extreme care in choosing the words they speak to patients. A larger subject is the problem of making doctors more conscious of the power projected onto them by patients and the possibilities for reflecting that power back in ways that influence health for better rather than for worse, that stimulate rather than retard spontaneous healing. As I said earlier, we have thrust medical doctors into the roles served by shamans and priests in more traditional cultures, but doctors are poorly trained to play out those roles constructively. The good shamans I have met in my travels have been master psychotherapists who know both intuitively and by their training how to take projected belief and turn it back to patients in the service of healing.

On rare occasions a medical hex may motivate an exceptional patient to prove the doctor wrong by getting well. I remember one old woman who had survived uterine cancer years before telling me with a toothless grin, "That doctor told me I had less than a year to live, and now he's dead and here I am!" Unfortunately, that is the exception. The usual effect of a medical hex is despair, and I cannot believe that despair has beneficial effects on the human healing system. It is not a good idea to stay in treatment with a doctor who thinks you cannot get better.

It seems most strange that practitioners of the so-called healing art should have such little faith in healing. What are the roots of medical pessimism? One that I identify is the lopsided nature of medical education, which focuses almost exclusively on disease and its treatment rather than on health and its maintenance. The preclinical portion of the medical curriculum is top-heavy with detailed information about disease processes. Here the word "healing" is used rarely, if ever; the term "healing system" not at all. As I will explain in the next chapter, we already know some of the mechanisms of healing, but without the concept of a healing system, we cannot take this knowledge and put it together into any useful constructions.

The biomedical model from which conventional medical theory and practice derive makes it very difficult to present a view of the healing system to doctors-in-training. Its materialism leads to emphasis on form rather than function. The healing system is a functional system, not an assemblage of structures that can be neatly diagrammed like the digestive or circulatory systems. Here again, Eastern medicine has the advantage over its Western counterpart. Traditional Chinese medicine emphasized function over structure and, as a result, was able to understand that the human organism had a defensive sphere of function that could be stimulated, long before Western doctors realized that the "functionless" organs of the body—tonsils, adenoids, thymus, and appendix—were components of the immune system.

Worse, the biomedical model discounts or entirely writes off the importance of the mind, looking instead for purely physical causes of changes in health and illness. My experiences and observations of healing suggest that the mental realm is often the true locus of cause. Despite growing public interest in mind/body interactions, professional interest remains at a low level.

It is not only teaching that suffers as a result of these limitations but also research. Research produces the information that enters the medical curriculum; without research there is just anecdotal evidence. The disease focus of medical inquiry is obvious. Look at our National Institutes of Health. Really they are National Institutes of Disease: the National Cancer Institute, the National Institute of Allergy and Infectious Disease, the National Institute of Arthritis and Skin Diseases, the National Institute of Diabetes and Digestive and Kidney Diseases, the National Institute of Neurological Disorders and Stroke, and so on. Where is the National Institute of Health and Healing?

Very little research exists on healing, and what has been done is too narrow in scope. Investigators have paid some attention to one impressive phenomenon, spontaneous remission, but remission is not synonymous with healing. The word "remission" implies a temporary abatement of a disease process that may well recur. Moreover, remission is strongly associated with cancer, and cancer, in my view, is a special case. If we look only or mostly at spontaneous remission of cancer, we come away with a distorted picture of the healing system that in no way reveals its full range of activities and potentials.

The first comprehensive search of the medical literature for case reports of spontaneous remission was published in 1993 as a thick, annotated bibliography, containing hundreds of references. Fully seventy-four percent of them concern cancer, and the authors note that "a review of the remission literature reveals that almost all, if not all, the papers on remission have been about cancer." A first—and only—World Conference on Spontaneous Remission took place in 1974 at Johns Hopkins University School of Medicine. It was exclusively about cancer.

Healing is a researchable phenomenon. For years I have been asking my colleagues to look at and study folk cures of warts as examples of healing responses. Wart cures are common, dramatic events in which the healing system, activated by belief, rids the body of virus-infected tissue precisely and efficiently, making conventional treatments for warts look clumsy and barbaric. Still, the whole subject is regarded more as an amusement by medical scientists than as a serious field for investigation.

When medical students finish their preclinical studies and go on to work in the wards of teaching hospitals, the lopsidedness of their education is reinforced by their experience of illness. Third- and fourth-year students, along with interns, residents, and fellows, are immersed in the world of hospital medicine. The patients they see there are not representative of the total spectrum of illness. Rather, they constitute a skewed sample—the very sick. In that group, healing responses occur less frequently than in the general population. If you treat predominantly people with life-threatening crises and end-stage chronic disease, naturally you are going to be pessimistic about outcomes.

These facts of life of medical training—its unbalanced focus on disease rather than health, the limitations of its conceptual model, the deficiencies of research, and its skewed experience of illness toward the very worst possibilities—are sufficient to account for medical pessimism. Yet underlying all this are deeper motivations, never discussed and rarely considered, that have to do with why people become doctors in the first place.

When I ask students why they chose medical school, the usual kinds of answers I get have to do with helping others, enjoying prestige and power, and having job and financial security. I believe there is another reason that is less conscious. The practice of medicine provides an illusion of control over life and death. One way to deal with fears of life and death is to seek comfort in that illusion. But every time a patient fails to get better or, especially, dies, doctors must confront the fact that their control is illusory. The prediction of a negative outcome may offer psychological comfort to the physician: if the patient gets better, the doctor can be pleasantly surprised and take credit for it, whereas if the patient gets worse or dies, the doctor predicted it and therefore still seems to be in control. Medical pessimism may thus be a psychological defense against uncertainty, which does not excuse it or lessen its impact on patients. The fact is that we live in an uncertain universe, and do not have controlling power over life and death. What we do have is the ability to understand how the human organism can heal itself, a subject that is inherently comforting and gives reason for both doctors and patients to be optimistic.

THE FACES OF HEALING: JOHN

THE ONLY REMNANT John Luja has of his disease is a two-inch patch of itchy skin on his right lower leg, and he thinks that might not even be related to his prior problem. Now seventy-five, John runs a landscaping business outside St. Louis. He says he doesn't go to doctors and he has always used home remedies, probably because he grew up in Lithuania in a culture that was much more self-reliant than ours in matters of health.

In 1980 John developed an unusual problem: the skin on the front of both his lower legs became red and itchy. After four weeks it turned "kind of yellow and dead looking," and he did go to a doctor, who told him the problem looked like scleroderma, a potentially serious autoimmune disease. The doctor performed a skin biopsy to be sure, and the biopsy result was indeed scleroderma. To be absolutely sure, he sent John to a specialist, who did another biopsy and confirmed the diagnosis. "They told me there was no real cure," John recalls. "They said I could use cortisone cream to control the itching, and they said I should take cortisone pills, too, because it would give me some insurance against involvement of my internal organs."

John found that the cortisone cream worked immediately to make the skin on his legs feel better. "Then after two weeks, it stopped working; in fact, it made things worse. I think I might have been allergic to it. I found a cortisone lotion that seemed to be better." He also started taking prednisone pills. Now the skin started to harden, and new affected areas appeared on his back, arms, and chest. "The doctor told me the scleroderma would probably start inside me and that I'd probably die from it."

On learning this, John's daughter and son-in-law, then living in Arizona, decided to move back to the St. Louis area to be near him. Mike, his son-in-law, says that much of John's skin at that time "looked and felt just like plastic, like the surface of a mannequin. They had told him that he had a fatal illness, and we just accepted that."

In fact, John never accepted the doctors' prognosis. He had little faith in the prednisone and stopped taking it after six weeks. Instead, he decided he would research the subject himself. "I thought what I had was something like arthritis," he says, "because I noticed that I would get worse before it rained. About three or four days before rain, the itching would get real bad. I also thought it had something to do with nerves, because I was having a lot of trouble with the business and was very nervous when it started. And I figured it had something to do with too much calcium."

So John started reading about home remedies for arthritis and excess calcium in the system. He decided to try vinegar and lemons, washing the affected skin with vinegar and eating fresh lemons. I asked him how he ate the lemons. "I just ate them straight," he said. "The other thing I tried was aloe vera juice. I bought it at the health food store and started drinking it every day. Soon the itching was gone. I never used the cortisone lotion again.

"Still, I thought something was wrong inside me. I felt I needed to shock my system, and I got the idea from a book of using a high dose of vitamin E. I took 5,000 units of vitamin E a day for two weeks." That is definitely a high dose of vitamin E, since the recommended daily allowance is 30 international units, and a megadose, advocated by proponents of antioxidant therapy, is 800 to 1,000 units a day.

John says: "I think that really started something."

His disease had been present for six months. Two months after he started his home remedies, it stopped spreading. Then the hardened skin began to soften. "The doctor was surprised to see the change. He told me, 'I don't know what you're doing, but whatever it is, keep doing it!' After six months, the condition started to disappear on my arms and chest. After two years it was gone and has never come back."

I asked John what he had done about the nervous component of his illness. "I just settled down," he replied. "Whenever your nerves are involved in a disease, you've got to make a change in your life; you've got to change your thinking."

Mike thinks his father-in-law's attitude had a lot to do with the outcome. "I think it was the way he was raised, in a culture that valued home remedies more than professional treatment. He never bought into the doctors' pessimism. And he really had faith in his aloe juice. He always had a gallon of the stuff with him and drank it by the glass."

"My health today is pretty good," says John Luja. "I still use vinegar if I get any itching. I still eat lemons from time to time. And I try not to go to doctors."

5

THE HEALING SYSTEM

IF THE HEALING SYSTEM is invisible or difficult to see from the vantage point of clinical medicine, its existence is clear from other points of view. Simply as an evolutionary necessity, organisms must have mechanisms of self-repair to counteract the forces that create injury and illness. For most of our existence as a species, we have not had doctors, whether conventional, alternative, or otherwise. The survival of the species alone implies the existence of a healing system.

My purpose in writing this book is to convince more people to rely on the body's innate potential for maintaining health and overcoming illness, but I cannot easily give you a picture of this system. Lacking organized research, we know few of the details of its components and mechanisms. Also, the human organism is dauntingly complex, and its ability to repair itself is one of its most complex functions. Mind/body interactions frequently appear relevant to peoples' experiences of healing, but we lack a model that integrates mind into biological reality.

There is an aphorism that I find useful in such situations: "As above, so below; as below, so above." This means that patterns of truth observed at any level of reality will be true at every level of reality. Therefore, if we can discern the operation of the healing system at any level of biological organization, we should be able to infer the nature of its operations at other levels. I will describe what we know about mechanisms of self-repair at a few key points of the human organism, beginning with DNA, the macromolecule that defines life. The tone of this chapter will be a bit more technical than that of the previous ones. Do not be discouraged if you cannot absorb all the details presented here, because what matters are the general principles.

DNA takes the same form in all organisms, from human beings to viruses—an enormous molecule with a double-helix structure made up of two chains of sugar molecules, twisted about each other, with "rungs" linking the two chains. The rungs form between complementary pairs of nitrogen-containing subunits (nucleotides), whose specific sequences differentiate the DNA of one organism from that of another. Only four different nucleotides occur in DNA; they are the "letters" of a genetic code spelling out "words" of information that direct the construction and operation of all forms of life. The so-called Central Dogma of modern molecular biology states that DNA *replicates* itself in order to pass its genetic information on from one cell to another and from one generation to the next; DNA also *transcribes* its information into another macromolecule, RNA, that can travel out of the cell nucleus; RNA, in turn, *translates* this information into the manufacture of specific proteins that determine the structure and function of organisms. These three processes—the replication, transcription, and translation of genetic information—are the most basic processes of life. They are also amazingly intricate and risky, because there are so many points at which things can go wrong.

For example, in order for DNA to replicate or transcribe itself, the long double helix must unwind and separate, so that each strand can act as a template on which a new, complementary strand can form. During this process, DNA is susceptible to injury from certain forms of energy (ionizing radiation and ultraviolet light) and matter (chemical mutagens). Also, mistakes can occur in the assembly of the new strands, such as the placement of wrong nucleotides. Damage to DNA can have disastrous consequences for organisms. Therefore, sophisticated mechanisms have evolved for the repair of this molecule in order to assure nearly error-free transmission of genetic information from one generation to the next, even in the simplest forms of life.

All of the mechanics of replication, transcription, and translation are directed by a special class of proteins called enzymes. A great deal of the genetic code specifies the manufacture of enzyme molecules, which, in turn, oversee the chemical reactions that develop the genetic code into biological reality. In a sense, enzymes are the "hands" that carry out DNA's instructions. It was not until 1965 that scientists, using a technique called X-ray crystallography, were able to picture the three-dimensional structure of an enzyme (one in the white of a hen's egg), but since then our knowledge of enzymes has expanded rapidly. The more we know about them, the more magical they seem.

Enzymes catalyze the chemical reactions of life—that is, they speed up the rates at which these reactions reach equilibrium but are not themselves changed in the process. Enzymes are necessary because if left to themselves, the reactions would not take place fast enough to support life. Chemists can speed up indolent reactions by subjecting them to high temperatures and pressures and by creating extreme conditions of acidity or alkalinity (pH). They can also add chemical catalysts to reactions, but these, too, often work best under physical conditions far removed from those of cells, which live at relatively low temperatures, at atmospheric pressure, and at nearly neutral pH. By contrast, enzymes in cells are able to catalyze reactions under the mild conditions of life and do so with much greater efficiency than their inorganic counterparts. They may be thought of as highly complex and efficient molecular machines.

How do enzymes work? The answer has to do with their three-dimensional configurations, which give them the ability to bind with great specificity to other molecules—substrates—and accelerate their tendency to react. The binding takes place at a particular site on the enzyme, which is both geometrically and electronically complementary to a portion of the substrate. Many enzymes will bind only to one substrate and not to any other molecule, even a very close relative. Once bound to an enzyme, the substrate may find itself in physical proximity to another reactant or it may be forced into a new configuration that strains particular chemical bonds, making them more likely to break or reform in ways that favor a desired reaction. Enzymes have diverse mechanisms by which they cause chemical bonds of substrates to change. In practical terms, they function as ingenious machines that alter substrate molecules: cutting them apart, putting them together, snipping particular pieces off them, adding others back, all with astonishing precision and speed.

One very interesting class of enzymes binds to DNA itself in order to direct the step-by-step replication of genetic information and to ensure that it is error-free. For example, enzymes called endonucleases cleave DNA at specific sequences, while exonucleases can cut off the ends of single strands. (Names of enzymes always end in -*ase*.) DNA gyrase catalyzes the "unzipping" and unwinding of the double helix in order for transcription to begin. A family of enzymes called DNA polymerases then directs the assembly of the new strands.

The first DNA polymerase to be identified was polymerase I, discovered in *E. coli* bacteria, which are widely used in genetics research. Scientists assumed that this enzyme was the sole director of replication, but thirteen years after its discovery, a mutant strain of the bacteria was found that had almost no detectable polymerase I. Although it reproduced at a normal rate, suggesting the existence of another form of the enzyme, this strain was unusually susceptible to the damaging effects of UV radiation and chemical mutagens. This was the first piece of evidence that polymerase I, in addition to directing replication, plays a central role in repairing damaged DNA.

If I were to forget to take my hat when walking from my office to my car on a sunny day, my bald head would receive a dose of UV radiation. If the sun were high in the sky and it was summer, the UV rays would be more energetic and more numerous. In even a few minutes, many of them would penetrate into living cells beneath the epidermis of my scalp, and some of them would strike the nuclei of cells. Some of those strikes would hit DNA, and some of those might hit crucial points of the DNA molecule during the process of replication or transcription, altering a nucleotide in a way that caused it to bond abnormally to its neighbor. This change would result in a kink in one strand of the double helix, a genetic error. When you consider that of the 300 trillion cells in an average body, some ten million die and are replaced every second, you get an idea of the number of cells at risk even from very brief exposure to agents that can chemically alter DNA.

What happens in the nucleus of a skin cell whose DNA sustains this kind of injury from UV light? Very probably and almost immediately, an endonuclease would recognize the defect and snip the affected strand on one side of the injury. Then an exonuclease would snip the other side, cutting off the damaged end. Polymerase I would then fill in the gap with undamaged nucleotides, and finally, a DNA ligase would connect the broken ends. This is a very elaborate, molecular version of cut-and-paste. (As efficient and effective as this kind of healing is, it is not a substitute for wearing a hat as protection from the sun.)

If, during replication, polymerase I accidentally incorporates the wrong nucleotide into a growing strand, the enzyme can recognize the error, excise it, and restore the correct sequencing. Therefore, polymerase I actually proofreads its own work, editing mistakes as it directs the synthesis of new copies of DNA.

Many variations exist on these themes, with many different enzymes available for the healing of DNA from the myriad kinds of damage it is likely to sustain. We know the details of some of them; the details of others are obscure. One very elaborate system, the "SOS response," has been discovered in *E. coli*. Agents that damage DNA induce a complex of changes in these bacteria that stop cells from dividing and increase their ability to repair damaged DNA, probably by stepping up production of healing enzymes.

Here, then, are basic activities of the healing system, discernible at the level of macromolecules, which are an interface between living and nonliving matter. At this level there is no immune system, nor are there nerves to carry messages from the brain. We are far below the world of organs. Even without knowing more about the details of self-repair of DNA, it is possible to draw a few conclusions:

- Healing is an inherent capacity of life. DNA has within it all the information needed to manufacture enzymes to repair itself.

- The healing system operates continuously and is always on call.

- The healing system has a diagnostic capability; it can recognize damage.

- The healing system can remove damaged structure and replace it with normal structure.

- The healing system not only acts to neutralize the effects of serious injury (as in the SOS response in *E. coli*), it also directs the ordinary, moment-to-moment corrections that maintain normal structure and function (as in the proofreading and editing activity of DNA polymerase I).

- Healing is spontaneous. It is a natural tendency arising from the internal nature of DNA. The occurrence of a lesion (such as a kink created by misbonding as a result of a hit by UV radiation) automatically activates the process of its repair.

In larger patterns of biological organization in the human being these same characteristics obtain. As above, so below; as below, so above.

The next stop on our tour is at the single cell, in particular the membrane surrounding the cell, the *plasma membrane,* a boundary and interface with the extracellular environment. DNA is now far below us in a distant nucleus, and we are in a world of interactions between large surfaces.

When I took high-school biology thirty-five years ago, plasma membranes were thought of as passive containers that kept cells' contents from spilling out. By the time I was in college, membranes appeared to be more interesting. They had a distinctive layered structure composed of lipids (fats) and proteins, with the proteins embedded in and attached to a kind of flexible, fluid lipid matrix. When I got to medical school, researchers had recognized the dynamic, active nature of plasma membranes. They are sites of active transport of substances from outside the cell to inside the cell, with receptors on their outer surfaces, specialized protein structures designed to bind to particular hormones and nutrients. Moreover, it was discovered that membranes connect to vast systems of tiny channels within cells and that they help cells take in wanted, and expel unwanted, materials. New membrane is constantly being synthesized within the cell, and old membrane is constantly being absorbed.

One of the most dynamic aspects of membrane biology is a process called endocytosis—the pinching off or budding of plasma membrane within a cell to form hollow structures called vesicles. In recent years, investigators have clarified some of the details of endocytosis and in so doing have revealed—to me, at least—another aspect of the healing system.

The best studied example of endocytosis involves receptors for LDL—low-density lipoprotein—a carrier molecule that transports cholesterol from the bloodstream to cells. When bound to LDL in the bloodstream, cholesterol is in the "bad" form that tends to deposit in arterial walls, causing atherosclerosis and coronary heart disease. A high level of serum LDL cholesterol is a risk factor for heart attacks, but many cells are equipped with receptors to bind LDL and remove it from the circulation.

When an LDL receptor on the external surface of a cell membrane binds to an LDL molecule, the receptor moves to another special structure on the membrane, a depression lined with a distinctive protein coat, called a "coated pit." Once in the pit, the occupied receptor undergoes endocytosis and winds up inside the cell in a vesicle, which then merges with other, similar vesicles. The materials in the coalesced vesicles are then sorted and sent in different directions. Once inside cells, LDL cholesterol cannot do our arteries any harm; cells actually need some cholesterol in their metabolism and can dispose of any excess. In the sorting process, the LDL receptor is recycled back to the surface of the membrane, while LDL (and excess cholesterol) is sent for disposal to a structure called the lysosome. Lysosomes contain powerful enzymes that can chop up large molecules into small, disposable pieces.

On the outside surface of the plasma membrane, the recycled LDL receptor is ready to bind more LDL and take another trip through the interior of the cell. Studies show that LDL receptors recycle every ten to twenty minutes. Since their lifespan is ten to thirty hours, they can make many trips in and out of the cell, transporting many molecules of LDL. Then, at some point they wear out. When an LDL receptor's structure and function deteriorate, it, too, goes off to a lysosome for destruction, and its place is taken by a newly synthesized receptor.

As researchers clarify the ins and outs of endocytosis, a picture is emerging of plasma membranes that is dizzying. It appears that at many points on the cell surface, membrane is forever being sucked into the cell ("invaginated" is the technical term), examined, sorted, and recycled back up to the surface. One phase of this process is the recognition and elimination of defective membrane structures via lysosomes.

Here again, as at the level of DNA, we can see the operations of an inherent, spontaneous healing system, in continuous operation, capable of recognition (diagnosis) as well as removal and replacement (treatment) of defective structure and function. Here at the cellular level, we can also see a capacity for regeneration of structure that allows the healing system to perform moment-to-moment maintenance. Healing at the membrane level is especially important, because cell surfaces are subject to much abuse and are also the sites of communication between cells through the interaction of receptors with molecules produced elsewhere.

Let us jump to a higher level of organization. Aggregates of cells form tissues, tissues form organs, organs form systems. At the tissue level, healing becomes more complex but shows the same general characteristics. The process of wound healing is well known and well studied; even so, many of us fail to see its larger significance. Suppose you cut your finger with a knife. Your immediate concerns are pain and bleeding. The pain will subside quickly; it is how you perceive the activity of peripheral nerves notifying your brain of the injury. Unless you have a clotting disorder, the bleeding will also stop soon with the formation of a clot that will harden to a protective scab. If you are attentive, you will notice the appearance of inflammation around the edges of the wound beginning within twenty-four hours of the cut: slight but definite tenderness, redness, swelling, and warmth. This is an immune response, caused by the migration of white blood cells to the area to defend against the entrance of germs as well as to clear the area of dead and dying cells.

The first wave of immune cells to invade the area are neutrophils, the most common white blood cells, which are the "infantry" of the body's defensive forces. They are soon followed by macrophages ("big eaters"), which can engulf and digest great quantities of cellular debris. Concurrent with this immune activity is the beginning of cellular proliferation from the normal surface (epithelial) cells at the edges of the wound. Spurs of these cells grow out from the edges under the clot to fuse in the midline, forming a thin but continuous layer of what will become new skin. Then a more vigorous proliferation of cells occurs with the appearance of a soft, pink, grainy tissue called granulation tissue. It will eventually fill the space of the wound. Under the microscope, granulation tissue shows itself to be full of fibroblasts, cells that synthesize the proteins that give our bodies architectural integrity, as well as newly forming blood vessels. The new vessels first appear as buds or sprouts on existing vessels at the margins of the cut. Finally, the immune cells recede, new skin develops and thickens, making the scab unnecessary, and, unless the wound was unusually deep, your finger will be as good as new.

Research into the mechanisms of the many steps of wound healing has demonstrated the important role of chemical regulators called growth factors. Growth factors are very small proteins (polypeptides) produced by cells or present in the bloodstream that either stimulate or inhibit cell growth. For example, a family of polypeptides called fibroblast growth factors (FGFs) not only stimulate fibroblasts but also induce all the steps necessary for new blood vessel formation. Epidermal growth factors (EGFs) stimulate cell division by binding to a special receptor on the cell membrane; when bound to their receptor, they somehow increase synthesis of both DNA and RNA in the cell nucleus. Transforming growth factor alpha (TGFα) binds to the same EGF receptor and stimulates cell growth, but its beta relative, TGFβ, has an opposite effect: it inhibits the growth of most types of cells.

The balance between these opposing factors is critical to health and healing, because unopposed pressure on cells in either direction would be calamitous. EGF and FGF, without antagonism, could produce wild growth of cells and perhaps transformation to cancer. (Uncontrolled proliferation of new blood vessels is a common feature of rapidly growing malignant tumors, for example.) Unopposed inhibition would thwart healing, leaving wounds unrepaired and vulnerable to infection or further injury.

So at this more complicated level of biological organization, in addition to all the features that we saw at the levels of DNA and plasma membranes, we can also see that *the healing system depends on a coordinated interaction of stimulating and inhibiting factors affecting the growth and proliferation of cells.* Furthermore, this kind of balance appears to underlie the normal life of healthy tissue, not just healing responses to injury. Once again the healing system is responsible for moment-to-moment maintenance of health in addition to its special functions required to manage injury and illness.

Another well-studied case of healing at the tissue level is the repair of a simple bone fracture. The healing system is so good at this that a radiologist may not be able to tell where a bone was broken once the process is complete. Following a fracture, the first steps of healing are similar to those we just reviewed. A blood clot fills and surrounds the fracture cleft, sealing it off and providing a loose framework on which fibroblasts and new blood vessels can grow. Eventually, the organized clot becomes a mass of tissue called a soft callus. Now, the healing system takes a different path from the repair of a surface wound. The beginnings of new cartilage and bone appear in the soft callus by the end of the first week, eventually converting it into a large, spindle-shaped provisional callus that acts as an effective splint. This reaches its greatest size two or three weeks after the injury, then becomes increasingly strong as bone construction intensifies.

The actual creation of new bone again involves mutually antagonistic forces, mediated both by growth factors and by special cells called osteoblasts and osteoclasts. The former build bone up while the latter tear it down, with muscle and weight-bearing stresses on the bone dictating the fluctuations in activity of the two phases. Assuming the fracture was well aligned when the healing process began, reconstruction is often perfect.

Scientists have elucidated the finer details of bone healing at the cellular level. Robert Becker, an orthopedic surgeon and researcher, spent many years proving that tiny electric currents generated by the injury cause cells at the edges of the fracture to *dedifferentiate*—that is, to revert from mature cells to primitive ones with high capacities for growth and regeneration. These primitive cells regain potentials that mature cells have lost; they resemble the cells of embryos, and are able to redifferentiate into all the cell types needed to make a perfect, new bone. Becker's work led to the development of electrical bone stimulators, appliances that encourage the healing of complicated skeletal injuries and bone infections, which are now widely used. It also led him to look beyond bones to other sorts of healing, such as the spectacular ability of salamanders to regenerate amputated limbs.

After conducting many experiments, Becker concluded that limb regeneration in salamanders is not fundamentally different from bone healing in humans. It, too, depends on tiny electric currents that make cells dedifferentiate and then redifferentiate into all the components of a new leg. His general conclusion was that, in theory, humans should have this same ability. That is, all the circuitry and machinery is there; the problem is simply to discover how to turn on the right switches to activate the process.

Regeneration of lost or damaged structure, which we have seen to be a capacity of the healing system at every level so far, is an everyday event in some tissues, especially those at surfaces exposed to constant irritation. Our bodies are forever shedding their outer layers of skin, and new skin is constantly being made by the layers below. The entire lining of the intestinal tract sloughs off and is renewed every day, a spectacular regenerative feat.

Even more impressive is the ability of the liver—the largest organ in the body and one of the most active—to regenerate lost tissue. You can cut away most of the liver—up to eighty percent of it—and the remaining portion will restore the lost substance in a matter of hours, as long as the tissue is normal. Similar restoration of structure and function can occur after partial destruction of liver cells by viral hepatitis and by chemical toxins.

Other organs of the body seem unable to regenerate. Heart muscle that is lost as a result of interruption of blood supply in a heart attack is not replaced by muscle. Healing occurs in the form of a fibrous scar, but there is no regeneration of the original tissue. The same is true of neurons in the brain. Heart muscle cells and nerve cells are so specialized in function—so differentiated—that they seem to have lost the capacity for new growth. Yet perhaps even in these vital cells there are switches waiting to be discovered that might turn on the appropriate sequences of DNA in the nucleus. If science begins to focus on the healing system, isolating and understanding its mechanisms, both electrical and chemical, for regulating cell growth and differentiation, it is not impossible that doctors will one day be able to spark the regeneration of damaged hearts and brains and severed spinal cords. That will truly be a new era of healing-oriented medicine.

If we look at the level of whole body systems, like the circulatory, digestive, and immune systems, healing appears no less prevalent or powerful but more diffuse and mysterious. When I was in medical school I was taught that atherosclerosis was irreversible. Once coronary and other arteries were stiffened and narrowed by cholesterol deposits, inflammation, and calcification, they could never improve, said the books and professors, only worsen. In fact, this pessimistic view was based on no experimental evidence, because no one had yet tried to reverse atherosclerosis.

Once, as a college newspaper editor, I interviewed an expert on rivers, long before ecology and environmental concerns were fashionable. His words made a great impression on me because they sounded right and resonated with my own experience. He told me that rivers are like living organisms in that they have many different mechanisms to keep themselves healthy. You can dump sludge into a river and, up to a point, the river can detoxify itself and remain in good health. For example, turbulence in a river mixes water with oxygen, a powerful purifier and germicide, as is ultraviolet light from the sun. Also, many of the plants that grow in rivers, both algae and higher plants, can remove contaminants from water. But if you keep dumping sludge, at some point you will exceed a critical level where natural purification mechanisms become overwhelmed and break down. Plants and beneficial microorganisms die, flow patterns change, the river becomes sick.

I was busily taking all of this down in my notebook for the story I was going to write. What I heard next so caught my attention that I stopped writing. The expert continued, saying that a river that appears hopelessly polluted is not beyond help. If you will simply stop putting bad substances into it, eventually the levels of contaminants will drop to a point where the natural healing mechanisms revive. Oxygenation increases, sunlight penetrates to deeper levels, beneficial organisms return, and the river cleans itself up.

Why shouldn't arterial systems behave the same way? In fact, we now have clear evidence that atherosclerosis *is* reversible, if you simply stop putting into your body the substances that cause it (mainly saturated fat) and stop obstructing the healing system with your mind (by cultivating anger or emotional isolation, for example). We do not yet know what mechanisms the system uses in this case, but we can observe regression of atherosclerotic plaques in coronary arteries, with corresponding increase of blood flow, in patients who follow programs to lower serum cholesterol greatly and learn to process stress and emotions differently. Moreover, the response to changes in lifestyle is rapid. Using sophisticated tests of cardiac perfusion (like thallium scanning), doctors can demonstrate increased flow through coronary arteries in some patients within a month of starting a program of lifestyle change.

I have seen equally rapid and dramatic responses in patients with many kinds of illnesses who stopped living in ways that promoted disease and switched to lifestyles that supported natural healing. I am not a medical researcher. I am a medical practitioner. Researchers and practitioners have very different outlooks and goals. As a practitioner my chief concern is to keep healthy people healthy and help sick people to get well; I haven't focused equally on why people get better. Still, I am convinced that just because we have not yet discovered a mechanism does not mean that none exists. I am confident that mechanisms of healing at complex levels of biological organization will emerge when investigators begin to search for them.

I DO NOT WANT to end this discussion of the healing system without at least a cursory look at its operations in the realm of mind. Because we know so little of the mind and because our science is so ill equipped to approach it, there is no possibility of seeing mechanisms. Still, it is interesting to observe the process of healing of psychological injuries, using grief as a model. Grief over loss is a universal experience, and its quality is the same whether the loss is of a pet, a job, a relationship, a spouse, or a child. Each loss ties in to all loss; each death reminds us of our own death. Yet the forms of grieving vary greatly from person to person and depend also on the nature and symbolism of each particular loss. Grieving is a kind of work we are required to do, a process of coming to accept loss and reaching a new emotional equilibrium with changed circumstances. Grieving itself is a variety of healing, an operation of the healing system.

Therapists and counselors who work with grieving clients recognize different stages of the process, which may or may not occur sequentially; perhaps it would be better to call them facets of grief rather than stages. One, often the first, is shock and denial ("No, this can't be happening!"). Denial is a natural anesthetic, and while it has a bad reputation (and, of course, is unhealthy if it persists), it may be very useful as a temporary mechanism to permit a basic level of functioning when the full impact of grief would be devastating. Denial may be succeeded by or alternate with anger and rage ("How dare this happen to me?"), which I can't help likening to the inflammatory response that comes soon after the initial pain and bleeding of a wound subside. Anger may give way to a stage of wishful fantasy ("If only I had been a better mother [father, husband, wife, son, daughter, person], this wouldn't have happened"), which often gives way to depression ("I can't go on"). Although it may look like illness, depression is actually a progressive stage of the grieving process, because it represents unconscious acceptance of the loss and release of the fantasy of being able to recover it. When acceptance becomes conscious, grieving can end, the loss is assimilated (in some cases even perceived as a gift that opens a new phase of life), and emotional ease is again possible. By understanding the natural contours of emotional healing, therapists may be able to help clients through it, encouraging appropriate expressions of emotion to facilitate movement toward completion.

We might argue about where emotional healing fits into the subject at hand. Is it higher or lower than healing at the level of body systems? Is mind the highest expression of genetic information encoded in

DNA or a manifestation of a field of consciousness underlying matter, including DNA? As above, so below; as below, so above. It makes no difference. The point is: wherever we choose to look in the human organism, from DNA to the mind, healing processes are evident.

Are there limits to what the system can accomplish? Some of the reported cases of complex healing indicate potential for repair and regeneration that is far beyond ordinary experience. Here is one example, taken from the roster of miraculous cures at Lourdes and reported in an article that appeared in the *Canadian Medical Association Journal* in 1974. The author wrote:

> In order for a healing to be classified as miraculous, five criteria must be met. First, it must be proved that the illness existed, and a diagnosis established. Second, it must be shown that the prognosis, with or without treatment, was poor; third, that the illness was serious and incurable; fourth, that the cure happened without convalescence, that it was virtually instantaneous; and finally, that the cure was permanent. These criteria must be met by the Medical Bureau of Lourdes, the Church, and the diocese in which the "miraculée" lives.
>
> At Lourdes, each case presented is reviewed by three panels of physicians. Since 1947, only 75 cases have been accepted at the first level. Of these, 52 were accepted by the second level, and only 27 were pronounced as scientifically inexplicable by the third level. After the panels of physicians have made their decision concerning the miraculous healing, the Church then makes a judgment as to whether these inexplicable cases are the result of divine intervention. The case is then sent to the local diocese where the local bishop sets up a commission to examine the evidence. These commissions are frequently more stringent than the medical panel at Lourdes, since out of the 27 cases mentioned above, only 17 were pronounced as miracles by the local diocese.

The story of Vittorio Micheli, born February 6, 1940, is one of the seventeen cases of latter-day miraculous healing:

> Vittorio Micheli was inducted into the Italian army in November 1961, being pronounced physically fit, albeit he had noticed minor pains in March of that year. In April 1962 he presented to the Verona military hospital complaining of pains in the region of the

left ischium [the bone of the pelvic girdle that supports weight in sitting] and haunch. Extensive clinical examination, X-ray investigations and biopsies led to the diagnosis of sarcoma [primary bone cancer] of the left pelvis.

By June the condition had worsened and X-rays in August showed "almost complete destruction of the left pelvis," according to army records. Micheli was put in a hip-to-toe cast, with which he was able to stand and move around. In August the army medical service sent him for radiological treatment but after three days concluded the case was not treatable by irradiation. The treatment was switched to chemotherapy but after two months no improvement was discerned and it was discontinued. In November X-rays showed luxation of the femoral head and by January the femur had lost connection with the pelvis.

The following May Micheli decided to go to Lourdes. His cast was exchanged for a stronger one and examination then showed the left hip to be deformed. The patient had totally lost control of his left leg. Pain was severe and continuous, requiring analgesics. He could no longer stand. The patient also suffered loss of appetite and digestive problems.

At Lourdes Micheli, still wearing his cast, was plunged into the baths. Immediately he felt hungry, a characteristic of Lourdes cures. His pains disappeared and he said later, under intensive examination, that he had the feeling his left leg had reattached itself to the pelvis. He felt well.

But he didn't jump straight out of the bath and run off to the grotto. His cast was still enclosing him. Indeed, although Micheli believed he had received a cure, the army doctors didn't. They kept the cast on him. But within a month Micheli was walking, still with the cast. In August radiographs showed the sarcoma had regressed and the bone of the pelvis was regenerating. The improvement continued and today [in 1974], although there is some distortion, the sarcoma has disappeared. Micheli works in a factory, standing for eight to ten hours a day. Articulation of his left hip and leg is "the same as normal" according to bureau records.

If this kind of healing can happen in one human being, I believe it can happen in all. All the circuitry and machinery is there. The challenge is to discover how to turn on the right switches to activate the process.

THE FACES OF HEALING:
OLIVER

AT EIGHTY-SIX Oliver Walston of Pemberville, Ohio, is still in good health. He walks with a limp, a residue of the rheumatoid arthritis that plagued him for much of his adult life, but it has been a long time—twenty-two years—since his arthritis was active, and he now has no pain. Oliver is a retired farmer and businessman who was the director of an insurance company, a constable, and the president of a school board. He says that until now, doctors have shown no interest in the story of how he lost his arthritis.

Oliver's joints began to bother him in his mid-thirties. "I first noticed it in my feet," he says. "Then my knees began to swell and ache badly, and soon after that it settled in my fingers, elbows, shoulders, neck, and spine. In the winter I could not purchase gloves large enough for my swollen hands, so I had to settle for big mittens. I also had to wear shoes two sizes larger than I used to."

Oliver tried all kinds of medication, both prescription and over-the-counter, but nothing gave him consistent or lasting relief. He also tried heat treatments and various topical remedies with no success. At the time of this story, when he was sixty-four, he was resigned to his condition and was managing the pain by taking twelve buffered aspirin tablets a day, six extra-strength and six regular strength. Here is what happened, in Oliver's words:

"On this particular day, my wife had washed my pajamas and hung them on the clothesline to dry. When dry, they were folded and put on the bed. I retired at 10 p.m. and put them on. About 1:30 a.m. I got up to go the bathroom and felt a sting on the inside of my left knee. I slapped it hard, shook my leg, and out fell a honeybee. Two days later the bee sting was still swollen and sore, but the arthritis swelling in that knee began to go down. The next day, the pain from the sting subsided, and I stopped taking the extra-strength aspirin, because the pain and swelling in all my joints began to recede. Two weeks later I stopped all the medication. Within five or six weeks, the swelling and inflammation were gone from all the joints. I've never been bothered by arthritis since, and I even went back to my old shoe size."

I asked Oliver Walston what he thought had happened. "I don't know," he replied. "Mother Nature does some wonderful things. I don't want to encourage people with arthritis to go out and get stung by bees. Maybe it will help some people, but it might make others worse."

In fact, bee-sting therapy has a long history of use for rheumatoid arthritis and other inflammatory and autoimmune disorders. Even some doctors practice it, usually under the name apitherapy or bee-venom therapy. Bee venom is a mixture of very powerful bioactive compounds, some of which have remarkable anti-inflammatory effects. For example, both adolapin and mellitin are more potent than common steroids, and another compound, apamin, currently under investigation in France, shows great promise as a new treatment for multiple sclerosis, another disease with a prominent autoimmune component. Purified bee venom is available for injection under the skin, but many apitherapists prefer to apply living honeybees to the patient, holding them with tweezers to the sites to be stung. They say the risk of this procedure is very slight, even when many stings are applied. Commonly, bee-sting therapy is repeated at frequent intervals.

But Oliver Walston did not really undergo apitherapy. He got one isolated sting, and somehow that changed the dynamics of an autoimmune problem of long standing, activating a complete and permanent healing response. He has some limitation of mobility in joints where extensive destruction of cartilage occurred, but there has been no active inflammation or progression of arthritis in the past two decades.

"Haven't any of the doctors you've seen over the years looked into the cause of your cure?" I asked him.

"No," was his succinct reply. "I think some of them were sorry I was no longer buying all the medicines."

6

THE ROLE OF THE MIND
IN HEALING

"I'M GOING TO fight this thing!"

How often I have heard patients declare their resolve to struggle against a life-threatening illness. They are supported in this stance by conventional wisdom and by societal norms. We are very comfortable with the symbolism and imagery of warfare in our approaches to disease. We fight wars against cancer and drug abuse. We look to medical scientists to develop new weapons against germs and other agents of disease. Doctors commonly refer to the pharmacopeia as the "therapeutic arsenal." It is not surprising that individual patients try to regain health by assuming warrior roles.

Over the years that I have been interviewing men and women who have experienced healing, I have come to feel that "fighting this thing" may not be the best way to obtain the desired result. Although there is no one state of mind that correlates exactly with activation of the healing system, a consistent theme in the interviews is acceptance of illness rather than struggle. Acceptance of illness is often part of a larger acceptance of self that represents a significant mental shift, a shift that can initiate transformation of personality and with it the healing of disease.

I find it difficult to talk to medical scientists about this possibility, because of the great gulf that exists between scientific understanding of mind/body interactions and public perceptions of the subject. Just recently I received a letter from a woman who attended a talk I gave on the future of medicine. She writes:

I am a medical technologist and after working in the hospital environment for a number of years, I became disillusioned with the traditional medical model. It just seemed to me that medicine as it is currently practiced is completely one-dimensional. I became interested in mind-body aspects of healing, and I continue to pursue learning everything I possibly can about the mind-body connection. I have since expanded my concept of True Health to include mind, body, and spirit. I really believe that we will, as a society, make a quantum leap in our true healing potentials once this mind-body-spirit complement is accepted and understood by all.

The writer speaks for many people today in her enthusiasm for mind/body medicine. There has been an enormous surge of books, magazine articles, and television shows on the subject, many of them featuring doctors and researchers who are dedicated to advancing knowledge of the mind's role in health and illness. What the public does not understand is that these visible efforts are not representative of medicine and science in general. In fact, relatively few in the medical establishment take the field of mind/body medicine seriously; and the most prestigious researchers, those who set priorities and influence funding, are contemptuous of colleagues who work in it. What research there is is often of poor quality. Mind/body medicine is not taught in medical schools, except occasionally as an elective course. Meanwhile, proponents of the biomedical model are rejoicing about what they see as imminent conquest of the final frontier: human consciousness. There is increasing consensus in establishment science that mind is merely the product of the brain's circuitry and biochemistry, which we are on the verge of clarifying to the last detail. From this perspective, where mind is always an effect rather than a cause, scientists are unlikely to come up with ideas for studying how the mind might affect the body.

From my vantage point as a medical school faculty member, I see movement backward, away from some of the progressive approaches of the recent past, and, as a result, a widening division between professional attitudes and public expectations. For example, when I was a student in the late 1960s, the entire medical community acknowledged four diseases to be psychosomatic (literally, "mind/body") in origin: bronchial asthma, rheumatoid arthritis, peptic ulcer, and ulcerative colitis. Today, that short list has been whittled down to two—asthma and rheumatoid arthritis—with researchers busily challenging those assumptions as well.

Nine years ago, I saw an unusual and difficult patient, a man in his early fifties who worked as a wholesale produce manager. Except for mild hypertension that had not required medication, he had been in good health—until he quit smoking. He had been a two-pack-a-day cigarette smoker for most of his adult life, but, increasingly, his family had put pressure on him to stop. Finally, he did. "It wasn't that hard," he told me. "I just put my mind to it and only really suffered for the first three days." But two months after he stopped, he developed ulcerative colitis "out of the blue," never having had any digestive problems. He went to a gastroenterologist, who started him on medication, told him not to drink milk, and sent him on his way. The medication did not control the patient's cramping and diarrhea and produced unpleasant side effects. After a month, he decided to follow his intuition that if he resumed smoking, his colitis would disappear. He did, and it did—very promptly. By the time he came to see me, he had repeated this pattern three times. Each time the colitis appeared faster after he quit smoking and took longer to disappear when he resumed. Now he feared he was going to be an addicted smoker with ulcerative colitis.

When I presented this patient to a group of second-year medical students at the University of Arizona, I was dismayed to find that they had learned nothing about the psychosomatic nature of ulcerative colitis. They had learned many facts about cellular and biochemical abnormalities in the disease but nothing about any involvement of the mind in its origin and possible remission. Shortly afterward an article in the *New England Journal of Medicine* reported for the first time on an increased incidence of ulcerative colitis in ex-smokers, but not in current smokers. After reviewing the pathophysiology of the disease and the pharmacology of nicotine exhaustively, the authors concluded that they could find no mechanism to explain the correlation.

If you work from the premise that ulcerative colitis is psychosomatic, it does not take a great deal of intelligence to surmise that smoking is an effective outlet for stress and that if you shut that outlet, the stress is going to go somewhere else. Why in some people it goes to the colon, while in others it produces compulsive eating or nail biting, must be a matter of individual susceptibility. My advice to the patient was not to make another attempt to quit smoking until he had mastered techniques of stress management. I sent him to a biofeedback therapist and a hypnotherapist and also gave him a number of suggestions about improving his lifestyle. (He was a major consumer of coffee, which irritates the colon, and was not eating in a way to make his digestive system happy.)

In this way I learned that ulcerative colitis was no longer one of the classic psychosomatic ailments; that concept had gone out of fashion.

I was much more aware of the successful attempt to eliminate peptic ulcer from that category. It is fashionable today to regard ulcer as an infectious disease, due to the activity of a bacterium, *Helicobacter pylori*. The discovery of the ability of this organism to cause chronic irritation of the lining of the stomach and the duodenum has led many doctors to conclude that ulcers are unrelated to stress and to rely entirely on antibiotics to treat the disease. I have no doubt that *H. pylori* is a factor in gastritis and ulcer (and, almost certainly, stomach cancer), but that admission does not negate the influence of mind. Most people infected with this germ do not get ulcers or other symptoms, and some people with ulcers do not have the infection. Might not stress change the chemistry of the stomach in ways that allow the germ to follow an aggressive, invasive course? All of my experience with infections suggests that the mere presence of a bad germ is not the whole story. Variations in host resistance determine the behavior of microorganisms capable of causing disease, whether they live in balance with their hosts or injure them.

I remember listening to a radio report of dramatic increases in stress-related disorders among children in the war zones of Bosnia. Two of the diseases doctors there are seeing increasingly are hypertension and ulcer, both normally rare in this age group. Evidently, Bosnian doctors still cling to the old-fashioned view that ulcer is a stress-related disorder.

Actually, some of the indifference toward mind/body interactions that I complain about is peculiarly American. In other countries psychosomatic medicine is more viable (though still marginal), and investigators are working to expand the list of stress-related disorders rather than eliminate it. In Japan, more than twenty conditions are recognized as psychosomatic. I am delighted to see among them "autonomic nervous system imbalance," a disorder I recognize and diagnose frequently but one that does not officially exist in the United States. I diagnose it by taking a careful history and by simply feeling hands. Cold hands (in warm rooms) are the result of reduced circulation due to overactivity of the sympathetic nervous system, which causes small arteries in the extremities to constrict. People with chronically cold hands often have disturbances of digestion and other body functions rooted in internal tension; if it persists, this imbalance of autonomic nerves can lead to serious problems. It is best treated by mind/body approaches rather than by prescribing drugs to suppress symptoms.

A German colleague who works at a hospital devoted to psychosomatic medicine surprised me recently by describing the success his institution has in treating tinnitus—ringing in the ears—a common symptom that can be quite debilitating. American medicine has no specific treatments for tinnitus, no understanding of its cause, and little success in alleviating it. My German friend thinks tinnitus results from chronic muscle tension in the head and neck, often associated with poor posture and stress. He prescribes yoga and relaxation training along with body work and says he is frequently able to help rid patients of it.

Because I am not a researcher I will not waste words speculating about mechanisms to explain the role of the mind in healing. I can see many possibilities, not only in the operations of the autonomic nervous system, but also in the panoply of interactions between receptors and the many neuropeptides' that we classify variously as neurotransmitters, hormones, and growth regulators. Candace Pert, one of the pioneer investigators of these regulatory substances, suggests that each one might be associated with a particular mood state and might affect behavior in addition to its actions on body functions. She notes that receptors for many of the neurotransmitters cluster in the gut and in the brain, especially in areas concerned with emotion. Endorphin receptors certainly have this distribution; they affect intestinal function as well as produce euphoria and tolerance for pain. This gives deep biochemical meaning to the commonly referred to "gut feelings." Perhaps our guts are also seats of emotion. What goes on in our guts might influence deep brain centers and vice versa.

Since cells of the immune system have receptors for many of these same peptide molecules, it is likely that our defenses are also part of this web or net that connects the nervous system and the endocrine system, suggesting mechanisms that explain how host resistance to infection varies with host state of mind. Pert writes: "Clearly, the conceptual division between the sciences of immunology, endocrinology, and psychology/neuroscience is a historical artifact; the existence of a communicating network of neuropeptides and their receptors provides a link among the body's cellular defense and repair mechanisms, glands, and brain." In short, the mechanisms are there to be discovered if researchers will look for them. In the meantime, practitioners should not be constrained by the lack of research.

Let me share with you a few experiences that have strengthened my own long-standing belief in mind/body interactions and have made me pay even closer attention to the mental and emotional lives of patients who consult me for physical problems.

In August 1991, when my wife, Sabine, was seven months pregnant with her fourth child (my first), we were in British Columbia, where I was teaching a workshop on health and healing. One of the participants was a friend and colleague, Marilyn Ream, a family-practice doctor from Spokane, Washington, who works in a women's health clinic. Marilyn was completing training in interactive guided imagery therapy, one of my favorite mind/body approaches. I wanted her to give a demonstration of the method, and Marilyn asked Sabine if she would consent to be a volunteer subject in front of the group. Sabine agreed.

My wife has a history of back trouble associated with pregnancy. Usually, around the seventh month her lower back goes out—two vertebrae move out of place—and she is in the habit of getting weekly chiropractic adjustment to help. On this occasion we had been traveling for several weeks, no one was available to adjust her, and she was living with steady pain. Marilyn asked her if she wanted to work on her back in a guided imagery session. Sabine said no; she thought it was a mechanical problem needing a mechanical solution. Instead she wanted to work on issues around the birth. She wanted the baby to come on time, because I was scheduled to leave the country a week after the due date and she wanted the labor to be quick, because she had had long and difficult labors with her previous pregnancies.

Marilyn asked Sabine to lie on the floor, loosen her clothing, and take a series of deep breaths. Interactive guided imagery uses the forms of hypnotherapy to induce a state of light trance and openness to the unconscious mind; but, more than standard hypnotherapy, it empowers patients by encouraging them to develop their own strategies for managing illness. It assumes that the unconscious mind comprehends the nature of disease processes and how to resolve them, an assumption consistent with the healing system's diagnostic capability. The problem is to make that information accessible to waking consciousness and to encourage patients to act on it. Marilyn began the process by asking Sabine to picture herself in a familiar place where she felt completely secure, then to describe it. Sabine described a site in the canyon country of southern Utah. Marilyn directed her to focus on small details, to try to hear sounds and smell scents as well as see the place. Sabine warmed to the task and quickly became very relaxed.

Marilyn then asked her to shift her focus to her uterus and to the baby inside it. Sabine was soon in contact with the baby. Marilyn guided her through a dialogue with the baby, in which Sabine asked her (we knew the sex by this time) to come on time (she agreed to do so) and to help make the labor quick and uneventful. In this dialogue, Sabine would speak the words she "heard" the baby use in reply to her questions. After a time, Sabine felt she had completed this work, and Marilyn told her to return to her spot in southern Utah.

"How do you feel?" Marilyn asked.

"Great. Very peaceful."

"Is there anything else you'd like to work on? How about your back?"

"Mmmm. Okay."

"Good. Then put your attention on the part of your back that hurts and tell me what you find there."

Sabine gave a little gasp.

"What is it?" Marilyn asked.

"It's . . . it's all black."

"Go to the blackness and see if it has anything to say to you," Marilyn suggested.

"It says it's really angry," Sabine answered, sounding surprised. "It's angry at *me*."

Sabine was quite unprepared for the intensity of her back's anger at her. With Marilyn's guidance she entered into a tentative conversation with it and discovered that it was angry at her for being angry at it, and for not taking care of it.

"Ask it what it wants." Marilyn directed.

"It says it wants me to put warm towels on it."

"Will you do that?"

"Yes, but I've been putting cold on it. I thought cold was better for it."

"Tell it you'll put warm towels on it and ask it if it will stop hurting."

"I did. It says it will stop."

"How does it feel now?" Marilyn asked.

"Better," Sabine replied. She moved around on the floor. "Definitely better. That's the first time in weeks it's been any better."

"Is it completely gone?"

"No."

"Ask it if it can go away entirely."

"It says it can."

"Ask it to please do so."

"Okay. I did. And I think it did."

"Now how does it feel?"

"My God, I think it's gone."

"Is it gone?"

Sabine moved this way and that. "Yes, it's really gone."

When Sabine returned to normal consciousness, the pain was still gone. It remained absent that night and the next day. (Nonetheless, Sabine kept her promise to put warm towels on her back.) In fact, the pain did not return for the remainder of the pregnancy, even though Sabine got no further chiropractic work. She had never before been free of back pain in the last two months of a pregnancy.

I will tell you what happened with the labor and delivery in a moment. Meanwhile, on the way home from British Columbia, I too had an interesting experience with this technique. Sabine and I drove back to Tucson, stopping first to visit a friend in Olympia, Washington, who had a hot tub. Usually I am quite discriminating about hot tubs: some I get into and some I don't. I had my doubts about this one but soaked in it anyway. Two days later, I had a skin infection. Hot-tub folliculitis is now a recognized disorder, a bacterial infection of hair follicles, caused by an organism called *Pseudomonas* that is notoriously resistant to treatment. In my case, it produced several painful red lesions on the left lower leg and knee. I could not take proper care of myself on the drive, but each morning and evening I would put hot compresses on these sites of infection, try to squeeze material out of them, and sop them with hydrogen peroxide. They looked as if they contained pus, but nothing came out. Then new lesions appeared on my thigh and left arm.

As the infection progressed upward, I became more anxious about it. By the time we arrived home a week later, it had spread to my face, and I began to feel generally unwell. I was contemplating going to a doctor the next day, when Sabine, still flushed with enthusiasm about her pain-free back, said, "Why don't you call Marilyn and have her do a guided imagery session with you on the phone?"

"Oh, come on," I said. "This is a bacterial infection." Sabine looked at me in a knowing way. "My back was a mechanical problem," she reminded me.

I called Marilyn, more for Sabine's sake than for mine. Marilyn said she had never worked over the phone but was willing to try. I curled up on a couch with the phone cradled by my right ear and under Marilyn's guidance went to a favorite spot in New Mexico's Gila Wilderness. After I was settled in, Marilyn asked me to pick the one lesion that was bothering me the most. I picked the one on my face.

"Put yourself there," Marilyn directed, "and tell me what you see." I saw a mass of swirling, trapped, angry, red energy.

"Listen to see if it has anything to say to you." I put my attention on the spot and "listened." Immediately words popped into my mind.

"It says it can't leave my body by going outward," I reported excitedly. "I've been wanting it to go out, but it can't. The only way it can leave is by going inward and being absorbed."

"If that's the case, what should you be doing?" Marilyn asked.

My conscious mind supplied the answer. "Well, I suppose I should stop squeezing these things. Soaking them with compresses is all right, but I should be resting more."

"Does it have anything else to tell you?"

"I don't get anything else, except a thought that I should be eating hot peppers to stimulate my circulation."

"Then let's go back to that wilderness place you started off in."

When I hung up the phone, Sabine said she could see a difference in the lesions. "They don't look as purple," she told me. I could not see any difference, but I went to bed relaxed and confident that my body could take care of itself. The next morning, without my having eaten peppers or done anything else, I could see that the problem had clearly begun to diminish. Within twenty-four hours, all of the sites of infection were obviously on the mend, much to my delight.

If a pure mind/body approach like interactive guided imagery can cure back pain associated with misaligned vertebrae and a bacterial skin infection, why shouldn't it be able to turn around anything? These experiences left me convinced that no body problem is beyond the reach of mental intervention, especially since mind/body techniques are very time- and cost-effective and are unlikely to cause harm.

Three weeks before Sabine's due date I asked a friend and colleague, Dr. Steve Gurgevich, who practices hypnotherapy, to do a session with her, again in the interest of a timely, quick, uncomplicated birth. The baby was in a posterior presentation at this time, which worried us. Sabine's last baby had been posterior, causing long, painful labor. Steve did an hour-long session with her at the end of an afternoon, encouraging Sabine to talk with the baby, asking her to turn around before the beginning of labor and help make the labor quick. When he brought Sabine out of her reverie, she looked supremely relaxed. After Steve left, Sabine and I went to the kitchen to start dinner. Suddenly, she clutched her belly and bent over.

"What is it?" I asked.

"I think the baby's turning," she said, amazed.

It happened that our midwife was coming for dinner that night. She examined Sabine and reported that the baby was now in an anterior presentation, having turned within twenty minutes of being asked to do so. The baby came right on her due date, October 4. Labor lasted a mere two hours and six minutes, which was, if anything, a little too brief in that we barely had time to prepare. Needless to say, Sabine and I are both true believers in the effectiveness of mind/body approaches, and when we hear doctors and researchers dismissing the role of the mind in health and healing, we exchange knowing smiles.

In taking a history from a new patient, I ask many questions about lifestyle, about relationships, hobbies, ways of relaxing, patterns of eating and exercising, sex, and spiritual interests. In a formal history, all of these questions are grouped in a section called the "social history"; many practitioners omit it, because they consider it unimportant. The first time a medical student sits down with a patient to take a history, the process takes over an hour. Students follow a prescribed form, ask questions by rote, then painstakingly write up the lengthy answers. By the third year of medical school, under the pressures of the wards, students learn that they must speed up the process in order to get their work done. By internship and residency, histories become streamlined, mostly by eliminating questions. Unfortunately, the social history gets jettisoned first, since doctors put higher priority on questions about symptoms, past health problems, and current medications. I call it unfortunate because in my experience the social history most frequently contains clues to the origins of patients' problems as well as possibilities for their solution.

I am convinced that stress is a primary cause or aggravating factor in many conditions that bring patients to doctors. Suppose a patient comes in complaining of frequent headaches, and physical examination and blood tests are normal. If I want to determine whether the headaches are stress-related, I can usually do so by asking one simple question, namely, "What happens to the headaches when you go on vacation?" Symptoms that disappear on vacations are likely to arise from stressful circumstances in a person's workaday life. To determine which of the circumstances is the problem—job, marriage, children, lack of relationships, or something else—requires a bit more probing.

Because I take extensive social histories and work from a model of health and healing predicated on mind/body interaction, I am keenly aware of correlations between mental/emotional events and healing responses. These correlations are important, because they suggest ways that people can keep their healing systems in good working order and can use their minds to promote healing rather than obstruct it. I present this information in detail in Part Two of this book.

First, some caveats. Healing sometimes just happens in the absence of any profound change of heart or mind. Some scoundrels are healed of serious illnesses, while some saints die agonizing deaths. At the level of DNA repair by enzymes, the influence of mind on the healing process may be negligible, as it may be at other levels. Nonetheless, I see a clear role of the mind in healing, visible in correlations of healing responses with mental and emotional changes.

For example, a healing response may immediately follow the resolution of some intolerable situation, such as ending a bad marriage or quitting a miserable job or making peace with an estranged family member. A colleague wrote me that the most dramatic case of healing he has seen was "a bank president with chronic hypertension, whose blood pressure normalized one day after his wife filed for divorce. It dropped to 120/80 and stayed there."

Another correlation is disappearance of a serious medical problem with falling in love. I have seen this with autoimmunity—rheumatoid arthritis and lupus particularly—and also with chronic musculoskeletal pain and chronic fatigue. I wish I could arrange for patients to fall in love more often. If I could figure out how to do that, I would be a very successful practitioner indeed.

I have also seen healing mobilized by expressions of anger. New Age therapists who teach people to rid themselves of negative emotions may not like to hear this, but facts are facts. One example is a patient I worked with over a long period, a man in his thirties with chronic autoimmune disease that attacked his blood platelets and red blood cells. Through a complete reworking of lifestyle and the use of several mind/body approaches, including visualization, he was able to get off the steroids and other suppressive drugs he had been taking for years. Becoming aware of and then expressing anger toward doctors and hospitals was part of the change. Finally, his health improved so much that he felt able to fulfill a long-standing desire to make an adventurous trip through Australia and New Zealand. One day I received an emergency call from down under. My patient had been thrown from a horse and had cracked two vertebrae (weakened in the recent past from long-term steroid use); the shock had set off an episode of autoimmune destruction of blood cells, and he was being air-evacuated to a hospital in Arizona.

Despite the accident and the reactivation of the disease process, he looked better than I had ever seen him, and he said that he had enjoyed a year of unprecedented good health. As he checked into the hospital, I told him not to be discouraged, that setbacks were to be expected. The goal, I said, was to make the relapses less and less frequent and get through them faster with less drastic intervention. The patient was started on steroids, but his blood counts fell so low that the hospital doctors wanted to give him transfusions. He refused, and I supported him in his refusal. In the past, he had been able to turn falling blood counts around by working with his emotions and by visualizing his white blood cells protecting his platelets and red cells from immune attack. The doctors put ever greater pressure on him to take the transfusions. Finally, one night, as he lay sleepless in the hospital, he felt a surge of rage at his predicament and his dependence once again on hospital medicine. He experienced this as a body sensation as well as an emotional wave that he directed at the whole attending staff. Within hours, his platelet and red cell counts started to climb, making transfusions unnecessary, and he was discharged from the hospital within days. He also ended his steroid use following this episode faster than he ever had in the past. I have no doubt that appropriate, focused expressions of anger can sometimes activate the healing system, New Age therapists notwithstanding.

Belief in the healing power of some person, place, or thing can also be a key to success. This is the realm of placebo responses and miracle shrines. We do not seem to be able to will healing responses to occur, because our will does not connect directly to the autonomic nervous system and other controlling mechanisms of the healing system. Yet we can circumvent that obstacle by projecting belief in healing onto something external and interacting with it. I have already noted that if physicians understood this process and were better trained to work with projected belief, they would better fulfill their roles as shaman/priests and be much more effective at helping sick people get well.

Finally, the most common correlation I observe between mind and healing in people with chronic illness is total acceptance of the circumstances of one's life, including illness. This change allows profound internal relaxation, so that people need no longer feel compelled to maintain a defensive stance toward life. Often, it occurs as part of a spiritual awakening and submission to a higher power.

I will summarize one case history as an example. A Japanese friend of mine, Shin-ichiro Terayama, who is an executive director of the Japan Holistic Medical Society, is a cancer survivor. By training Shin is a solid-state physicist and management consultant. Now fifty-eight and radiantly healthy, he is an international networker for the cause of holistic medicine, an accomplished cellist, and a counselor of the sick, especially those with cancer. I do not think I would have liked him if we had met ten years ago, before he was diagnosed with cancer. In photographs from that time he appears pinched and unpleasant, nothing like the warmhearted, spiritually awake man I know.

Back then he was a workaholic, on call twenty-four hours a day. He slept little, drank between ten and twenty cups of coffee a day, was much enamored of beefsteaks and sweets, and had no time for music in his life. In the fall of 1983 he had a fever lasting a month and could not stand or walk, but medical tests were normal. In those days, Shin says, he had complete faith in doctors and hospitals. A few months later he had three episodes of blood in his urine and became very tired. A friend who was a lay practitioner of Oriental medicine and macrobiotics told him something was wrong with his kidney, a diagnosis he based on observation and a check of the acupuncture meridians. He recommended a radical change of diet, but Shin was not interested, and the doctors still told him nothing was wrong.

Early in the fall of 1984, Shin's fatigue increased so markedly that he could not work. He wanted only to rest. When he returned to a clinic for additional tests, an abdominal mass was discovered, and a subsequent sonogram revealed the right kidney to be enlarged by thirty percent. Still, Shin did nothing. In November 1984, at the urging of his wife, a physician, Shin went to a hospital. X-rays revealed a tumor, and the doctors pressed him to consent to surgical removal of the kidney. Shin asked if the tumor was benign or malignant and was told it was "something in between." In fact it was renal cell carcinoma—kidney cancer—and had already metastasized to his lungs.

In Japan, the diagnosis of cancer is still routinely withheld from patients lest it depress them unduly. This leads inevitably to subterfuge. After the surgery, Shin's doctor said that he wanted to give him a series of injections as a "preventive measure." In fact, the treatment was cisplatinum, a strong chemotherapy agent, but Shin did not know it. He did know that the shots made him vomit, turned his beard white, and caused his hair to fall out, and he refused to complete the series. His doctor next ordered "ray treatments" to the kidney area, which he said were like "artificial sunlight." After the first few of these, Shin became very tired, lost his appetite, and had to remain in bed all day. One night he had a powerful dream about attending his own funeral, which made him feel for the first time that he was very sick and might die and had been deluded about the real nature of his illness. He also developed an unusual symptom, a hyperacute sense of smell.

"I was on the second floor of the hospital," he recalls, "but I could smell food being prepared on the fourth floor. I could smell the body odors of all the nurses. I was in a ward with six patients, and the smells became intolerable. I had to get away from them; they reminded me of death." Shin waited until after dark, got out of bed unseen, and followed his nose to safety. The only place that smelled all right to him was the roof of the hospital, where he drank fresh air into his lungs. Meanwhile, a nurse discovered him missing from his bed and raised an alarm. When a search party found him on the roof, their immediate thought was that he was about to commit suicide, which would bring the hospital bad publicity. Eventually five nurses came and carried him bodily back to his room. Next morning his doctor scolded him, saying, "You caused a big commotion last night. If you want to stay here, you must follow the rules; otherwise you can go home." This was music to Shin's ears. He promptly signed out of the hospital and went home. He then consulted his macrobiotic friend, who urged him to adopt a strict brown rice diet. "I couldn't imagine it," said Shin.

When Shin awoke the next day, he was amazed to find himself alive. The morning seemed to him unbearably beautiful, and he was aware of a great desire to watch the sun rise. He went to the eighth-floor rooftop of his apartment house, where he could look over the skyline of Tokyo. He recited Buddhist mantras and poems, put his hands together to pray, and awaited the sun. When it rose, he felt a ray enter his chest, sending energy through his body. "I felt something wonderful was going to happen, and I started to cry," he says. "I was just so happy to be alive. I saw the sun as God. When I came back down to my apartment, I saw auras around all my family members. I thought everyone was God."

During the next few weeks Shin observed the strict diet and performed daily the important ritual of watching the sun rise from his roof—the one thing he looked forward to each day. His condition fluctuated. His doctor tried to warn him off the macrobiotic diet, urging him to eat more meat and fish, and also tried to get him to take oral chemotherapy. Shin refused. He then checked into a new healing retreat a friend had opened in the Japan Alps, with hot spring baths and excellent natural food. He rested, took daily walks in the forests and mountains, and began to play the cello, something he had not done for years.

"The clean air and water invigorated me," he recalls, "and I became aware of the natural healing power that was in me and around me. Gradually, I began to realize that I had created my own cancer. I had created it by my behavior. And as I came to that realization, I saw that I had to love my cancer, not attack it as an enemy. It was part of me, and I had to love my whole self."

Today Shin Terayama is not merely a cancer survivor. He is a transformed being, who neither looks, acts, nor thinks like his old self. I have been privileged to hike with him in the mountains of Japan and America, sit with him in hot springs, attend his concerts and lectures, and listen to him counsel dozens of newly diagnosed cancer patients. "You must love your cancer," he always tells his clients. "Your cancer is a gift. It is the way to your transformation and new life."

Many doctors might not agree that Shin's is a case of spontaneous healing. After all, he underwent all three standard treatments for cancer: surgery, chemotherapy, and radiation, even if he did not complete the latter two. Renal cell carcinoma is fascinating: for kidney cancer with lung metastases, the five-year survival rate is only five percent, yet it is one of the types of cancer most strongly associated with spontaneous remission. The feature of Shin's story that I find most impressive is his psychospiritual transformation, symbolized by the sun ray penetrating his chest on a rooftop in Tokyo, and summed up in his statement "I saw that I had to love my cancer, not attack it as an enemy." That is true self-acceptance.

Most people do not go through life in an accepting mode. Instead they are in a state of perpetual confrontation, trying by the imposition of will to shape events and control situations. According to Lao-tzu, the ancient Chinese philosopher, such an attitude is directly opposed to the way of life (the Tao), and those who cling to it are doomed:

> *As the soft yield of water cleaves obstinate stone,*
> *So to yield with life solves the insoluble.*
>
> *It is said, "There's a way where there's a will,"*
> *But let life ripen and then fall,*
> *Will is not the way at all:*
> *Deny the way of life and you are dead.*

Acceptance, submission, surrender—whatever one chooses to call it, this mental shift may be the master key that unlocks healing.

THE FACES OF HEALING:
MARI JEAN

IN 1978 Mari Jean Ferguson, then thirty-eight, was diagnosed with hypertension—high blood pressure. She had just given birth to her first child after a difficult pregnancy, during which she had experienced irregular heartbeats and bad respiratory allergies. Her doctors wanted to medicate her for all three conditions, but she refused.

"My then father-in-law was a pharmacologist who had worked for a drug firm," she says, "and I never took medications without first checking with him. In this case, he told me the drugs they wanted me to take were pretty heavy-duty and advised against them. He told me to wait a year and see what happened. I did continue with allergy shots, which I'd been taking for some time. Allergists had made a lot of money off me since I was a teenager, and being allergic was still my biggest medical problem. By using stress-management techniques and breathing exercises and by controlling my weight I was able to keep my blood pressure in the high-normal range for several years without drugs."

Mari Jean needed all the help with stress management she could get. Her career was in doubt, since she was up for tenure review as a professor at a prominent midwestern university. Having a child at age thirty-eight was frowned upon by the tenure committee, and eventually she was turned down. Also, her marriage was on the rocks. Following her daughter's birth her husband became "overtly abusive," disclaiming responsibility for the child on the grounds that it was not his.

It was Mari Jean's second marriage. Her first had ended in divorce when her husband fell into a pattern of binge drinking and psychiatric hospitalizations. That was in Berkeley, California, where Mari Jean had earned her Ph.D. in sociology in the late 1960s. She had come a long way from her home in northern Alberta, "where I wasted a lot of time in rebellion against my family. I was into a lot of truancy in high school, went to business college, got married early, and was always doing the wrong thing. My brother was the family hero and got all the approval." In 1970, her father died of cancer at age sixty, leaving her mother distraught.

When Mari Jean lost her academic job in 1981, she enrolled in a program to become a family therapist and went through therapy herself for two years. "I began to realize how dysfunctional my family had been, and I began to grow, but, ironically, that created more problems in my second marriage, because my husband stayed in place. Then out of the blue, he filed for divorce and cleared out all of the money."

Another blow came in 1984, when her brother died suddenly of myocarditis, a viral infection of the heart. Her mother, brokenhearted, had a series of strokes that required Mari Jean to make frequent trips to Alberta to care for her until she died in 1986. Mari Jean's blood pressure crept up until it was no longer manageable without medication; she started on the drugs just before her mother's death. Mari Jean, who was overweight and smoked cigarettes, now became clinically depressed. She took antidepressant drugs for a time and got back into psychotherapy. In 1989 she moved to Pittsburgh to start a new life, having accepted a job as an associate professor of sociology at a small college.

"I was very overqualified for this place," she says, "and I knew I didn't fit in, but I decided to keep my mouth shut and try." She now came under the medical care of Dr. Amy Stine, who maintained her on a combination of two antihypertensive drugs. "Despite my best intentions, I found myself getting into trouble again," Mari Jean recalls. "My department chairman is on a vendetta to get rid of me when I come up for contract renewal, and I've had to get a lawyer."

In October 1993, Mari Jean saw Dr. Stine for a checkup. Dr. Stine was surprised to find her patient's blood pressure way down: 90/60. "You're overmedicated," she told her, and eliminated one of the drugs. When Mari Jean visited Dr. Stine again, early in 1994, her pressure was still 90/60. "What are you doing?" Dr. Stine asked. Mari Jean paid little attention. "I've learned over the years that most doctors aren't that interested in you," she says. Dr. Stine took her off medication completely.

At the next visit, Mari Jean's blood pressure remained 90/60, an unusually low value. This time Dr. Stine demanded an explanation. "You haven't lost weight. You haven't changed your diet. You haven't stopped smoking. You haven't increased your activity. You haven't done any of the things people are supposed to do to get their blood pressure down. What did you do?"

"Do you really want to know?" Mari Jean asked. "I'll give you the short version. I saw myself repeating the same patterns I've done all my life, always putting myself before God, always saying, '*I'm* going to do this, *I'm* going to do that.' Last fall, for the first time in my life I said, 'Just let go—let whatever happens happen.' And that's it."

Dr. Stine says she has never seen anything like this case. Mari Jean Ferguson's blood pressure is still low normal and stable. "I'm awed that my mind alone could do this," Mari Jean says.

7

THE TAO OF HEALING

If the body is so good at healing, why do we get sick?

The healing system is always there, always operative, always ready to work to restore balance when balance is lost; but at any given moment its capacity to restore may be inadequate for a required task. Consider the example of DNA injury by ultraviolet light. If only one strand of the double helix is damaged, repair by enzymes is the norm. In the process of repair, polymerase I uses the intact strand as a guide to replace the damaged nucleotides. But what if both strands are injured? If two rays of UV happen to strike both strands in the same place, the injury will be beyond the repairing capacity of polymerase I. The change becomes fixed in replicating DNA—a mutation, and much more likely than not to have deleterious effects.

Or consider LDL cholesterol and the body's ability to remove it from the bloodstream by the activity of LDL receptors on the surface of cell membranes. As long as output of cholesterol by the liver remains below a certain level, serum LDL cholesterol will stay within safe limits, but if the owner of the liver eats a steady diet of bacon cheeseburgers, production of cholesterol will likely exceed the capacity of the system, and serum LDL cholesterol will rise to levels where arterial damage occurs.

Also, some people do not have enough LDL receptors. In one well-studied, inherited disorder of cholesterol metabolism, LDL receptors are lacking, and serum cholesterol remains dangerously high regardless of dietary manipulations. Unless they take cholesterol-lowering drugs, people with this problem will develop cardiovascular disease at very young ages.

In other cases, the activities of the healing system may be frustrated by complicating circumstances. Wound healing cannot be completed if a foreign body remains in the wound or if infection develops. If you are malnourished or have an abnormally low metabolism or are weakened by chronic illness, the healing system may not have enough available energy to deal with wounds and broken bones.

Some years ago I saw a young woman who complained of fatigue and inability to concentrate. Doctors had found nothing wrong with her, and she had embarked on a fruitless round of consultations with alternative practitioners. She had tried various homeopathic remedies to no avail. On the advice of a naturopath she had eliminated all sugars from her diet. Acupuncturists and herbalists had worked on her without success. She had spent a small fortune on psychotherapy but could not discover an emotional reason for lack of energy. When I saw her, she appeared droopy, listless, and depressed, frequently becoming tearful as she told me about her symptoms and her failure to find someone to treat them effectively. Her symptoms included disturbances of digestion and menstruation as well as a marked deterioration of her ability to heal. A year before the visit she had suffered a broken leg in a car accident. Despite proper treatment, the broken bone failed to heal; the medical term for what happened is a *nonunion* of the fracture. She showed me her right big toe, which was discolored, black and blue. "It's been that way since I stubbed it four months ago," she told me. "Cuts and bruises just don't heal the way they used to."

This woman had severe hypothyroidism, which doctors had failed to detect because her thyroid function tests were normal. Thyroid function tests are not always reliable, especially in young women. I suspected this patient's immune system was making antibodies to thyroid hormone, neutralizing it before it could exert its effects. As a result, her metabolism was greatly slowed, even though blood tests showed her thyroid functioning properly. Her healing system simply did not have enough metabolic energy available to it to do the required work. When she began to take supplemental thyroid hormone, her metabolism slowly normalized, as did her ability to heal.

So the short answer to the question "Why do we get sick?" is that the capacity of the healing system to restore balance can be exceeded by the forces or circumstances of imbalance. A longer answer would have to address the issue of why forces of imbalance exist, and that would take us deep into the realms of philosophical inquiry. My belief is that health and sickness are complementary opposites, that we cannot have one without the other, any more than good and evil can stand alone. The challenge is to use sickness as an opportunity for transformation.

Does healing necessarily mean complete disappearance of disease on the physical level?

No. The literal meaning of "healing" is "becoming whole." It is possible to have an inner sense of wholeness, perfection, balance, and peace even if the physical body is not perfect. I have known persons with missing limbs who seemed to me more whole than some persons with all their limbs. (See the story of Jan on page 115 for another example.) Of course, it is desirable to restore physical wholeness, and the healing system will do it if it can, but when physical disease is fixed and immovable, healing can occur in other ways, including adaptation to and compensation for any loss of structure or function.

Is it possible to die in a healed condition?

Why not? Death and healing are not opposites. To die as a healed person would mean being able to view one's life as complete and accept the disintegration of the physical body. There are many reliable accounts of the last days of sages, especially from Buddhist traditions and extending up to the present day, that illustrate the possibility of healing into death. They bear little resemblance to what goes on in modern hospitals, where doctors often see death as the ultimate enemy to be fought with all the weapons of modern medical technology. Trapped on this battleground, patients usually have no opportunity for final healing, nor do people in our culture have ready access to practical information about using life to prepare for death.

In other cultures and other times, the "art of dying" was a popular theme of books and discourse. I would like to see it revived.

What is the relationship between treatment and healing? If I want to pursue healing, should I forgo treatment?

Suppose I come down with bacterial pneumonia, a serious, possibly life-threatening infection of the lungs. I go to a hospital, receive intravenous antibiotics, recover, and am discharged, cured. What caused the cure? Most people, doctors and patients alike, would say it was the treatment. But I want you to consider a different interpretation. Antibiotics reduce numbers of invading germs to a point where the immune system can take over and finish the job. The real cause of the cure is the immune system, which may be unable to end an infection because it is overwhelmed by sheer numbers of bacteria and whatever toxic products they might make. Of course, the immune system is itself a component of the healing system.

I maintain that the final common cause of all cures is the healing system, whether or not treatment is applied. When treatments work, they do so by activating innate healing mechanisms. Treatment—including drugs and surgery—can facilitate healing and remove obstacles to it, but treatment is not the same as healing. Treatment originates outside you; healing comes from within. Nonetheless, to refuse treatment while waiting for healing can be foolish.

I am reminded of the story of a religious man caught in a flood. As the waters rise around his house, he resorts to prayer, confident that the Lord will save him. Eventually he is forced to go to the roof of his house, but he continues to pray. Two men in a rowboat pass the deluged house and call out to him, offering rescue. The man declines. "The Lord will save me," he says. Later, with the water swirling about his knees, a motorboat comes by with another offer of help. "No thanks," the man replies, "I trust in the Lord to save me." Finally, a National Guard helicopter flies over and drops a rope ladder. Although the water is now up to his neck, the man waves the chopper on. "The Lord will save me," he calls up to the guardsmen. But moments later the water closes over his head, and after a brief struggle, he drowns. The next thing he knows, he is in heaven, standing before his Maker. "Why didn't you save me, Lord? My faith in you never wavered. How could you let me down?" he asks. "Let you down?" thunders the Lord. "I sent you a rowboat. I sent you a motor-boat. And then I sent you a helicopter. What were you waiting for?"

How do I know when treatment is appropriate?

You must learn what medicine can and cannot accomplish, which diseases respond to conventional treatments and which do not. It may be better to rely on the healing system than on medicine. Consider infectious disease, for example. The greatest medical advance of the twentieth century has been the reduction of infectious disease by means of improved public sanitation, immunization, and antibiotics. In the early part of this century, infectious disease was a common killer of children and young adults. In the latter part of the century, chronic degenerative disease, mostly in older people, has replaced infectious disease as the category of illness doctors are called upon to treat most often. With this shift, people in our society have become quite complacent about infectious disease, at least about bacterial infections, believing that antibiotics—"wonder drugs"—give us total protection.

This view is not shared by infectious-disease specialists, who are witnessing a relentless rise of organisms resistant to our strongest drugs. Diseases thought to be conquered, like tuberculosis, are resurgent. Organisms thought to be incapable of resistance, like the one that causes gonorrhea, are now resistant. Worse, the rate of development of resistance is increasing, as is the speed of its transmission. A new antibiotic might work for only a few months now before germs learn how to neutralize it; and once resistant strains appear in Chicago, they turn up in Beijing within weeks. The hard fact is that we are losing the arms race with bacteria.

These alarming developments raise an important question. Is it better to put our faith in weapons against external agents of disease or in internal resources that can make us less vulnerable? Experience with antibiotics and bacteria suggests that exclusive reliance on weapons, however effective they may appear to be at first, gets us into worse trouble down the road. The weapons themselves influence the evolution of bacteria in the direction of greater virulence, making them more dangerous adversaries. On the other hand, if we concentrate on improving host resistance, the germs stay as they are, and we are protected. So it is probably wiser to rely on the healing system than on drugs and doctors.

If I fail to get better, is it my fault?

I have always found it interesting to ask people why they think they got sick. When I was a medical student I asked that question of a number of older women with breast cancer, women of my grand-mother's generation. The answers all had to do with past injuries: "Twenty years ago, I fell against a table and badly bruised my breast." "When I was in my early forties, I was in an accident, and my breast got hurt." When I pose the same question to patients today, there is no mention of injury. Instead they say things like, "I bottled up my anger at my husband for all those years," or "I never expressed the grief I felt," or "I've never been in touch with my feelings." Clearly, this is a significant change, but what does it signify?

Our cultural fascination with mind/body interactions, along with the popularity of self-help books and New Age philosophies, has fostered a sense of personal responsibility for illness. We make ourselves sick by certain habits of mind, by failing to discharge negative emotions, by not leading spiritual lives. People who promote these ideas are well intentioned. They want us to be more responsible for our own well-being and to recognize that we can use our minds to help the healing process, all of which is fine. But an unintended result of their message is to create a great deal of guilt. "I gave myself cancer." "If I don't get better, I must be a bad person." Guilt about illness is destructive; it cannot possibly help the healing system.

The once-popular idea that breast cancer results from an old injury has no scientific validity. It may be that the new formulations about bottled-up feelings are just as wrong. I think breast cancer results from a complex interaction of genetic and environmental factors, in which lifestyle choices, such as diet, use of alcohol, and exposure to estrogenic toxins, may have much more influence than emotions. I do believe that grief and depression may suppress immunity, giving malignant cells the chance to grow into perceptible tumors; but I reject the idea that people give themselves cancer by failing to express anger and other emotions. And I emphatically reject the notion that failure to heal represents any kind of judgment about a person's state of mind or spirituality. Dr. Larry Dossey, one of the few doctors who has looked into the relationship between prayer and healing, has compiled an impressive catalog of saints, both Eastern and Western, who have died of cancer, so many that cancer seems almost to be an occupational hazard of sainthood. Keep this in mind if you are tempted to believe that healing depends on enlightenment and transcendence of negative emotions.

Is spontaneous remission of cancer the best example of the activity of the healing system?

Because they are rare and dramatic occurrences, and because cancer is a feared disease that resists most attempts to cure it, spontaneous remissions attract attention and make good stories for the media. In my view they are not the best examples of healing responses. Cancer is a special case, unlike other diseases (see Chapter 19), and these cases distract us from the healing system's less glamorous but much more important work. Spontaneous remissions of cancer represent extraordinary activity of the system. The system's ordinary activity is really more remarkable.

Zen Buddhism urges practitioners to experience the extraordinariness of the ordinary, to discard the gray filters of habitual perception and see the miraculous nature of everyday experience. Beginners at meditation often imagine the goal to be attainment of unusual states of consciousness: out-of-body experiences, visions, celestial choirs heard with the mind's ear, psychic powers, and so forth. Zen masters teach that such experiences are irrelevant to the process of spiritual development and should not be given special attention if they occur. Instead, they direct students simply to sit and pay attention to the most ordinary aspects of existence, such as the rising and falling of the breath.

We hardly notice—let alone appreciate—the ordinary activities of the human body's healing system. Given all of the potential agents of injury and illness that surround us, all of the changes that occur within and around us from moment to moment, it is amazing that we survive at all. Think for a moment of all that can go wrong: constant bombardment with radiation that can damage DNA; millions of cell divisions each second, any one of which could result in a genetic accident; countless molecules of irritants and toxins that get into our systems through every possible point of entry; forces of wear and tear that abrade our tissues; pressures of aging; the sea of viruses, bacteria, and other potential agents of disease in which we live; not to mention emotional assaults that stress our nerves and threaten mind/body equilibrium. To make it from one day to the next without serious incident is nothing short of miraculous.

Each day in which we enjoy relatively normal health testifies to the activity of the healing system. Its inestimable value lies not in its ability to produce remissions of disease but rather in the maintenance of health through the vicissitudes of daily life. Here is a real opportunity to appreciate the extraordinariness of the ordinary.

Is it possible to enhance the activity of the healing system in order to protect health?

Yes. How to do that is the subject of the next part of this book.

THE FACES OF HEALING: JAN

JAN BARNETT HAS a big spleen, so big that it makes buying clothes difficult for her. "I look like I'm five months pregnant," she says with a laugh. Except for that, and occasional shortness of breath on exertion (a symptom of anemia), she leads a normal life—better than normal, actually, because she considers herself a very happy, lucky woman. "If I were to die today, I'd have no regrets," she told me. "It's been a full, wonderful life, and I have a great sense of inner peace."

Ten years ago, when she was forty years old, Jan went to a doctor for a well-person checkup. The doctor felt the enlarged spleen, and the results of Jan's blood tests looked bad. The doctor recommended splenectomy, once a common operation, as the spleen was considered an expendable organ, and sent Jan to a surgeon. Fortunately, the surgeon's views were more up-to-date. "We don't do that anymore," he told the patient, "at least not till we find out the reason for the enlargement." He sent Jan to a hematologist.

It turned out that Jan Barnett has a rare, poorly understood disorder called primary myelofibrosis, or agnogenic myeloid metaplasia; removal of her spleen would have killed her. "Myeloid metaplasia" means that marrowlike tissue is growing in a different place from where it should be—in this case, in the spleen. "Agnogenic" is a choice word meaning "of unknown cause" (or, perhaps better, "We haven't a clue as to why you have this condition or what we can do to fix it"). The root problem is replacement of functioning marrow by fibroblasts, the cells that make connective tissue. In response to this life-threatening process, the spleen takes over the job of manufacturing blood cells; its enlargement is a compensatory—or healing—response to the disease, which is why splenectomy would be disastrous.

The prognosis in primary myelofibrosis is uncertain. Most people who acquire it are older than Jan, often in their sixties or seventies, and they may die of other causes. In some people, the marrow disorder turns into leukemia. "They told me it was rare in my age group and that the average life expectancy was ten years," Jan recalls. "But they gave me some other statistics that were more hopeful, like twenty-five percent of people had no further problems. I thought, 'That's not so bad. I can be in that twenty-five percent.' " No treatment was offered or recommended. "I'm actually grateful for that," Jan says. "Since there were no drugs or surgery to help me, it left me to do all the work on my own." She was told to have regular blood counts to determine whether the condition was progressing.

In the few months after diagnosis, Jan made a number of changes in her life. "My eating was always healthy, so my diet didn't have to change much, but I began a committed exercise program that has become an important part of my life. Originally, I swam; now I do power walking. Exercise gave me an unanticipated, wonderful benefit in addition to the ones you'd expect. It gave me time to begin doing psychological work, to think about my inner life."

Jan says the most significant changes were psychological. "First of all, I gave myself permission to take care of myself. I resolved never to apologize for nurturing myself. I dropped out of an overtaxing school program in nursing and went instead for a master's degree in experiential education. (My experience was living with this diagnosis and coming to a holistic philosophy of health.) I made sure I always got plenty of rest and sleep. And I began to look at my inner turmoil.

"I grew up in an awfully dysfunctional family. My mother became mentally ill with manic depression when I was nine, and my stepfather was alcoholic. I remember seeing a doctor at the Mayo Clinic for a second opinion about the diagnosis of primary myelofibrosis. He asked me if I had ever had any exposure to toxins that might explain my getting this unusual disease, and I laughed, because what flashed into my mind was all the emotional toxicity of my family life. Most of it was centered around my mother. I didn't want to see her at all. Just saying or thinking the word 'mother' triggered a storm inside me. I didn't know that healing this attitude would be the key to moving toward wholeness.

"About five months after the diagnosis, I came to understand that the only way my relationship with my mother could change was for me to see her with different eyes. I remember the exact moment when I achieved this. It was like a rebirth, the beginning of my being a well person. You have no idea what life can be like when that kind of toxicity is removed. Ever since then I've lived with inner peace instead of inner turmoil, and I really don't worry about the physical condition. My family has been incredibly supportive; we've all grown from this. We're all aware of the preciousness of each day and the need to work out issues as they come up. We have our problems, but we work on them."

Jan works today as a bereavement coordinator for a hospice in Mankato, Minnesota. Her blood counts have been remarkably stable for the past ten years. The hematologists she has seen usually do not comment on her stability, but recently one did allow that she has "really done amazingly well." Jan says she gets out of breath if she climbs a lot of steps but otherwise has no limitations. "I get interesting feedback from my family," she says. "They tell me I'm just kind of different, that they feel a great sense of peacefulness around me."

THE FACES OF HEALING:
ETHAN

THE FIRST TIME Ethan Nadelmann had trouble with his back was in the summer of 1981, when he was twenty-four years old. There was no triggering episode, just severe lower back pain that seemed to appear out of nowhere. Ethan, who was physically fit and liked to play basketball, was suddenly disabled; in fact, he could barely walk. Ten days later, however, the pain slowly eased away, eventually disappearing as mysteriously as it had come.

Ethan is a political scientist, an internationally known expert on drug policy. In 1981, when he had his first experience of back pain, he was studying for general exams for his doctorate in government at Harvard, as well as contemplating entrance to Harvard Law School in the fall. Two years later, when he was under a great deal of stress from schoolwork—he was now in his second year of law school and third year of graduate school—Ethan had another episode of back pain, this one precipitated, he thinks, by working out with weights. Now the pain went into his right leg and was very severe, forcing Ethan to seek medical help from an orthopedic surgeon. A CT scan revealed a herniated disc in the lower lumbar spine. The doctor prescribed indomethacin (Indocin), a strong anti-inflammatory drug. The pain lingered for months. Finally, the orthopedist recommended that Ethan get a second opinion from another surgeon, who told him, "If you're not better in a month, you'll have to have surgery." Ethan got better in a month, eventually weaning himself off the Indocin. The experience left him shaken. "I became wary of playing basketball, stopped doing overhead presses on the weight machine, and generally became more cautious," he says.

For the next few years, Ethan's back caused him no major problems. "I had little flare-ups from basketball, racquetball, and heavy lifting," he recalls, "usually lasting a few days, maybe a week at most." He married in 1986, and became a father two years later. I first met him at that time, when he was leading an active, stressful academic life as an assistant professor at Princeton University.

In June 1991, when Ethan returned from a trip to Europe, his back was bothering him "a little," but the pain was omnipresent and increased throughout the summer. In late August, following a basketball game, the pain "got really bad and didn't go away." A week later, in early September, his condition deteriorated, and he sought help from massage therapists, including a shiatsu practitioner. She told him he would be uncomfortable after her treatments, and he was. A few days later, he woke up very early, which was unusual for him, and felt restless. He took a walk and shortly after returning home developed chills and a fever of 102 degrees. The next morning the fever and his back pain were gone, but instead there was right sciatic pain. He revisited the massage therapists.

Just at this time, he had to run an important, three-day meeting of a working group on drug policy reform. I happened to be a member of the group and was distressed to see Ethan in such obvious pain. On the second morning he told me he had awakened with severe pain in his right calf. The pain kept increasing. "I'm waking up in tears in the middle of the night," Ethan said. A few days later he went to the local hospital, where he received an injection of Demerol, which gave him one night of relief.

Massage therapy now gave only temporary relief, and Ethan went to the orthopedist for X-rays and an MRI scan. By now he could not even stand up straight. The MRI showed two ruptured discs, one of them "shattered into multiple fragments." The orthopedist recommended immediate surgery and prescribed oral narcotics and Valium.

Ethan called me for advice, but he was in such pain and on such high doses of narcotics and Valium that I found it hard to have a conversation with him. He himself says he does not remember some conversations from this period. I told him to get a second opinion before he consented to surgery. I also urged him to read a book, *Healing Back Pain,* by John Sarno, a New York doctor who makes a strong case that most back pain is the result of the mind's interference with normal functioning of nerves and blood circulation to muscles, a situation he calls tension myositis syndrome, or TMS. Ethan, through his drug-induced grogginess, made it clear that he did not want to hear anything about his problem being psychosomatic.

Shortly afterward, Ethan called to say he had obtained a second opinion and that it was the same as the first: immediate surgery to remove the shattered disc and relieve pressure on nerves. Again, I found it very difficult to talk to him. He said he was so disabled by pain that he was thinking of going in for the operation within the next few days. I told him to try to hold off, to see if he could get temporary relief from acupuncture or hypnotherapy, and to try to make an appointment to see Dr. Sarno.

I had several reasons for recommending Dr. Sarno's book. I had met a number of patients who had tried every imaginable treatment for back pain, then had gone to Dr. Sarno and been cured. The cure consisted simply of reading his book, going for an individual appointment, and attending evening lectures in which he explained how the mind produced pain in the back. This sounded too good to be true, but I remembered the one disabling episode of back pain I had had; it was clearly related to my emotional state—grief over the simultaneous loss of two close relationships—and it disappeared suddenly after three weeks. It never returned. Then I saw two cases of men with severe chronic back pain that disappeared as if by magic when the men fell in love. Finally, I had just attended an interesting professional conference of a group called the North American Academy of Musculoskeletal Pain, where I was invited to give a keynote address on the meaning of pain. The speaker after me gave a fascinating lecture on the lack of correlation between the subjective experience of back pain and objective measures of musculoskeletal dysfunction, such as X-rays and MRI scans. He showed X-rays and scans of patients that looked so awful you could not believe these people could stand or walk, yet they were free of pain and had normal mobility. In other cases, people were immobilized by pain, yet their spines looked normal. To my mind, all of this information was consistent with Dr. Sarno's philosophy.

Furthermore, I knew something of the extraordinary stress Ethan was under. In addition to all of the academic pressures, his marriage was strained badly, and his baby girl was at a demanding age. He seemed to me an ideal candidate for TMS.

Ethan did not visit a hypnotherapist, nor did he receive acupuncture; but he did read Dr. Sarno's book. He says he paid attention to it for several reasons. "First of all, I recognized that I was under a lot of stress. Second, the fact that the pain had suddenly jumped from my lower back to my leg seemed peculiar. Third, I remembered my experience in 1983, when an orthopedist told me I would get better in a month or have to have surgery, and I got better. And Dr. Sarno presented a very compelling analysis and argument."

Now the surgeon was pressing for an operation, and he was armed with MRI scans that showed a badly shattered disc. Ethan was worn down by pain and mentally clouded by opiates and Valium. Still, he managed to resist. "I saw another doctor, who gave me one cortisone shot. It gave only minor relief. Sometimes hot baths helped, but mostly the pain in the lower leg was agonizing." He read in Dr. Sarno's book that herniated discs by themselves do not cause pain. They can cause muscle weakness and other symptoms of nerve dysfunction, but not pain; the pain is TMS, caused by the mind, even though it might attach itself to an area of mechanical injury. Ethan made an appointment with Dr. Sarno and dragged himself to New York to keep it.

"Sarno wasn't very interested in the MRI," Ethan recalls, "only in the results of muscle testing in the leg, which showed no nerve dysfunction. He did a quick physical exam and told me it was a clear case of TMS, that I should get off the painkillers because I didn't need them. And he told me I would definitely get better and would be playing basketball again. All I had to do was accept his diagnosis. His evening lecture happened to be that evening, so I attended. There were maybe forty people there, mostly upper middle-class. I heard a lot of talk of people getting better. One guy talked about how his back pain had jumped into a finger. Anyway, as I was sitting there, listening to all this, my pain subsided. Afterward I went to dinner at a friend's. There was no pain.

"Sarno told me I shouldn't do any kind of physical therapy. He thinks any interventions directed at the back reinforce the mistaken idea that the pain originates there. Instead he wants you to figure out what kind of psychological pain is going to the body. Well, I wasn't completely ready to abandon physical approaches, so the next morning I kept an appointment I had made with an osteopath. He told me Sarno was partly right but that I should still get physical therapy. The pain started to come back a little that day. That night I dreamed about Sarno having an argument with the osteopath over the issue of physical therapy. When I woke up the pain was less, and I decided not to go to physical therapy. I had some mild opiate withdrawal when I stopped the painkillers."

Ethan says the pain then assumed a new pattern. "It would nudge me awake early in the morning, then fade and become insignificant later in the day. Over the next six weeks it disappeared entirely." He then began looking seriously at his marriage and the possibility of ending it, setting a time limit for trying to make it work.

One month later Ethan resumed exercise with weights and basketball without worries. One month after that, he had a "major personal breakthrough" that left him feeling highly invigorated and fitter than ever. A year later, he and his wife separated, and he felt satisfied to have come to a resolution. "It was the pain and my experience of healing that provided the impetus to do it," he recalls.

Ethan's brother, a doctor, does not accept Ethan's interpretation of events. "He tells me the cortisone shot did it. But, according to my reading, that should last three to six months at best, and I've now been pain free for almost three years, except for occasional muscle soreness related to exercise. Once I had a period of pain in my side, which made me worry briefly about an ulcer. Then I decided it was my mind looking for yet another physical focus for pain, and as soon as I did that, it went away. I've since met many other people who have had similar success with Sarno's approach, people of diverse backgrounds. He is a combination of a scientist and a faith healer. His intellectual arguments made great sense to me; they rang true. I also had little faith in surgical solutions, having seen too many people whose pain returned a few years after having back surgery."

I asked Ethan what he would tell others who suffer from back pain. "Read Sarno's book and see if it rings true for you," was his answer. "People seem to have a hard time accepting the theory until they've exhausted all other remedies or, like me, are facing the knife."

THE FACES OF HEALING: EVA

"IT'S BEEN FIFTEEN years," says Eva Forrester proudly. "Fifteen years. Look at me! If I can do it, you can do it." Eva works as a clerk in the largest health food store in Tucson, Arizona, and this is what she says to many of the customers who come to her for advice. Eva had breast cancer fourteen years ago. Today she is a healed woman, who tries to inspire others to overcome life-threatening diseases.

In 1979, at the age of fifty, Eva Forrester found a lump in her left breast. X-rays gave no cause for alarm, and the first doctor she saw told her the lump felt benign. When another doctor tried and failed to get a needle aspirate of the lump, a biopsy was scheduled. "Before the nurse said anything about the result, I knew," Eva recalls. "I knew it was cancer. They wanted to do a mastectomy. I refused. I panicked. I told them I wanted to wait, although I don't know what I thought I was waiting for. I liked my doctor, an osteopathic surgeon. He said, 'We have to do something.' I decided to consult with my family in Mexico."

Eva is Mexican-American, born in Chihuahua, the child of a Mexican mother and a Lebanese father. "My father was a dental surgeon, and my nephew is an M.D., so I come from a medical background. I have a real extended family; I'm very blessed in that way. When I told them the news, they were all scared. But I'm a Christian—I believe in God, and I've studied all other religions. I believe that what is supposed to be will be. So, finally, I consented to surgery." In 1980 Eva underwent a modified radical mastectomy. Her tumor was large, and had already spread to local lymph nodes, putting her in a high-risk category. She was sent to an oncologist at the University Medical Center, who wanted to start chemotherapy.

"I couldn't do it," Eva says. "Something in me said, 'No!' It was very sad how they treated me. First they sent a woman M.D. to try to persuade me. Next they said, 'You're going to be back here in no time at all and then we'll have to use higher doses on you.' Still, I said no. My own doctor finally agreed to respect my wishes. There would be no chemo, no radiation."

Instead, Eva embarked on a course of natural healing under the guidance of a chiropractor/naturopath. "I used all the herbs that were supposed to have anticancer properties, but I knew that what I really had to do was change my entire being, and I guess I'm still doing that. I changed my way of thinking, trying to see better things in others, getting closer to Christ, getting closer to the Indian way of life. (You know, I have some Aztec blood.) I worked to turn it all into a positive experience, and there have been many good results. I can relate to people much better than I used to, for example."

Seven years after the surgery, Eva went through a divorce. Her marriage, which had been strained at the time she discovered the lump, did not survive the mastectomy. "My husband could only see me as something less than a whole person," she says. "Some men just can't get beyond that. But I grew through that experience, too. I'm thankful to the Great Spirit for my journey, not bitter about it. I'm very close to my three children, all now in their early forties, and very close to my extended family."

I asked Eva if she had returned to the doctors for tests. "I've had some tests, but I don't go overboard," she answered. "I don't like X-rays, so I try to avoid them. The first few blood tests were kind of scary, but I just applied myself harder and used purely natural treatments. Now everything looks fine.

"Still, I have some hard days—you know how that is. But then I go to the store and the Great Spirit sends me a person who says, 'Eva, what you gave me is working,' and it's all worthwhile. So many young women have come into the store who have the same thing. They are so scared. I know many who have died—too many. It's very personal for me. I get involved with each one."

It is a fact of life in the America of the nineties that health food store clerks have replaced pharmacists as dispensers of practical advice to many sick people, especially those with difficult problems or ailments that do not respond well to conventional treatment. The change is another indicator of widespread disaffection with standard medicine. I have often watched Eva Forrester play this role behind the counter of the New Life Health Center. She stands in front of shelves of vitamins and supplements and engages clients with an open, nonjudgmental, comforting manner. She explains patiently the basics of natural healing, of helping the body rely on its own resources. And frequently, she leans closer to a client and says, "Look at me! Fifteen years! If I can do it, you can do it."

"I come from a culture that values healers," Eva explains. "Everyone knows how to find men and women who have this knowledge: *curanderos* and *curanderas*. That's the path I'm on. I want to become a very good *curandera*."

PART TWO

❦

OPTIMIZING THE
HEALING SYSTEM

8

OPTIMIZING YOUR HEALING
SYSTEM: AN OVERVIEW

HOW WOULD YOU experience optimal efficiency of your healing system? Very likely you would not be aware of it, because we tend to pay little attention to our health when it is good. You would recover speedily from illness and heal from injuries uneventfully. Ordinary stresses of everyday life might annoy you but would not derange your digestion or blood pressure. Sleep would be restful, sex enjoyable. Aging of your body would occur gradually, allowing you to moderate your activity appropriately and live out a normal life span without undue discomfort. You would not contract heart disease or cancer in middle age, be crippled by arthritis in later life, or lose your mind to premature senility.

This scenario is realistic and, I think, worth working for. Actually, the body wants to be healthy, because health represents efficient operation of all of its systems. A useful analogy is the engine of a car. When all components are doing what they should be doing in just the right way, efficiency is maximal, and operation is quiet, producing a "contented" purr that you rarely notice. An engine that calls attention to itself by sounding noisy and rough, knocking, and expelling black smoke is not efficient. Since efficiency is the ratio of work done to energy supplied, the sick engine is working harder to accomplish less. In a similar way it takes less energy to be a healthy person than to be a sick one, and just as a driver may not pay attention to the sound of a well-running engine, people may not be aware of the condition of good health until it breaks down. A program to boost the efficiency of the healing system will not necessarily produce immediately noticeable changes. It is a long-term investment in the future of the body. If you are seeking boundless energy, eternal happiness, an ageless body, or immortality, please look elsewhere. I will be writing only of real possibilities, consistent with the findings of medical science.

I propose to introduce this subject by asking you to consider obstacles to healing. If you understand the general kinds of problems that interfere with healing, you will know what kinds of preventive and corrective action you can take.

LACK OF ENERGY

Healing requires energy. Energy is supplied by metabolism, the process of conversion of caloric energy in food to chemical energy that the body can use for its various functions. Malnourished and starving people are not good candidates for spontaneous healing. Even people who eat enough may not metabolize well for one reason or another; despite their caloric intake, they may suffer deficits of energy that impede healing.

Recall the story I told of the young woman who came to me complaining of fatigue and who had suffered a nonunion of a broken bone in the leg (see page 108). Over the years, a number of (male) doctors had written her off as a complaining female, but to me the nonunion of a fractured bone and a persistent bruise on a big toe suggested a physical problem; and given her other symptoms and history, I suspected hypothyroidism even though her thyroid function tests were normal. The patient came from a distant city, and I found it very difficult to put her under the care of a physician who was willing to attempt thyroid hormone replacement. When she did start treatment, there was no change in her condition for quite some time. But finally, after ten weeks, her symptoms began to recede. Depression lifted, energy increased, and menstruation and digestion improved as metabolism slowly returned to normal. With these changes, her healing ability returned as well.

Hypothyroidism provides a clear illustration of the dependence of the healing system on the availability of energy from metabolism. More common reasons for insufficient metabolic energy are inadequate diets, impaired digestion, and improper breathing, all of which are within your control.

An adequate diet means one that provides not only enough calories but also all of the nutrients necessary for efficient metabolism without any excesses that promote disease. What constitutes a good diet is a matter of controversy, and much of the controversy is based on emotion rather than reason. In the next chapter I will summarize my views of leading-edge nutritional research to tell you how you can modify your diet in a manner that will increase your healing potential.

The term "impaired digestion" covers a wide range of ailments, from esophageal reflux to hemorrhoids, with a variety of stomach and intestinal complaints in between. But, until proved otherwise, most digestive problems should be assumed to be rooted in stress, because the mind has an unlimited capacity to interfere with normal operation of the gastrointestinal system by disturbing the balance of the autonomic (involuntary) nerves that regulate it. I will advise you how to neutralize stress and harmonize the functioning of the autonomic nervous system in order to avoid these problems.

When I say that improper breathing can lead to deficits of metabolic energy I have a picture in mind of an extreme example: a man I know in his late forties who suffers from emphysema and lifelong bronchitis and asthma. Despite a healthy appetite, he is no more than skin and bones, unable to store up reserves of metabolic energy simply because he cannot take in enough oxygen to burn the fuel he eats. Even in the absence of chronic lung disease, poor breathing can limit metabolism and the amount of energy available for healing. Poor breathing is correctable, and I will tell you how to change it.

Finally, I should mention that lack of energy can also result from immoderate expenditure of energy as a result of overwork, overexertion, lack of rest and sleep, and addictive use of stimulant drugs. Obviously, these problems are also correctable.

POOR CIRCULATION

The healing system depends on the circulation of blood to bring energy and materials to a malfunctioning or injured area. You can see graphic examples of impaired healing due to poor circulation in persons with diabetes whose arteries are subject to premature and rapid progression of atherosclerosis as a result of their altered metabolism. Diabetics must be careful not to cut or nick their feet, since even a slight break in the skin may turn into a large ulcer that refuses to heal. The body just cannot supply enough nourishment, oxygen, and immune activity to the area because of insufficient circulation.

You can maintain your circulatory system in good working order by following a healthy diet, by not smoking, and by exercising, and I will give you more specific suggestions in the following chapters.

RESTRICTED BREATHING

I have already mentioned that restricted breathing can reduce efficiency of the healing system through its dampening effect on metabolism, but I believe it can interfere in other ways as well. The operations of the brain and the nervous system depend on adequate exchange of oxygen and carbon dioxide, as do those of the heart and the circulatory system and all organs of the body. Breathing may be the master function of the body, affecting all others. Restrictions in breathing can be the result of past traumas, both physical and emotional. Most of us have never received instruction about breathing and how to take advantage of it as a harmonizer of mind and body. For that reason I devote a portion of Chapter 13 to the subject.

IMPAIRED DEFENSES

Spontaneous healing is unlikely to occur if the body's defenses are weak. Defense is the responsibility of the immune system, whose main job is to distinguish between self and not-self and take action against the latter. When immunity is crippled, as in AIDS, it is easy to see how much of a problem this creates for the healing system. When immunity is weakened in more subtle ways, impairment of healing may be less obvious.

There are three main categories of weakening influences on the immune system: (1) persistent or overwhelming infections; (2) toxic injury by certain forms of matter and energy; and (3) unhealthy mental states. You can protect yourself against all of these influences and, in addition, learn techniques to enhance immunity through adjustments in diet, exercise, and judicious use of vitamins, minerals, and herbs. You will find the information you need in this part of the book.

TOXINS

Toxic overload is one of the commonest reasons for diminished healing responses, but the subject is immensely complicated, emotionally charged, and highly political. We take toxins into our body with the food we eat, the water we drink, and the air we breathe, as well as in the form of drugs we use, whether we obtain them on medical prescription, buy them over the counter, or use them recreationally. I am concerned about toxic forms of energy as well as matter; electromagnetic pollution may be the most significant form of pollution human activity has produced in this century, all the more dangerous because it is invisible and insensible.

Whether energetic or material, toxins can damage DNA, which contains the information needed for spontaneous healing; disrupt the biological controls on which the healing system depends; weaken defenses; and promote the development of cancer and other diseases that already represent failures of healing by the time they make themselves known. Toxic overload may be a significant cause of allergy, autoimmune disease, and a variety of degenerative diseases (like Parkinson's disease and ALS [amyotrophic lateral sclerosis]), whose causes now seem obscure.

The medical profession and the scientific research community have been remarkably slow to pay attention to this issue, which I consider to be one of the greatest threats to health and well-being in the world today. You have probably read stories in the press about clusters of leukemia cases in neighborhoods near power lines, about the increasing incidence of lymphoma among farmers who use agricultural chemicals, and about a worldwide increase in asthma and bronchitis as air pollution gets worse. Recently, I have followed news stories about a mysterious cluster of lupus cases in the border town of Nogales, Arizona, not far from my home near Tucson. Systemic lupus erythematosus is a potentially serious autoimmune disease not known to be communicable or to have environmental causes. Yet the incidence in Nogales is many times the national average. In 1994 reporters found that a ranching operation on the Mexican side of the border had been dumping pesticides into streams and burning manure contaminated with pesticides because it could not afford to build a proper disposal facility. No causal link is yet established, but I predict one will be.

If you want to increase the likelihood of spontaneous healing, it is imperative that you learn to guard against toxic injury. That means limiting exposure, protecting your body from the effects of pollution, and helping your body eliminate any toxins that do get in.

AGE

We assume that age is an obstacle to healing, that old people do not heal as readily as young people and have lowered immunity and resistance in general. Actually, there is little research to support those assumptions, but observation suggests that they are true. It is impressive to watch how quickly children heal from simple surgeries, like hernia repairs and appendectomies. This is not to say that old people are incapable of spontaneous healing, just that it may take more time. Moreover, methods may exist to protect the healing system from the effects of aging as well as to stimulate general resistance and vitality in the elderly.

Traditional Chinese medicine has identified a number of natural substances that act as tonics of this sort. As a group they appear to be nontoxic and effective. Some of them are now available in this country. I have reviewed the literature on these substances, have tried some of them myself, and with patients, and will give you suggestions for how to use them. You cannot stop the changes of time, but you can modify lifestyle and activity as you age, and it is good to know that help is available to maintain the efficiency of your healing system.

OBSTRUCTION BY THE MIND

After reading Part One of this book and looking over the case histories presented throughout, you should have a firm conviction that the mind is a major influence on healing, for better or worse. Spontaneous healing can be triggered by mental events; it can also be frustrated by habitual ways of using the mind. I have already noted that the mind can depress the immune system and can unbalance the autonomic nervous system, leading to disturbances in digestion, circulation, and all other internal functions. You must know how to use the mind in the service of healing.

SPIRITUAL PROBLEMS

During my travels throughout the world I have met many healers who believe that the primary causes of health and illness are not physical but spiritual. They direct their attention toward an invisible world assumed to exist beyond the ordinary world of the senses. In this realm they search for reasons for illness and ways to cure it. Some of these people believe in karmic causes of illness (actions in the past or in past lives); others, in the ability of deceased ancestors to affect one's life and health; others, in possession by spirits; and still others, in the possibility of psychic attack by malevolent shamans. It is impossible to talk to most scientists about an invisible world, since scientific materialism looks only for physical causes of physical events. I have learned not to try to discuss the possibility of non-physical causation of physical events with most doctors, but I do discuss it with some patients and think about it a lot. Therefore, I would not consider this part of the book complete without some information about the spiritual dimension of healing and what you can do to make sure all is well on that level.

This completes my inventory of obstacles to spontaneous healing and identifies those subjects about which I need to give you information. Let's begin with diet.

9

A Healing Diet

At a recent workshop I taught on natural health a man was wearing a T-shirt that said, "Eat Right, Exercise, Die Anyway." There is truth in that motto. We will all die, and our life span may be genetically programmed. Nevertheless, our choices about how we live may interact with genetics to determine the quality of life we experience as we age. I believe that lifestyle significantly influences our risks of contracting common diseases and certainly affects our ability to heal. Of all the choices we make, those concerning food are particularly important, because we have great potential control over them. But, as you probably already know, there is great disagreement as to what constitutes a healthy diet.

I have seen too many people who have lived to ripe old ages on "bad" diets to believe that food is the sole or even chief determinant of good health. It is simply one influence, one that we can do something about. Books about diet and health appear with great frequency, many of them contradicting each other. Even on the Big Questions, such as the health hazards of dietary fat, major disagreements exist among experts. Some doctors extol a low-fat diet as the key to health and longevity, while others say that cutting fat in the diet may add at best a few weeks to one's life span. There is similar disagreement about the benefits of vegetarianism. Many surveys find that vegetarians have lower rates of heart disease and cancer, but doctors argue about the reasons for that, with some maintaining that vegetarians tend to be more health conscious and take better care of themselves in general, while others say animal foods are hazardous, and still others say that if nonvegetarians ate the same amount of fat (less) and fiber (more) as vegetarians, there would be no differences.

I do not have time or space to enter into these kinds of arguments, and I do not wish to add to your confusion. Instead I want to outline simple, practical suggestions for modifying diet in ways that I believe favor healing responses. You will have heard some of this before, but essential truths cannot be repeated often enough. I am not interested in nutritional fads and will concentrate only on what I see as key areas of consensus emerging from studies of diet and health. These findings concern (1) total calories, (2) fat, (3) protein sources, (4) fruits and vegetables, and (5) fiber.

TOTAL CALORIES

An unexpected research finding that may have great practical significance is that experimental animals live longer with much lower rates of disease when they consume less than the recommended daily allowance of calories. The health and longevity benefits of "undernutrition" are clearly established for laboratory rats and mice, but remain unproved for humans, although there is every reason to believe they apply. The finding is unexpected because we associate less-than-optimal nutrition with poor growth and health, and common sense tells us that we do better if we are well nourished. In fact, most of us may be overnourished, and too much of a good thing may be doing us harm.

If we all lived in controlled environments and had measured portions of monotonous food dispensed to us at regular intervals, none of us would be overweight, I am sure, and I suspect many of us would live longer and experience spontaneous healing more frequently than we do now. Fortunately or unfortunately, we live in a world that tempts us with a great variety and abundance of food, and many of us eat not to satisfy physical hunger but to allay anxiety, depression, and boredom, to provide a substitute for emotional nourishment, or to try to fill an inner void. Most of us are not voluntarily going to embark on programs of undernutrition; I wonder if there might be other ways to take advantage of the research findings.

Two possibilities occur to me. The first is to modify diet to lower caloric content without greatly reducing the amount or appeal of food we consume. The second to is restrict caloric intake, either by fasting or by eating a limited diet at regular intervals—say, one day a week. I have experimented with both of these techniques, and think both are useful.

The easiest way to reduce calories in dishes you like is to cut the fat content. Fat has almost twice as many calories per gram as protein and carbohydrate, so it is the major contributor of calories to our diets. It is remarkably easy to cut fat by one-half, three-quarters, or more in dishes you prepare at home, and it is getting easier all the time with the appearance of low-fat cookbooks and low-fat or fat-free versions of popular foods, like chips, mayonnaise, and sour cream. Of course, fat also contributes taste and pleasure to food, and you do not want to sacrifice those qualities totally. Nor do you want to eat such great quantities of lighter foods that you wind up taking in more calories than before. (I know people who formerly ate ice cream only occasionally but now eat large helpings of nonfat frozen yogurt every day. I think their caloric intake has increased rather than decreased as a result of the change; this and similar adjustments may explain why obesity in America continues to increase, even as total fat in the American diet declines.) In short, it is possible to reduce caloric intake and still eat plenty of satisfying foods by using less fat, which is one way to reap some of the health benefits of undernutrition.

At different times in my life I have experimented with fasting one day a week, usually on Mondays. When I fast, I consume nothing but water or herb tea, sometimes with lemon in it, and I find this to be a useful physical and psychological discipline. It feels healthy. If you are very skinny and sensitive to cold, I do not recommend fasting in this way. Instead you might want to try drinking fruit juice or clear liquids one day a week. Not only do these practices give your digestive system a rest, they decrease total caloric intake and, again, may provide benefits of undernutrition without forcing you to give up the pleasures of eating. There are many secondary benefits as well, such as greatly increased appreciation of food following a fast and greater ability to eat consciously rather than unconsciously.

In any case, watch for further research reports on the health benefits of undernutrition. If the findings hold up and continue to look applicable to humans, it will be worth trying to cut your intake of calories in order to realize more of your body's healing potential.

FAT

I will devote more time to a discussion of fat than to any other aspect of diet, because I believe the implications of research on how fat affects the body are vitally important. Eating too much of the wrong kinds of fat can seriously impair your healing abilities and may be the biggest dietary mistake you can make.

Fats are mixtures of fatty acids, which are chains of carbon atoms with hydrogen atoms attached and a distinctive acidic chemical group at one end. Fatty acids can be classified by the lengths of the chains and by whether all of the available chemical bonds of the carbon atoms are occupied or saturated with hydrogen atoms. Unsaturated fatty acids have one (mono-) or more (poly-) links in the chain consisting of double or triple bonds between adjacent carbons. Points of unsaturation alter the configuration of the molecule, and its physical and chemical characteristics.

Fats composed mainly of saturated fatty acids are solid at room temperature, and the greater the saturated fat content, the higher will be the temperature of melting. Animal fats are highly saturated, as are two vegetable fats: the oils of coconuts and palm kernels. At the opposite end of this chemical spectrum are the polyunsaturated vegetable oils, all of which stay liquid in colder temperatures. The lower the temperature at which solidification occurs, the greater the degree of unsaturation. Corn, soy, sesame, sunflower, and safflower oils are examples of polyunsaturated fats. In the middle of the spectrum are vegetable oils composed primarily of monounsaturated fatty acids, those with just one double or triple bond in the chain of carbon atoms; examples are olive, canola, peanut, and avocado oils.

At the moment, conventional medical doctors who are concerned about nutrition are giving us two general kinds of advice about dietary fat. They are telling us to cut way down on the total amount of fat we eat and also way down on the amount of saturated fat we eat. In my view, this is only part of the story.

Evidence for the health risks of saturated fat is overwhelming. In most people, a high percentage of saturated fat in the diet stimulates the liver to make LDL (bad) cholesterol in quantities greater than the body can remove from the circulation. The result is damage to arterial walls (atherosclerosis), impairment of the cardiovascular system, increased risk of premature death and disability from coronary heart disease, and reduction of healing capacity through restriction of blood flow.

Evidence for the health risks of total fat is much less convincing. Given the popular prejudice against fat in our society, many people would like to believe that very low-fat diets will make us live longer, prevent cancer, and boost our immunity, but we do not have hard data to support these ideas. Very low-fat diets—around ten percent of total calories from fat, as compared with forty in the average American diet—are of great therapeutic benefit to persons with established cardiovascular disease, but they are hard to adhere to and may not do much for the rest of us. I believe it is worth cutting fat to moderate levels—say, twenty to thirty percent of total calories—but that it is much more important to concentrate on reducing saturated fat and the other unhealthy fats that I will write about in a moment.

The main natural sources of saturated fat are beef, pork, lamb, unskinned chicken, duck, whole milk and products made from whole milk (especially cheese, butter, and cream), and processed foods made with tropical oils (palm and coconut). Of all of these, beef fat may be the greatest threat to health. In addition there are unnatural sources of saturated fat: margarine, solid vegetable shortening, and all processed foods made with partially hydrogenated oils. In these products, liquid vegetable oils have been artificially saturated with hydrogen to make them solid or semisolid at room temperature and increase their resistance to spoilage. No matter how good the oils are that go into this process, what comes out is saturated and hazardous to cardiovascular health.

Obviously, the easiest way to remove saturated fat from the diet is to cut way down on animal foods, especially meat and whole milk products—a strategy I recommend. In addition, you should eliminate sources of tropical oils and artificially solidified oils, which are dangerous for another reason, which I will explain below.

Not long ago, doctors recommended replacement of saturated fats like butter with polyunsaturated vegetable oils, like corn and safflower, in the belief that these oils would lower cholesterol and benefit the heart and arteries. During this period, margarine, whose only virtue in the early part of this century was its low cost, changed in the public mind from a cheap substitute for butter to a healthy alternative to it. Sales of safflower oil, the most unsaturated of all the vegetable oils, boomed. I hope this era has now come to an end. Polyunsaturated oils are bad for us in other ways. They are chemically unstable, owing to their content of fatty acids with energetic double and triple bonds that tend to react with oxygen, resulting in toxic compounds that can damage DNA and cell membranes, promoting cancer, inflammation, and degenerative changes in tissue. I strongly recommend eliminating them from the diet.

Moreover, when unsaturated fatty acids are heated or treated with chemical solvents and bleaches, they tend to deform from a natural, curved shape (called the *cis*-configuration) to an unnatural, jointed shape (called the *trans*-configuration). Trans-fatty acids, or TFAs, may be extremely toxic, even though medical scientists have been very slow to recognize the danger. Even now, as they are finally beginning to admit that margarine may be worse for the heart than butter, they are still focusing solely on margarine's content of saturated fat rather than on its abundance of TFAs. The body builds cell membranes out of cis-fatty acids and also uses them in synthetic pathways for hormones. We do not know what it does with TFAs; if it tries to use them in the same ways, the result might be defective membranes and hormones. I believe that TFAs in the diet damage the regulatory machinery of the body, significantly compromising the healing system. Remember that TFAs are rarely found in nature, only in fats that have been subjected to unusual chemical and physical treatment. Some researchers refer to them as "funny fats," but there is nothing funny about what they may do to us. You can avoid any danger by eliminating from the diet all margarine and solid vegetable shortening and products made with them, all products listing "partially hydrogenated" oil of any kind on the label, and all commercial brands of polyunsaturated vegetable oils (corn, soy, sesame, sunflower, safflower), since these have been extracted with heat and solvents that promote formation of TFAs. (I refuse even to consider cottonseed oil as a food. It has a high percentage of saturated fat, may contain naturally occurring toxins, and is likely to be contaminated with pesticide residues.)

What then *can* we eat? Vegetable oils that are predominantly monounsaturated—olive, canola, peanut, avocado—do not pose the

cardiovascular risk of saturated fats or the cancer risks of polyunsaturates. The individual oils within this category differ significantly
from one another, and it is important to know the advantages and
disadvantages of each.

Olive oil appears to be the best and safest of all edible fats. The
body seems to have an easier time handling its predominant fatty
acid, oleic acid, than any other fatty acid. Replacing saturated fat in
the diet with olive oil leads to a reduction of bad cholesterol (whereas
replacement with polyunsaturated vegetable oils lowers good cholesterol as well). Olive oil is delicious and has been used as an edible oil
for thousands of years. The best-quality, called extra-virgin, is
extracted with gentle pressure rather than with heat or solvents; you
can buy it in almost any supermarket for a reasonable price. Olive
trees are extraordinarily long-lived and beautiful, inspiring reverence
in cultures that cultivate them; they produce well without heavy
applications of pesticides and agricultural chemicals. Moreover, in
populations that use olive oil as their main cooking fat, rates of cardiovascular disease are lower than expected for the amount of total
fat consumed, and rates of degenerative diseases and cancer are also
lower than in many other populations. Olive oil is the outstanding
element of the Mediterranean diet that has attracted so much
research attention in the past few years. Mediterranean peoples eat
plenty of fruits and vegetables, whole grain breads, substantial quantities of fish, and moderate amounts of animal foods, but when all of
these factors are analyzed, olive oil has the highest correlation with
better health.

As a result of my own research, I have come to rely on olive oil as the
principal fat in my diet, using it for almost all cooking in which I use
fat, for all salad dressing, and occasionally as a dip for bread (though I
usually eat bread without anything on it). If you do not like the taste of
olive oil, you can buy "light" varieties that lack the distinctive odor
and flavor; although these might be useful in some dishes, like Oriental stir-fries and baked goods, they are probably less healthful because
they have been processed. If the only change you make in your diet is
to replace butter and margarine with olive oil, you will have made a
tremendous step toward better health and healing.

Canola oil (the name is a contraction of "Canadian oil," because
the product was developed in Canada) is a modern version of a traditional cooking oil of India and southern China extracted from

rapeseed. Rape is a mustard relative, whose seed contains an oil with very little saturated fat and a high percentage of monounsaturated fatty acids. It also contains a toxic fatty acid, erucic acid. Modern growers have reduced the erucic acid content of rapeseed oil and improved it in other ways; but despite its current popularity—canola oil has eclipsed safflower oil as the darling of the health food industry—I am much less enthusiastic about it than I am about olive oil. We have no comparable epidemiological data for canola oil of the sort we have for olive oil to suggest that health is better in populations that use it. The canola oil you find in supermarkets has all been extracted in ways that deform fatty acids, and rape is heavily treated with pesticides that probably find their way into the oil. You can buy organic, expeller-pressed canola oil in health food stores at considerably higher cost, and this is the only kind I would use. I keep a bottle of it in my refrigerator for occasional recipes where I want a perfectly neutral-flavored oil, but I find that I use it up very slowly. In my opinion it is a distant runner-up to olive oil.

Peanut oil, once the preferred choice of Chinese cooks, has a much greater percentage of polyunsaturated fatty acids than olive oil and may also contain toxins, both natural and unnatural. I see no reason to use it. Avocado oil, available only in health food stores, is too expensive and has nothing to recommend it for use in the kitchen. Avocados are interesting additions to the diet but, given their fat content, should be used with great moderation. If you cannot give up the idea of spreading fat on your bread, try a little mashed, seasoned avocado instead; it is a way of replacing a highly saturated fat with a monounsaturated one.

There are three other oils in my refrigerator that I use in small quantities as flavorings: roasted (dark) sesame oil, walnut oil, and hazelnut oil. These are polyunsaturates that must be kept cold and not used in foods heated to high temperatures. They have strong odors and tastes that I like in soups, salad dressings, and marinades; in small amounts they are delicious and not unhealthy.

Before I leave the subject of fats, I want to mention one other category that seems to promote health and healing. These are the omega-3 fatty acids found in some fish and a few plants. Omega-3s are highly unsaturated fatty acids with special properties. They appear to reduce inflammatory changes in the body, protect against abnormal blood clotting, and, possibly, protect against cancer and degenerative changes in cells and tissues. A great deal of research suggests that optimal diets should include sources of these hard-to-find compounds. Here are your choices:

You can eat the fish that contain omega-3s in their fat, mostly oily fish from cold northern waters: sardines, herring, mackerel, bluefish, salmon, and, to a lesser extent, albacore tuna. (I will have more to say about fish in the next section of this chapter.) Or you can take omega-3 supplements as capsules of fish oils. Canola and soy oil provide tiny amounts, but two less common vegetable oils from flax and hemp are rich sources: the seeds of these plants have high concentrations of omega-3s. You can buy flax seeds, flax meal, and flax oil in health food stores. Hemp oil is becoming available in some health food stores. Finally, one wild green—purslane—is an omega-3 source. Mediterranean peoples use it in soups, and it is easily grown in the garden; in fact, it tends to be a persistent weed.

I do not recommend taking fish oil capsules. They may be contaminated with toxins and may not provide the same benefits as eating the right fish. My personal preference is to eat salmon, sardines, or herring two or three times a week. (Mackerel is harder to get, bluefish is often contaminated with mercury, and albacore tuna is not a rich enough source.) If you choose not to eat fish, your best bet is hemp oil or flax, since purslane is not easy to come by. Hemp oil is greenish and nutty, quite good mixed with olive oil in salad dressing. Flax oil is sweet and nutty when fresh, but it deteriorates quickly and often tastes unpleasantly like oil paint (for which it is used as a base) by the time it gets to the table. If you can find good-tasting flax oil and like it, by all means use it. Otherwise, I would recommend adding flax meal to the diet. My suggestion is to buy whole flax seeds, which are quite cheap, keep them in the refrigerator, and grind enough for a few days or a week at a time, using a coffee grinder or blender. You can sprinkle flax meal over cereal or salad or add it to breads and cookies. It tastes good. A tablespoon of hemp or flax oil a day or two tablespoons of flax meal will give you a good helping of precious omega-3 fatty acids.

Here, then, are my recommendations about dietary fats:

- *Cut total fat* by eliminating deep-fried foods, moderating consumption of chips, nuts, avocados, butter, cheese, and other high-fat foods, and learning to modify recipes to reduce fat content of favorite dishes. Read labels of products you buy to determine fat content, and try to keep your fat intake in the range of twenty to thirty percent of total calories.

• *Make a special effort to cut saturated fat in your diet* by cutting down substantially on meat, unskinned poultry, whole milk and whole milk products, butter, margarine, vegetable shortening, and all products made with tropical oils and partially hydrogenated oils.

• *Eliminate polyunsaturated vegetable oils from your diet* by avoiding safflower, sunflower, corn, soy, peanut, and cottonseed oils and products made from them.

• *Learn to rely on olive oil as your principal fat,* preferably a flavorful brand of extra-virgin olive oil.

• *Learn to identify and avoid all sources of hazardous transfatty acids:* margarine, solid vegetable shortening, and all products made with partially hydrogenated oils of any kind.

• *Increase consumption of omega-3 fatty acids* by eating the appropriate fish, hemp or flax oil, or flax meal regularly.

PROTEIN SOURCES

We need protein to make new tissue, to grow, and to maintain and repair our tissues. Proteins are complicated molecules, made up of a variety of amino acids, some of which are essential nutrients that the body is unable to manufacture and must receive in the diet. Protein deficiency results in stunted growth and dramatic impairment of healing ability; but in our society, protein deficiency is practically nonexistent. Instead, most people consume too much protein, which can also affect health adversely, and many of us get our protein from questionable sources.

Most people rely on animal foods for protein: meat, poultry, fish, milk, and milk products. Vegetable sources are beans, grains, and some nuts. An important difference between animal and vegetable sources is that the latter are less concentrated. For example, the protein in beans is diluted by edible starch and indigestible fiber, so that you have to eat a greater volume of a vegetable protein source to get the equivalent of a portion of an animal food.

When you eat more protein than your body needs to make and repair tissue, it will be used instead as an energy source, as fuel. But protein is not an ideal fuel for the body. Because protein molecules are big and complicated, their digestion and metabolism require more work than the digestion and metabolism of carbohydrates and fats. So proteins are less efficient fuels: the ratio of work in to energy out is not as favorable as for other nutrients. A practical consequence is that if you are eating a high-protein diet, your digestive system is doing a lot of work, and less energy may be available to you for healing.

There is another problem with protein as fuel: it does not burn clean. Carbohydrate and fat, being composed solely of carbon, hydrogen, and oxygen, burn to carbon dioxide and water. Protein contains nitrogen, and in the process of metabolism degrades to highly toxic nitrogenous residues. The burden of dealing with these falls on the liver, which processes them to urea, a simple compound that is also highly toxic. The kidneys must then take up the task of eliminating urea. Tying up liver and kidney function in this way reduces the contribution of those organs to the body's healing system. Furthermore, the nitrogenous-breakdown products of protein metabolism can also irritate the immune system, increasing the risk of allergy and autoimmunity, which represent derangement of body defenses. For all of these reasons, it is better not to consume too much protein. You want to give the body enough for growth, maintenance, and repair, but not so much that it becomes a significant source of metabolic energy.

How much protein is too much? Remarkably small amounts are enough to satisfy the minimal requirements of the average adult—perhaps two ounces, or sixty grams, of a protein food a day. Many people in our society eat much more than that at every meal. Certainly four ounces (less than 120 grams) is plenty. In general: if you have a protein meal once a day—that is, a meal organized around a main course of meat, chicken, fish, eggs, or tofu—that is probably enough. Try to design other meals around carbohydrates and vegetables: stir-fried vegetables with rice, say, or pasta and vegetables, or salads and bread. Cutting down on protein will free up energy, spare your digestive system and especially your liver and kidneys from extra work, and protect your immune system from irritation.

In addition to thinking about protein in general and how to cut down on it, you should consider the advantages and disadvantages of the common sources of dietary protein, another subject that I consider important. Your choices about what kind of protein you ingest may have great influence on your long-term health and capacity for healing.

One problem is that diets rich in animal protein put you high on the food chain, not a good place to be. The food chain is the pattern of dependence of higher organisms on lower organisms for energy. Plants make energy from the sun. Herbivorous animals get that same energy by eating the plants. Carnivorous animals get it further removed from the source by eating the flesh of herbivores. The bigger the organism and the more carnivorous it is, the higher it is said to be on the food chain. One consequence of eating high on the food chain is that you take in much larger doses of toxins, because environmental toxins concentrate as you move up from level to level. The fat of domestic animals often contains high concentrations of toxins that exist in much lower concentrations in grains, for example. An independent problem is that the methods we use for raising animal sources of protein further load them up with unhealthy substances.

Here is a quick review of sources of dietary protein:

Meat has several strikes against it. It is a major source of saturated fat in the diet, as well as a highly concentrated form of protein. Being high on the food chain, it accumulates environmental toxins. Unless it is raised organically, it is also full of added toxins: residues of growth-promoting hormones, antibiotics, and other chemicals used by all commercial ranchers and farmers. "White meat" is no better than red meat, except that veal has less fat than beef, and pork fat (lard) seems less hazardous for the human cardiovascular system than beef fat. Unless meat is cooked very well, it may transmit pathogenic viruses and bacteria to humans who eat it.

Chicken has one main advantage over meat: its fat is external to muscle tissue and can be removed with the skin. Otherwise, chicken presents the same toxic hazards as the flesh of cows, sheep, and pigs and may contain even more added hormones. Dangerous bacteria, particularly salmonella, often contaminate chicken and can sicken humans who eat it unless the chicken is well cooked.

Fish increasingly appears to be a very healthy source of protein. I am referring here to scale fish, not to shellfish. Populations that eat the most fish have the highest longevity and lowest disease rates, and within those populations, the healthiest individuals are those who eat the most fish. Why fish is good for us is not clear. Omega-3 fatty acids may be a part of the explanation, but they are in some fish only, and the answer may not have to do with any one component. Are fish eaters healthier because of the fish they eat or because of what they don't eat? Most of them eat much less animal flesh, for example. There are important cautions about fish today. Much of it is contaminated by toxins that have been dumped into rivers and oceans. Larger, more carnivorous fish and fish that live in coastal waters are most dangerous in this regard. I recommend against eating swordfish, marlin, and shark because their flesh is likely to contain toxins. Increasingly, fish are being farmed throughout the world, especially salmon, trout, and catfish. Farmed fish may not be as beneficial to health as their wild counterparts (farmed salmon have lower amounts of omega-3s) and may have residues of drugs used to control diseases in crowded conditions. But even with these drawbacks, fish are a good protein source.

Shellfish are much less attractive, because they are more likely to contain toxins. They live in coastal effluents and feed in ways that expose them to high concentrations of wastes. Raw shellfish can easily transmit diseases to humans.

Milk products tend to be very high in saturated fat, unless they are made from skim milk or low-fat milk. Many people cannot digest the sugar (lactose) in milk, and many more probably experience irritation of the immune system from the protein in milk. (This is a particular problem with cow's milk; goat's milk does not seem to bother the immune system nearly as much.) If you have allergies, autoimmune disease, sinus trouble, bronchitis, asthma, eczema, or gastrointestinal problems, it is worth eliminating all milk from the diet for at least two months to see what happens to the conditions. In very many cases, they will improve dramatically. Commercial dairy products are another source of environmental toxins, drugs, and hormones.

Eggs, at least the whites of eggs, are good sources of high-quality protein, but egg yolks contain fat and cholesterol that most of us should limit. Commercially raised eggs are produced under awful conditions, may contain toxic residues of drugs and hormones, and may be contaminated with salmonella. Avoid raw and undercooked eggs, and try to find eggs from free-ranging chickens raised without drugs and hormones.

Grains and beans contain carbohydrate and fiber along with protein, so you can eat more of them without suffering a protein overload. Since they are often treated with a variety of agricultural chemicals, I recommend looking for organically produced varieties.

Nuts and seeds, like almonds and sunflower seeds, are sources of vegetable protein, but their high content of fat (mostly polyunsaturated) argues for moderation in their consumption.

Soybeans have much more protein than other beans, along with significant amounts of polyunsaturated fat. Soy protein can be isolated and transformed into an astonishing variety of forms, including facsimiles of animal foods. You will find most of these in the refrigerator cases of health food stores, but also look in Oriental grocery stores. Many forms of tofu and tempeh are now available, along with better and better burgers, wieners, and lunch meats, including some excellent low- and nonfat versions. There may be great health benefits to soy foods that are just coming to light. They contain a group of chemicals called phytoestrogens that may offer significant protection against prostate cancer in men and estrogenically driven diseases in women, including breast cancer, endometriosis, fibrocystic breast disease, and uterine fibroids, as well as the discomforts of menopause. Low incidence of these conditions among Japanese women may be due to their high consumption of soy foods, especially tofu. Two of the best-known soy phytoestrogens—genistein and daidzein—are now being explored for their ability to moderate human hormonal imbalances.

Having reviewed the major sources of dietary protein, I will now give you my simplest recommendations for taking advantage of this information to change your diet in a direction that favors spontaneous healing:

- *Eat less protein.* Learn to recognize sources of protein in your diet and to cut down on them. Practice making meals that do not revolve around large servings of dense protein foods.

- *Begin to replace animal protein in the diet with fish and soy protein.* By doing so you will both reduce your exposure to toxins and other harmful elements in meats, poultry, and milk and gain the benefits of health-promoting components of fish and soybeans.

FRUITS AND VEGETABLES

Our mothers were right to tell us to eat our vegetables. Vegetables and fruits appear to offer significant protection against cancer, heart disease, and other common ailments as well as to help immunity and healing. Besides, perfectly ripe fruits and good-quality vegetables are some of the greatest delights of the table. What is better than slicing into an aromatic melon or a peach running with juice and flavor, or a creamy-ripe mango? How about a colorful bowl of mixed salad greens dressed with olive oil and balsamic vinegar; barely cooked, crisp sugar snap peas; or perfect ears of sweet corn? Many people miss out on these pleasures because commercial growers plant varieties chosen for resistance to shipping rather than for flavor, or because the crops are harvested before they are ready to eat, or because they have suffered in transit to stores. Other people think they do not like vegetables because they do not know how to cook them and have never tasted them properly prepared. Fresh fruits and vegetables probably deliver more health benefits than canned, frozen, or dried versions.

As researchers identify more and more protective compounds in fruits and vegetables, there is a tendency in our society to isolate the compounds and use them in the form of supplements. I am not sure this is a good idea. Beta carotene, for example, the water-soluble precursor of vitamin A (that is, the body makes vitamin A from it), is now used in capsule form by millions of people, who have heard that it is an antioxidant and may prevent cancer. There *is* strong evidence that beta carotene helps prevent cancer when we eat it in our food; evidence for its effectiveness as an isolated supplement is much less solid. Beta carotene is one member of a large family of carotenes, yellow and orange pigments found in many fruits (peaches, melons, mangoes) and vegetables (sweet potatoes, squash, pumpkin, tomatoes, and dark, leafy greens). Other carotenes, like alpha carotene and lycopene (in tomatoes), may be even more important contributors to the cancer-protective effect of these foods, or they may act synergistically with beta carotene. Until a mixed-carotene supplement appears on the market, people whose diets are low in fruits and vegetables may be wise to take supplemental beta carotene, but they would be wiser still to increase their consumption of carotene-rich foods.

Reductionism—the belief that properties of wholes can be reduced to effects of single components—is a common proclivity of Western science and medicine. When we find a plant in nature that has interesting biological effects, we want to identify and isolate the "active principle" of the plant and give it to patients in pure form. Traditional Chinese doctors think very differently. They do not object to scientific analysis of healing plants, but they do not believe in using isolated components. In their view the desirable effects of herbal medicine result from synergistic interactions of all components of each plant and of all the plants (often a dozen or more) used in a typical prescription.

Recently, scientists identified a compound in broccoli, sulphoraphane, that may be partly responsible for that vegetable's powerful cancer-protective effect. Should you eat broccoli or wait for capsules of sulphoraphane to appear in health food stores? I say broccoli, because parts are not equal to wholes. If you think you do not like it, try it cooked in new ways. Here is a simple way of preparing broccoli that is so delicious I cannot get enough of it:

Trim the end off a large bunch of broccoli, cut off the main stem, peel it beneath the fibrous layer, and cut into edible chunks. Separate the head of broccoli into bite-size pieces and peel a bit of the skin from the stems to make them more tender. Wash the broccoli and place it in a pot with ¼ cup cold water, 1 tablespoon of extra-virgin olive oil, salt to taste, and several cloves of chopped or mashed garlic. Bring to a boil, cover tightly, and let steam until the broccoli is bright green and very crunchy-tender, no more than five minutes. Remove the lid and boil off most of the remaining liquid. Serve at once. You can mix this with cooked pasta (penne or rigatoni), season it with red pepper flakes and parmesan cheese, or eat it as is. It is beautiful to look at, utterly delicious, low in fat, rich in vitamins and minerals, and filled with sulphoraphane too!

If you would like to try a more exotic preparation of broccoli, here is a modified version of a Chinese dish with black bean sauce, without all the fat (often cottonseed oil) used in many Chinese restaurants:

Prepare the vegetable as in the previous recipe. Put it in a pot with the following ingredients: 2 tablespoons of salted black beans

(available in Chinese grocery stores) that have been washed in cold
water and drained; 2 large cloves of garlic, mashed; 2 teaspoons of
finely chopped fresh ginger root; 1 tablespoon of dark sesame oil; 2
tablespoons of soy sauce; 2 teaspoons of sugar; 1 teaspoon of red
pepper flakes, 2 tablespoons of chopped scallions; and ¼ cup dry
sherry. Bring to a boil, cover, and steam, as in the previous recipe,
until the broccoli is just crunchy-tender. Uncover to evaporate most
of the liquid and toss broccoli well in the black bean sauce before
serving (over rice, if you wish).

Of course, there is a caution about supermarket produce: it may be
contaminated with toxins, put there not by nature but by agribusiness.
I discuss this subject in detail in the next chapter and will tell you how
to protect yourself. It is important to try to find chemical-free produce
and to know which crops are the most likely to be contaminated.

FIBER

Fiber is the indigestible residue in plants that we eat, made up of carbohydrates too complex chemically for our digestive systems. Adequate fiber in the diet promotes digestive health, allowing us to have
regular bowel movements and improving the biochemical environment of the large bowel. Some forms of fiber also benefit the cardiovascular system by helping the body eliminate cholesterol.
Populations that have very low intakes of fiber have high rates of
colon cancer and vice-versa. If you do not eat enough fiber, your
digestive system will not function at peak efficiency, which can compromise healing ability in several ways.

The main sources of dietary fiber are fruits, vegetables, and whole
grains. Insoluble fiber, such as in wheat bran, is an important bowel
regulator. Soluble fiber, such as in oat bran, helps eliminate cholesterol. Some people who require fiber to regulate the bowels take it in
supplementary form as bran or psyllium (a seed with a fibrous husk).
I think it is easier to eat more fruits and vegetables, whole grains, and
cereals and breads made from whole grains, which may have other
benefits as well.

.   .   .

HERE IS A BRIEF summary of my recommendations for a healing diet:

- *Try to eat fewer calories* by eliminating high-fat foods and modifying recipes for favorite dishes by cutting fat content. Also experiment with periodic fasting or restricted dieting.
- *Cut down appreciably on saturated fat* by eating fewer foods of animal origin and none containing palm or coconut oils, margarine, vegetable shortening, or partially hydrogenated oils.
- *Do not use polyunsaturated vegetable oils for cooking. Use only good-quality olive oil.*
- *Learn to recognize and avoid sources of trans-fatty acids* (margarine, vegetable shortening, partially hydrogenated oils, and common brands of liquid vegetable oils).
- *Increase consumption of omega-3 fatty acids* by eating more of the right kinds of fish or adding hemp oil or flax products to the diet.
- *Eat less protein of all kinds.*
- *Try to replace animal protein foods with fish and soyfoods.*
- *Eat more fruits and vegetables of all kinds.*
- *Eat more whole grains and products made from whole grains.*

These recommendations are practical, sensible, and probably familiar to you. They are also important enough to repeat because they are the bare essentials of a healthy diet. They do not require you to become a food faddist or to give up everything you like. And, based on my knowledge and experience, I can assure you that they will help your healing system work more efficiently.

10

PROTECTING YOURSELF
FROM TOXINS

SPONTANEOUS HEALING DEPENDS on the unobstructed, efficient operation of all components of the healing system. If any of those components are injured or preoccupied with other tasks, the process of healing will be impaired. One of the greatest threats to the system is toxic overload from the multitude of harmful substances in today's environment. The word "toxin" comes from the Greek word for "bow," as in "bow and arrow." Untold numbers of poisoned arrows must have pierced the bodies of Greek warriors for the word to take on its present meaning, and images of war are not inappropriate to this discussion, for in a sense our bodies are under attack.

Medical scientists, especially those in the employ of government and industry, have been very slow to recognize the threat to public health posed by toxic residues; instead they often downplay it. The following quotation from a review article on organic food that appeared in a journal of food science and nutrition is typical of the official response to consumer fears about toxic chemicals used on produce.

The substitution of "organic" for "chemical" fertilizers during the growth of plants produces no change in the nutritional or chemical properties of foods. All foods are made of "chemicals." Traces of pesticides have been reported to be present in about 20 to 30% of both "organic" and conventional foods. These traces are usually within the official tolerance levels. Such levels are set low enough to protect consumers adequately. Indeed, there is no record of a single case of injury to a consumer resulting from the application of pesticides to food crops at permitted levels.

Not long ago a full-page color advertisement for a leading manufacturer of agricultural chemicals appeared in national magazines, showing an orange with a long label affixed to it; printed on the label were hundreds of names of chemical compounds. The caption read, "Mother Nature Is Lucky—She Doesn't Have to Label Her Products," and the text of the ad went on to inform us that since all fruits and vegetables are composed of myriad chemicals, there is no reason to worry about the addition of a few more. Recently, a more insidious argument has begun to circulate: namely, that natural toxins—contained in many crops—pose a greater threat to health than manmade ones.

Proponents of these arguments assume that the main concern is "injury," some immediately identifiable, acute response to the ingestion of pesticides. In fact, such cases do occur:

Aldicarb in watermelon, 1985. Aldicarb is an extremely toxic systemic carbamate pesticide. Its illegal use on watermelon led to the largest reported North American epidemic of food-borne pesticide poisoning. Active surveillance ascertained reports of 638 probable cases and 344 possible cases. Another 333 probable and 149 possible cases were reported from other western states and provinces of Canada. Illness ranged from mild gastrointestinal upset to severe cholinergic poisoning [an effect similar to that of nerve gas]. Levels in the melons that caused illness ranged from 0.07 to 3 ppm [parts per million] of aldicarb sulfoxide. The epidemic ceased after melons in distribution chains were destroyed, an embargo was imposed, and an inspection program was instituted.

But my concern about pesticides and other environmental toxins has not so much to do with the possibility of acute injury as with long-term compromise of the healing system and increased risks of cancer, immune dysfunction, and a variety of chronic ailments (like Parkinson's disease) in which cause-and-effect relationships with toxins have not been adequately investigated. Such effects could result from cumulative exposure over time to toxins from various sources.

And of course it is nonsense to say that the existence of harmful compounds in nature in any way excuses adding more of them to the environment. It is true that black pepper, basil, tarragon, alfalfa sprouts, celery, peanuts, potatoes, tomatoes, and white button mushrooms contain naturally occurring toxic compounds, but our bodies have evolved along with those species and probably have a better ability to defend against any injurious agents they contain. Moreover, if our healing system is already occupied with the neutralization of natural toxins, it will have a reduced ability to deal with an added load of artificial ones. Similarly, certain locations on earth have high background radiation due to high altitude or emissions of radioactivity by surface rocks, but this does not mean we should be complacent about exposure to X-rays or to nuclear waste. Cancer risks from radiation correlate with cumulative totals over a lifetime; the harmful effects of exposure to manmade radiation added to those received from natural sources can easily overwhelm the body's defensive capabilities.

In short, do not believe people who try to allay your concerns about toxic exposures. This is a real threat, and you must learn to take protective measures. Your body's ability to eliminate unwanted substances depends on the healthy functioning of four systems: the urinary system, the gastrointestinal system, the respiratory system, and the skin; it can discharge wastes through urine, feces, exhaled air, and sweat. The liver processes most foreign chemical compounds, detoxifying them if possible or breaking them down to simpler compounds that can leave the body by one of those four routes. In order to maintain your eliminative capacity, those four systems must be in good working order. You can ensure they are by drinking enough pure water to help the kidneys maintain a good output of urine, by eating enough fiber to ensure regular bowel function, by exercising your respiratory system regularly, and by periodically increasing output of sweat through aerobic exercise or exposure to heat (as by taking saunas or steam baths).

Some people sustain most of their exposure to toxins in the workplace. If you work in a chemically hazardous occupation (such as the manufacture of plastics, rubber, leather, textiles, dyes, poisons, or paper, or in a mine or dry-cleaning facility, or on a farm that uses agrichemicals), you should inform yourself about the dangers of products you come in contact with (by contacting the Environmental Protection Agency or consumer groups concerned with environmental toxins, for example) and take all precautions to minimize exposure. The rest of us are most likely to contact toxins in the air we breathe, the water we drink, and the food we eat, as well as from a few other sources. Let me review those sources, giving suggestions for self-defense.

AIR POLLUTION

Truly clean air has become a rarity as the twentieth century ends. Even in the Arctic, haze from industrial pollution now darkens the atmosphere, and many of us have had the experience of watching air quality deteriorate in places we have lived in over time. When I was working as a medical intern in San Francisco in 1968–69, I never saw smog in that city. From my apartment on a hill, I could see smog over Oakland, across the bay, where it was held by prevailing westerly winds. Ten years later, pollution increased to a point where it overwhelmed the atmosphere of the whole region, and today heavy smog in San Francisco is a common occurrence. In some locations, pollution is so much the rule that people's standards of air quality have changed: I was recently in Los Angeles on a day following high winds when pollution was low and heard radio commentators describe conditions as "smog free."

Some air pollution does come from volcanoes, forest fires, and dust storms, but to that background human activity has added an immense amount of industrial waste and automobile exhaust. Many of the compounds in smog are irritating to the respiratory tract; I have no doubt that worsening air pollution is the major cause of worldwide increases in asthma and bronchitis as well as a contributing cause to the rising incidence of chronic sinusitis, respiratory allergies, emphysema, and lung cancer. Some components of smog are known to be carcinogenic, while others probably damage cell membranes and other structures that make up the body's healing system. Researchers are also busily documenting the health hazards of secondhand tobacco smoke, which is a major problem in offices, shops, trains, planes, and restaurants.

It is much harder to protect yourself from pollutants in the air than from contaminated food and water. If you live in a city that is subject to bad smog, moving elsewhere may seem too drastic a remedy; however, you might consider moving to a less polluted district of your city, as there are usually microclimatic variations in any region that cause smog to concentrate more in some areas than others. In the most polluted cities of the world—Mexico City being the worst example—it is not uncommon for people to experience chest pain and breathing difficulty on bad days and for city governments to cancel school and issue warnings to keep very young and very old people indoors. If this is a preview of the future of our cities, it is a most unsettling one; but even if you live in a city with dirty air, you can protect yourself significantly by paying frequent visits to parks and groves of trees. Trees have a marvelous capacity to purify air; you can sense it even in the middle of the worst urban sprawls. When I visit Japan, which I do frequently, I usually have to spend a few days in Tokyo; I always seek refuge in the Meiji Shrine, a forested oasis in a desert of steel and concrete. Within a few moments of stepping inside the great *torii,* the wooden gates that mark the boundary of sacred space, I notice a change in the air: it feels purer, healthier, more breathable, and even an hour's walk within the park recharges me and enables me to cope with Tokyo's irritating smog. Remember this strategy if you find yourself caught in a city at a time of bad pollution: seek out parks and trees.

Indoors, you should make every effort to remove sources of pollution, such as all chemical products that give off volatile fumes; move them outside. Gas appliances, like stoves and water heaters, can contribute to indoor air pollution (newer gas stoves have automatic sparkers that eliminate pilot lights and reduce this threat), as can aerosol sprays. The medical profession increasingly recognizes environmental illness, such as "tight building syndrome" or "sick building syndrome," in which persons working in sealed buildings with recirculated air suffer a variety of symptoms that may be due to inhaled toxins. A common culprit is new carpet; chemicals used in carpet adhesives may trigger immune depression in some sensitive people. Commercial airliners also provide unhealthy indoor environments, especially now that companies are adding less fresh air to cabins in an effort to conserve fuel (and most international flights still permit smoking).

You can protect yourself from particulate air pollution with filters installed in your home's ventilation system or placed in whatever room of your house you spend the most time in. High-efficiency particulate air (HEPA) filters are readily available and reasonably priced;

you can get information on them from heating and ventilation contractors. Because they can do wonders for people with respiratory ailments, I recommend them frequently to patients. You should definitely get one if you live in a heavily polluted area or are forced to live or work with people who smoke.

You can also help your body neutralize inhaled pollutants by taking protective antioxidants, nutrients that protect tissues by blocking the chemical reactions by which many toxins cause harm. Increasing consumption of fresh fruits and vegetables is the simplest way to go about this. You can also take antioxidants in supplement form, the most effective and safest ones being vitamin C, vitamin E, selenium, and beta carotene.

Here is a simple daily antioxidant formula that I use and recommend to my patients:

Take between 1,000 and 2,000 milligrams of vitamin C two or three times a day. Your body may absorb this vitamin more easily in a soluble powder form rather than as a large, compressed tablet. I take a dose of vitamin C with breakfast, another with dinner, and, if I remember, a third before bed. I know it is more difficult to take anything three times a day rather than twice, so I do not insist on the bedtime dose, but I do urge you to take vitamin C more than once a day. (If you take it only twice, use the higher dose.) Plain ascorbic acid may irritate a sensitive stomach, so you should take it with food or look for a buffered or nonacidic form. If you experience flatulence or loose stools, take less; people vary greatly in their bowel tolerance to vitamin C. Eating plenty of fresh fruits and vegetables will satisfy your basic requirement for this important vitamin; however, larger amounts will give added protection against toxic overloads, and since ascorbic acid is itself nontoxic, there is every reason to supplement the diet with it. For people who cannot eat ample amounts of fresh fruits and vegetables, supplemental vitamin C is essential.

Vitamin E is a second powerful, nontoxic antioxidant. Although it is naturally present in grains and seeds, it is impossible to get large enough amounts from dietary sources to give the kind of protection needed against the toxins we breathe and take into our bodies in other ways. People under forty should take 400 international units (IU) of vitamin E a day; people over forty, 800 IU. Since vitamin E is fat-soluble, it must be taken with a meal to be absorbed. Also, natural vitamin E (d-alpha-tocopherol) is much better than synthetic (dl-alpha-tocopherol), especially when it is combined with the other tocopherols normally present in plant sources. You can easily find natural vitamin E with mixed tocopherols in health food stores. I usually take this supplement with lunch.

Selenium is a trace mineral with antioxidant and anticancer properties. Selenium and vitamin E facilitate each other's absorption, so the two should be taken together, whereas vitamin C may interfere with the absorption of some forms of selenium and should be taken separately. (This is a problem with many antioxidant formulas I see in drug and health food stores; they combine selenium with vitamins C and E in the same capsule.) I used to recommend daily doses of 50–100 micrograms of selenium, but ongoing research on its cancer-protective value suggests that higher doses are more effective. I now recommend 200–300 micrograms of selenium a day, the higher amount for those with any increased cancer risks. Doses above 400 micrograms a day may not be healthy. You can buy selenium supplements in any drugstore. I take mine with vitamin E at lunchtime.

I mentioned beta carotene in the previous chapter with regard to possible differences between consuming protective nutrients in the form of whole foods and taking them as isolated supplements. I hope that we will soon be able to buy supplements of mixed natural carotenes, as these would probably work much better than isolated beta carotene. In the meantime, try to add yellow and orange fruits and vegetables, tomatoes, and dark, leafy greens to your diet. I also take 25,000 IU of beta carotene as a supplement with my breakfast. I recommend a natural form, such as that obtained from marine algae, over synthetic forms; you will probably most easily find it in a health food store.

In summary, then, here is a simple formula that will not cost you too much trouble or money and will definitely help your body neutralize the harmful effects of toxins, however you ingest them.

At breakfast: Take 1,000–2,000 milligrams of vitamin C and 25,000 IU of natural beta carotene.

At lunch: Take 400–800 IU of natural vitamin E and 200–300 micrograms of selenium.

At dinner: Take 1,000–2,000 milligrams of vitamin C.

At bedtime (if convenient): Take another 1,000–2,000 milligrams of vitamin C.

CONTAMINATED WATER

We have much greater control over the water we drink than over the air we breathe; bottled water is available everywhere, as are inexpensive water filters for the home. Public health agencies concentrate on disinfecting water to protect us from infectious diseases; they largely ignore the problem of toxic contaminants, one of which is the very chlorine commonly used for disinfection. Toxins get into drinking water from many sources, including waste runoffs from industry, acid rain, leaching of agricultural chemicals into water tables, and the dissolution of metals and plastics from pipes. It is important to know where your drinking water comes from and what it might contain. You can have water tested to get this information, but will probably have to take samples to a private lab, because government laboratories will only test for bacterial content and a few of the major inorganic toxins like lead and arsenic.

Bottled water may or may not be an improvement over tap water, depending on where it comes from and how it is handled. If you are going to buy bottled water, ask to see an analysis of it, and do not use any brands that do not taste delicious. Only buy bottled water in glass or hard (clear) plastic containers; soft (translucent) plastic bottles commonly give the water an off taste that represents dissolved plastic.

Filtering water is much more economical than buying bottled water, because you can install a filtration system for a reasonable price. The best, by far, is steam distillation, but home distillers are expensive and use power. The next-best system is reverse osmosis, in which water is forced through a semipermeable membrane that acts as a barrier to contaminant molecules. Reverse osmosis systems are one-fifth the cost of distillers; they remove more foreign substances from drinking water than activated carbon filters, but they require adequate water pressure and produce a fair amount of waste water. They can be installed under the sink or on the countertop. When shopping for a reverse osmosis system, find out how often the filters must be changed and how convenient and costly it will be to change them.

Activated carbon filters remove unpleasant odors, colors, and tastes from drinking water but not dissolved minerals. They are convenient for the elimination of chlorine, which I believe to be a major health hazard. As a strong oxidizing agent, chlorine is highly reactive, tending to combine with organic contaminants in water to form carcinogens. Chlorine in drinking water may also contribute to heart disease and long-term damage to components of the healing system. Try to avoid drinking water that has an obvious taste of chlorine. You can buy inexpensive, portable carbon filters to take with you when you travel. I use them in hotels and restaurants to filter chlorinated water by the glass.

My advice about drinking water is simple and concise:

- *Inform yourself about the source of your drinking water* and what contaminants it might contain.

- *Install a reverse osmosis filtration system in your kitchen.*

- *If you use bottled water,* buy only brands in glass or clear plastic containers from bottlers who are able to provide an analysis or certification of purity.

- *Do not drink water that tastes of chlorine.* When you travel, order bottled water or take a portable carbon filter with you.

You should not become paranoid about contaminated water, but you should exercise sensible precautions. Remember also that by eating fruits and vegetables, taking antioxidant supplements, and keeping your body's systems of elimination in good working order, you will be able to neutralize or discharge toxins you do consume.

TOXINS IN FOOD

Obtaining food that is free of toxic contamination is much more difficult than obtaining pure water—an indictment of our agricultural practices. Again, I do not want you to become unreasonably fearful. Eating is a major source of pleasure in life and should be indulged in without anxiety. But I do want you to be informed about real hazards and know what steps you can take to protect yourself.

I will repeat my warning in the previous chapter that eating high on the food chain exposes you to greater risk of concentrated doses of environmental toxins. If you eat meat or poultry, shop for brands certified to be free of added drugs and hormones. If you eat fish, try to avoid very large, carnivorous species (swordfish, marlin) and species that live mostly near coastal effluents (like shellfish). Here is one aspect of the problem:

DDT in fish, 1985. The findings on DDT in ocean fish in southern California are an example of the long-term implications of using persistent pesticides. For several years, a local DDT manufacturer had used the sanitary sewer for discharge of some of its industrial waste which contained DDT. A few million pounds of DDT were deposited on the ocean bottom around the sewage outfall. This waste discharge was halted many years ago but recent analyses of fish from this area have shown elevated levels of DDT (to over 1 ppm) in the edible flesh. In addition, some DDT was also dumped into the ocean by use of ocean dumping barges but the exact location is not known. Evidence indicates that the DDT levels are decreasing over time, but the levels found raise a health concern because DDT is considered a potential human carcinogen. The FDA [Food and Drug Administration] action level of 5 ppm for DDT in fish was set long ago and did not consider the carcinogenic risk associated with DDT exposure.

When you eat lower on the food chain, you minimize these risks but still have to worry about toxins in produce. I have already referred to the naturally occurring toxins. The best defense against this class of compounds is to cut consumption of foods with the highest content (black pepper, peanuts, celery, alfalfa sprouts, for example) while eating a highly varied diet. Eating a varied diet offers two advantages. It ensures that you will get all of the nutrients that you need, and it reduces the risk of getting too much of any unhealthy elements.

Manmade toxins are another matter. Fruits and vegetables are treated with a great variety of agrichemicals: pesticides, fungicides, ripening agents, fumigants, and so forth, all within regulated guidelines for "acceptable" levels of residues. Many of these chemicals cannot be removed by washing, because they adhere tightly to vegetable tissue or because they are applied in ways that carry them inside the products. I cannot emphasize too strongly that residues of toxic chemicals in foods we eat are major health hazards, affecting us in ways that current medical science and governmental policy often fail to recognize. Let me recount two stories that illustrate my concern.

During my travels to Japan I have been struck by the very high incidence there of atopic dermatitis—eczema. As many as fifty percent of Japanese babies are afflicted with this disease, and cases among adolescents and young adults are much more severe and extensive than in this country. Eczema is a discomforting and disfiguring disease, both physically and emotionally, since it produces itching and red skin eruptions, often on the face and hands. In Japan I commonly see patients with eczema over most of their bodies. Conventional medical treatment is inadequate, to say the least, since it relies on topical and systemic corticosteroids to suppress the dermatitis without curing it, and patients become dependent on this medication with all of its associated toxicity. The epidemic of atopic dermatitis in Japan is a recent phenomenon. What has changed in the Japanese population that might account for it? Not genetics, certainly. Eczema has an inherited component—it often runs in families—but no significant genetic change can have occurred among Japanese in the past fifty years. What has changed is diet. Japanese now eat much more meat and many more dairy products than they did in the past. These animal-protein foods may directly irritate the immune system, creating a predisposition to allergic reactions like eczema. They also contain more added toxins than the plant and fish-based foods of the traditional Japanese diet. In addition, the use of agrichemicals and additives to processed foods has increased enormously in postwar Japan. A Japanese friend who is an internist has seen dramatic cures of eczema in people who switch to organic foods; she reports that some of her patients are eventually able to discontinue steroid treatment. To me this suggests that allergy, as well as other sorts of immune dysfunction, may be one consequence of toxic overload produced by eating chemically contaminated food.

A young woman patient of mine who suffers from severe asthma, chronic sinusitis, and multiple inhalant and food allergies has also found that chemical-free food makes a great difference. She is so sensitive and so aware of her body's reactions that she can often tell within hours of a meal which foods cause her respiratory difficulty and which do not. She has learned that buying organically produced fruits and vegetables is necessary for her health.

Because organic fruits and vegetables are more expensive and not as easily available as conventional produce, it is worth knowing the crops that are most likely to contain residues of harmful compounds. For example, by any standards of measurement, apples top the list of most contaminated foods; knowing that, I no longer buy them unless they come from certified organic producers. The next-most-hazardous fruit crops are peaches, grapes (and raisins and wine made from them), oranges, and strawberries. Most heavily contaminated vegetable crops include potatoes, carrots, lettuce, green beans, peanuts, and wheat. I strongly advise you to seek out certified organic versions of these foods and products made from them (including products made from wheat flour).

The good news is that the organic agriculture movement is flourishing, entirely the result of rapid growth of markets for organic produce as consumers become more knowledgeable about toxins in food. Not long ago, agricultural experts insisted it was not feasible to use organic methods on a commercial scale; you could do it in home gardens, they maintained, but not on large farms. Now, inspired by market demand, producers can grow fruits and vegetables organically on any scale; moreover, they can do so more profitably than they ever imagined, both because they do not have to buy expensive agrichemicals and also because certified organic produce commands higher prices. Fully half of the producers in California have now converted or are in the process of converting to organic methods, a boon to consumers as well as to the earth. It will be easier to find organic produce in ordinary stores in the near future, and the cost will be more competitive. This is a consumer-driven trend; you can help accelerate it by letting store managers know what you want.

Additives used in processed foods comprise another category of toxins. Two kinds that I recommend avoiding are chemical dyes (identified on labels as "certified color," "artificial color," or by a specific name like "red no. 3") and artificial sweeteners, including saccharin and aspartame. In general, processed foods contain more fat and more salt than you might otherwise eat, as well as a host of preservatives, flavor enhancers, and other additives that may interfere with spontaneous healing. Therefore, it is wise to reduce the percentage of processed foods in your diet and to choose only products made without artificial additives.

In summary, here are my suggestions for minimizing exposure to toxins in foods:

- *Reduce consumption of animal products and buy only meat and poultry certified to be free of drugs and hormones.*
- *Minimize consumption of foods known to contain natural toxins,* such as black pepper, celery, alfalfa sprouts, peanuts, and white button mushrooms.
- *Eat a varied diet* rather than eating the same items every day.
- *Always wash fruits and vegetables* (even though that will not remove many contaminants).
- *Peel fruits and vegetables if possible,* especially if they are not organically produced.
- *Try to buy only organically produced* apples, peaches, grapes, raisins, oranges, strawberries, lettuce, celery, carrots, green beans, potatoes, and wheat flour.
- *Look for sources of organic produce, join cooperatives and buying clubs that distribute it, and let store managers know that you want it.*
- *Reduce consumption of processed foods and try to avoid those containing chemical dyes and artificial sweeteners.*

DRUGS, COSMETICS, AND OTHER SOURCES OF TOXINS

I consider drug toxicity to be a subcategory of chemical pollution. People take drugs for medical reasons and for social/recreational reasons, obtaining them on prescription, over the counter, or illegally. It is important to understand that no fundamental difference exists between drugs and poisons except dosage. All drugs become toxic in high enough dosage, and some poisons become useful drugs in low enough dosage. I have no objection to the use of medical drugs when they are the best treatments for diseases, but I also encourage both doctors and patients to explore alternative treatments that reduce or eliminate the possibility of drug toxicity, which is the most common sin of commission of conventional medicine today. Herbal medicines are dilute forms of natural drugs. Being dilute, they deliver lower doses of potential toxins but still should not be consumed thoughtlessly or without good reason. In whatever form and for whatever reason you take drugs, you are increasing the workload on your liver, since it is the task of the liver to metabolize most foreign substances. You can help your liver deal with other toxins by not also burdening it with drugs.

Of the recreational drugs in use in our society, alcohol and tobacco are the most toxic. Alcohol is directly toxic to liver and nerve cells; it is also a strong irritant of the lining of the upper digestive tract. It has beneficial effects as well, particularly as a relaxant (and promoter of social interchange), as a tonic to the cardiovascular system, and as a stimulant to production of HDL (good) cholesterol. Assessment of the influence of alcohol on health must, therefore, involve a risk-benefit analysis of the patterns of use of each individual. In persons with healthy livers, stomachs, and nervous systems, *moderate* consumption of alcohol may promote health and healing. In those with ailing organs, even moderate drinking may be harmful, and heavy consumption for anyone may be incompatible with optimal health.

The case of tobacco is less equivocal. Although tobacco may facilitate concentration and relaxation, nicotine is highly addictive, especially when inhaled deeply; it is also a very strong stimulant that constricts arteries throughout the body, interfering with blood circulation and thus with healing. In addition, addiction to nicotine exposes the user to the harmful effects of other elements of tobacco smoke, including many carcinogenic compounds. Inhaling smoke compromises respiration, which, as I have noted, is one of the main functional components of the healing system. If you are one of the lucky few who can use tobacco nonaddictively, I will not try to argue you out of it, as long as you do not expose me to your secondhand smoke. Otherwise, I urge you to make all possible efforts to quit.

Medical drugs, in addition to their main constituents, are often dyed with the same synthetics used to color food. If you consume a substantial quantity of brightly colored pills and capsules, they can be a significant source of those chemicals that cannot do you any good; here is another reason to look for alternative treatments. Another source, less commonly thought of, is cosmetics, especially shampoos, hair conditioners, and lotions that can be absorbed through the skin. I recommend avoiding all cosmetic products containing chemical dyes (read labels!); it is not that difficult to find brands that are colorless, white, or tinted with vegetable extracts, although you may have to shop for them in salons or health food stores.

Poisons of all sorts, especially pesticides and herbicides, are among the most hazardous toxins in the environment. Try not to handle these materials, do not keep them in the home, and try not to use them in or around your home. Be equally cautious about all dyes, solvents, and other chemical products that give off fumes and have strong odors. If you are exposed to any of these substances, wash yourself well, breathe plenty of fresh air, drink lots of water, sit in a sauna or steam bath, and don't forget to take your antioxidants!

TOXIC FORMS OF ENERGY

It is clear that life evolved on earth in spite of certain frequencies of radiation that can damage DNA. To the natural radiation that bombards us from outer space, from the sun, and from the earth itself, human activity has added a great deal of electromagnetic pollution whose long-term biological effects are not well understood. Despite the lack of information, it is worth taking sensible precautions.

One end of the electromagnetic spectrum includes short-wavelength (high-energy) forms of radiation, such as nuclear energy and X-rays, that can knock electrons out of their orbits around atomic nuclei, creating charged particles (ions). The dangers of ionizing radiation are well known: it can kill in high dosage and by causing mutations in DNA promotes damage to the immune system and the development of cancers that may not manifest themselves until years after exposure. You can protect yourself from ionizing radiation by not working in an occupation that exposes you to it (uranium mining, nuclear power plant maintenance, radiology); by not living near a source of it, either natural or manmade (such as a nuclear waste disposal site); and by not letting doctors and dentists X-ray you without good reason. Remember that there is no such thing as a safe dose of ionizing radiation, since every bit adds to the cumulative total you receive over your lifetime, and it is that cumulative total that correlates with damage to DNA. Another reason to eat fruits and vegetables and take antioxidant supplements is that they can block chemical reactions that mediate radiation injury to genes.

Ultraviolet (UV) radiation from the sun is not ionizing; its waves are longer and less energetic, just beyond the highest-energy (violet) form of electromagnetic energy that we can see as visible light. Still, UV radiation is powerful enough to damage DNA in skin cells, making it the major cause of skin cancer, the incidence of which is increasing at an alarming rate. One possible reason for the increase is weakening of the earth's protective ozone layer as a result of atmospheric pollution so that the intensity of solar radiation reaching the surface of the earth is greater now than in the recent past. This is all the more reason to protect yourself by staying out of the sun when it is at a high angle in the sky, by wearing protective clothing, using sunscreens, and not making the mistake of going to tanning parlors in the belief that they offer just the "healthful tanning variety of UV." *All* UV radiation is harmful; in addition to hurting the skin, it promotes the development of cataracts and macular degeneration, two common causes of loss of vision in older people. You can protect yourself from this hazard by wearing UV-protective eyeglasses when you are in the sun and by taking antioxidants.

Beyond the other (red) side of the visible light spectrum are still-longer wave forms such as microwave and ELF (extremely low frequency) radiation, much used for military communications. Microwaves can agitate molecules of plant and animal tissue, generating heat, which is the basis for their use in microwave ovens; but aside from the danger of being cooked if you stand in the path of a concentrated beam, microwave and ELF radiation have not been considered biologically hazardous. Now that view is changing, with a number of scientists warning that these forms of energy can disrupt delicate biological control systems involving small electrical currents and weak electrical fields. Earlier, I described the role of these systems in the healing of wounds and bone fractures (see page 80); they may be the basis of most forms of complex healing of tissues and organs.

Microwave ovens are not a problem, because they rarely leak radiation unless they are obviously damaged. (They can, however, alter the chemistry of protein-containing foods cooked in them for a long time and can also drive foreign molecules into food wrapped in plastic or cooked in plastic containers. Never microwave food in other than glass or ceramic containers, and never cover it with plastic wrap during cooking. Use these convenient appliances for rapid defrosting and heating of food rather than for long cooking of main dishes.) But it may be unhealthy to live near a microwave transmitter or in the path of military communications hardware.

In the home, a number of familiar appliances create electromagnetic hazards that may also interfere with healing. Electric blankets and heating pads are best avoided, since they generate large electrical fields and are used right next to the body. Electric clock radios are dangerous for the same reason. Do not keep one near your head while you sleep. If you work in front of a computer video display terminal, it is worth investing in a screen that eliminates any electromagnetic transmissions and fields; these are available from computer supply dealers.

IF ALL THIS SOUNDS discouraging, I am afraid it is also realistic. Toxins, both chemical and energetic, are more and more a fact of life in our industrial world, and you must know their dangers. My suggestions for self-defense are reasonable and practical; even if you implement only some of them, you will be protecting your healing system from harm. Fortunately, nature provides us with products that can strengthen our healing abilities and make our bodies more resilient and resistant. I discuss this more cheerful subject in the next chapter.

11

USING TONICS

ANYTHING THAT INCREASES the efficiency of the healing system or helps it neutralize harmful influences will increase the probability of spontaneous healing. Tonics are natural products that do just this, and they are one of my special interests. In the sense of a strengthening or invigorating medicine, the word "tonic" derives from a Greek word meaning "stretch." Tonics stretch or tone our systems in the way physical exercise tones our muscles. Working the body—subjecting it to graduated tension followed by relaxation—increases natural resilience, an essential quality of health, because it determines our responsiveness to environmental stress. The more resilient we are, the greater our ability to bounce back from any kind of stress or injury.

Tonic medicines are now in very low repute among most practitioners of conventional Western medicine. They conjure up images of snake-oil salesmen hawking nostrums from painted wagons, and antique posters advertising patent liquids containing opium and alcohol. Today's doctors prefer magic bullets—drugs that exert specific effects in specific diseases by known biochemical mechanisms. They do not like panaceas—remedies with very general effects, said to be good for whatever ails you, whose mechanisms of action are at best obscure. Attitudes are very different among practitioners of traditional medicine in the East, where tonics are held in high esteem and both doctors and patients are willing to pay large sums for natural products believed to augment internal resilience and resistance.

An outstanding example of such a product is ginseng, obtained from species in the genus *Panax,* whose name comes from the same root as "panacea," that is, "all-heal." (Panacea, incidentally, was another daughter of Asklepios, the god of medicine in Greek mythology.) Demand for ginseng has always greatly exceeded supply, with the result that many adulterated and imitation products are on the market while prices for the best qualities of authentic material are sensationally high. Many Asians esteem ginseng as an invigorating tonic; some say it should be reserved for old age. Used regularly, it increases energy, vitality, and sexual vigor, improves skin and muscle tone, and confers resistance to stress of all sorts. Since it is generally nontoxic, it meets all the requirements of a useful tonic. I often recommend it to chronically ill patients and to those who are debilitated or lacking in vitality.

I also use and recommend a number of other tonics, some of them more familiar than others. I will describe those I recommend most frequently, having selected them for effectiveness, safety, and availability. Even if you are not chronically ill, debilitated, or lacking in vitality, you might want to experiment with this interesting category of natural remedies. They cannot hurt you, and given the threat of environmental toxicity from so many different sources, it is worth knowing about substances that can enhance immunity and resistance, functions central to the efficient operation of the healing system. I begin with the familiar ones and move on to the exotics.

GARLIC

Garlic (*Allium cepa*), the most pungent member of the onion family, is a central flavoring ingredient in many of the world's cuisines. It is equally esteemed as a medicinal plant in many cultures, and recent research has documented some of the healing properties attributed to it in folk medicine. Garlic is a rich source of sulfur-containing compounds with biological activity; although a number of controlled experiments demonstrate the plant's health benefits, it is not yet known just which compounds are responsible. The effects of garlic are numerous and varied, affecting many systems of the body that participate in healing; in my view the breadth of garlic's actions justifies categorizing it as a true tonic.

Some of its most dramatic effects are on the cardiovascular system. It lowers blood pressure by more than one mechanism, mimicking some of the newest antihypertensive drugs without their tendency to cause impotence, headaches, and other toxic effects. I have known people who have controlled moderate hypertension just by eating garlic every day. In addition, garlic lowers cholesterol and blood fats (triglycerides) while increasing the protective (HDL) fraction of total cholesterol and reducing the susceptibility of LDL cholesterol to oxidize. (Oxidation of LDL cholesterol is the first step in the process by which it damages arterial walls.) Finally, garlic reduces the clotting tendency of the blood by inhibiting the readiness of platelets to aggregate—i.e., to clump together. Platelet aggregation on roughened walls of arteries damaged by atherosclerosis commonly initiates the formation of blood clots that lead to heart attacks and strokes. For all of these reasons garlic appears to offer significant protection from cardiovascular disease. (Epidemiologists think that its routine consumption in parts of Spain and Italy may contribute to lower-than-expected incidence of atherosclerotic disease in those regions.)

In unrelated activity, garlic also acts as a powerful antiseptic and antibiotic, counteracting the growth of many kinds of bacteria and fungi that cause disease in humans. Furthermore, it enhances activity of the immune system, increasing numbers of natural killer cells that check the spread of cancers. Several studies show garlic to be an anticancer agent, again suggesting several different mechanisms. In addition to stimulating immune activity, it appears to block the formation of some carcinogens in the gut and protect DNA from damage by other carcinogens. Miscellaneous effects of garlic include protecting liver and brain cells from degenerative changes (probably as a result of its content of antioxidant compounds) and lowering blood sugar.

You can get all of these benefits simply by adding garlic to your food in any form. You can also buy a variety of garlic supplements: oil-filled capsules, capsules of "deodorized" oil, or tablets. Although the safety of garlic as a culinary herb is clear, we have no data on the safety of long-term use of concentrated extracts. One caution is that they might lead to bleeding problems in persons being treated with anticoagulant drugs, including aspirin. The effectiveness of garlic supplements is also unknown; manufacturers make many claims and try to disparage competing products, but we really do not even know how many of garlic's health benefits depend on its odoriferous constituents, so it is difficult to say whether the deodorized products work well or not.

My personal recommendation is to eat more fresh garlic. Mash it raw into salad dressing, cook it lightly in olive oil to flavor pasta, and, in general, add it near the end of cooking to enjoy its flavor. I grow garlic in my garden, planting individual cloves in September and harvesting big bulbs in May that keep for many months. I cannot imagine life without garlic and consider it one of the best general tonics for the healing system.

GINGER

Like garlic, ginger (*Zingiber officinale*) is a familiar culinary spice that has long enjoyed a strong reputation as a medicinal plant. (The specific epithet *officinale* in a botanical name indicates the plant's official status in medicine of the past.) From ancient times doctors in both China and India regarded it as a superior medicine, adding it to combination remedies for its tonifying and spiritually uplifting properties. Today people in many different parts of the world value it for its warming effect and ability to stimulate digestion, settle upset stomachs, and relieve aches and pains. In recent years a great deal of medical research, much of it in Japan and Europe, has documented remarkable therapeutic effects of ginger and its components; American doctors tend to be unaware of these studies. The chemistry of ginger is quite complex, with more than four hundred compounds known to contribute to the plant's fragrance, taste, and biological activity. Much of the focus of research has been on two groups of these—gingerols and shogaols—that give ginger its pungent taste. In addition, the "root" (actually a rhizome) contains enzymes and antioxidants that are probably also key components.

The tonic effects of ginger on the digestive system are clear: it improves the digestion of proteins, is an effective treatment for nausea and motion sickness, strengthens the mucosal lining of the upper GI tract in a way that protects against formation of ulcers, and has a wide range of action against intestinal parasites. Chinese cooks use fresh ginger in most dishes because they believe it neutralizes undesirable qualities of other ingredients, especially fish and meat, that might produce indigestion.

Other well-studied actions of ginger affect the production and deployment of a group of biological response moderators called eicosanoids, which mediate healing and immunity. The body synthesizes these important compounds from essential fatty acids and uses them to regulate critical cellular functions. Three principal categories of eicosanoids—prostaglandins, thromboxanes, and leukotrienes—are much in the news as subjects of ongoing research. Imbalances in eicosanoid synthesis and release underlie many common illnesses, from arthritis and peptic ulcer to the increased platelet aggregation that can trigger heart attacks and strokes. Ginger modulates this system in ways that reduce abnormal inflammation and clotting. It may be as effective as some of the nonsteroidal anti-inflammatory drugs that are now so popular, but much less toxic because it protects the lining of the stomach instead of damaging it. It is as a modulator of eicosanoid synthesis that ginger may be most helpful to the healing system.

Additionally, ginger tones the circulatory system and has anticancer effects, blocking the tendency of some carcinogens to cause mutations in DNA.

You can take ginger in the form of the fresh rhizome or as candied slices, honey-based syrups, or encapsulated extracts. A simple and delightful preparation is ginger tea: for an individual serving, put one-half teaspoon of freshly grated rhizome into a cup of boiling water, cover the pot, and steep for ten to fifteen minutes. Strain, add honey to taste, and drink hot or iced. You can buy honey-based ginger syrups in health food stores and add them to hot or cold water for an instant beverage, or you can make your own by adding one part of fresh, grated ginger to three parts of raw honey; keep this in the refrigerator.

When ginger is dried, its chemistry changes; in particular, the gingerols, which are abundant in the fresh rhizome, convert to the more pungent shogaols. These two classes of compounds may have different properties, with shogaols having more powerful anti-inflammatory and analgesic effects. Therefore, it might be wise to use more than one form of ginger, and persons with arthritis and other inflammatory conditions might get more benefit from capsules of dried, powdered ginger, which are available in health food stores. Ginger is nontoxic, but you may experience heartburn if you take a large dose on an empty stomach. I suggest taking it with food.

GREEN TEA

Green tea, the national beverage of Japan, is made from the unfermented leaves of the tea plant, *Camellia sinensis*. In preparing more familiar black tea, leaves are piled up in heaps and "sweated," a natural fermentation process that darkens the leaves and changes their aroma and flavor. Recently, medical researchers have discovered a number of health benefits of green tea, having to do with its content of catechins, a group of compounds mostly destroyed in the fermentative conversion to black tea. (Oolong tea is somewhere in between. It is briefly sweated, resulting in a color, flavor, and catechin content intermediate between green and black tea.) Catechins lower cholesterol and generally improve lipid metabolism. They also have significant anticancer and antibacterial effects.

All tea contains theophylline, a close relative of caffeine; in high doses it can be quite stimulating, and people can become addicted to it just as they become addicted to coffee. In moderation, green tea, with its slightly bitter taste and delicate aroma, makes a pleasant and healthful addition to the diet. It is my favorite caffeinated beverage, one I associate with relaxation and good company. It seems silly to me to take green tea in the form of a supplement, but I see many tablets and products containing extracts of it in health food stores, all trying to take advantage of the publicity about protective effects of catechins against heart disease and cancer. There are even green tea underarm deodorants that rely on the herb's antibacterial properties.

One of my favorite varieties of green tea is *matcha,* a bright-green powder used in the Japanese tea ceremony and also served informally as a treat. It is prepared from very young, select tea leaves that are steamed, dried, and ground very fine. To prepare a beverage from it, you place a teaspoon of the powder in a ceramic tea bowl, add a small amount of boiling water, and whip the mixture to a froth with a bamboo whisk. *Matcha* is usually enjoyed with small sweets. It is definitely stimulating, having been used by Zen monks to maintain wakefulness during long periods of sitting meditation. You can buy *matcha* and ordinary green tea (*sencha*) at Japanese grocery stores; the latter is also now widely available in teabags in supermarkets.

If you are currently a drinker of coffee, black tea, or cola, you might consider switching to green tea. Not only is it a relatively benign form of caffeine, it offers impressive benefits as a general tonic.

MILK THISTLE

A most interesting tonic herb from the tradition of European folk medicine is milk thistle, *Silybum marianum*. The seeds of this plant yield an extract, silymarin, that enhances metabolism of liver cells and protects them from toxic injury. Although the pharmaceutical industry has produced many drugs that damage the liver, it offers nothing to match the protective effect of milk thistle, which is itself nontoxic.

Anyone who is a heavy user of alcohol should take milk thistle regularly, as should patients using pharmaceutical drugs that are hard on the liver, including cancer patients undergoing chemotherapy. I recommend this herb to all patients with chronic hepatitis and abnormal liver function, and have seen cases of normalization of liver function in persons who took it every day for several months and also worked to improve their diets and lifestyles. If you work with toxic chemicals or feel you have suffered toxic exposures from any source, take milk thistle. It will help your body recover from any harm.

You will find milk thistle products in all health food stores. My preference is to use standardized extracts in tablet or capsule form. Follow the suggested dosage on the product you buy, or take two tablets or capsules twice a day. You can stay on milk thistle indefinitely.

ASTRAGALUS

If you are Chinese you will recognize this tonic herb at once. Under the name *huangqi* it is widely sold both singly and in many combination formulas for the treatment of colds and flus. *Astragalus* is a large genus in the pea family, some species of which are toxic to livestock. (Locoweed of the American Southwest is an astragalus.) But the toxins are only in the above-ground parts, never in the roots, and it is the root of a nontoxic Chinese species, *Astragalus membranaceous,* that provides the herbal medicine. The plant is a perennial herb with long, fibrous roots, native to northern China and Inner Mongolia. Both wild and cultivated plants are sources of commercial astragalus, which is sold in bundles of thin slices that resemble wooden tongue depressors and have a sweet taste. Chinese herbalists recommend adding these slices to soups and removing them before serving because they are too tough to chew. You can buy dried astragalus in Chinese herb stores, or you can buy astragalus tinctures and capsules in health food stores. You will also find in health food stores many Chinese herbal products that contain astragalus as a principal ingredient.

Traditional Chinese doctors consider this plant a true tonic that can strengthen debilitated patients and increase resistance to disease in general. They also use it as a promoter of other herbs known to increase energy, aid digestion, and stimulate the production and circulation of blood. In contemporary Chinese medicine astragalus is also a chief component of *fu zheng* therapy, a combination herbal treatment to restore immune function in cancer patients undergoing chemotherapy and radiation. Research in China has demonstrated increased survival in patients receiving both herbal and Western therapies, as well as moderation of the immunosuppressive effects of the latter.

Pharmacological studies in the West confirm that astragalus enhances immune function. It increases activity of several kinds of white blood cells as well as production of antibodies and interferon. These properties have to do with the root's content of polysaccharides, large molecules composed of chains of sugar subunits. Polysaccharides are structural components of many organisms; until recently they did not excite much interest among Western pharmacologists, because they are not the types of molecules that act as magic bullets and because conventional wisdom holds that they cannot even be absorbed from the gastrointestinal tract. But polysaccharides are a common feature of many herbal medicines that enhance immunity, so we must not yet understand their properties.

I recommend astragalus to many patients, since I find it to be safe and effective. In particular, I suggest it for people with chronic infectious diseases, such as bronchitis, sinusitis, and AIDS. I also recommend it to many cancer patients, both those undergoing conventional treatment and those who have completed treatment. And I think taking astragalus regularly is beneficial for people who are debilitated, lacking in energy or vitality, or feeling vulnerable to stress. It is easy to find astragalus products in health food stores; follow dosages specified on the labels.

SIBERIAN GINSENG
(ELEUTHERO GINSENG, SPINY GINSENG)

The root of a large, spiny shrub native to northern China and Siberia, Siberian ginseng (*Eleutherococcus senticosus*) is now one of the most widely used tonic herbs in the world, so much in demand that authentic material may be difficult to obtain. *Eleutherococcus* is a genus in the ginseng family, different from *Panax,* the source of true ginseng. Soviet scientists discovered the remarkable "adaptogenic" (stress-protective) properties of this species in the course of searching for ginseng substitutes, and as news of its benefits spread, many Soviet athletes and military personnel began to use it to increase physical performance and endurance.

Much animal and human research has demonstrated the protective effects of Siberian ginseng as well as its ability to enhance immune function. Active components include polysaccharides and a distinctive group of compounds called eleutherosides. In buying Siberian ginseng products, look for alcohol extracts or dry extracts (in tablets or capsules) that have been standardized for eleutheroside content; this is your only assurance that you are buying genuine material.

Unlike most of the tonic herbs I will mention in this chapter, Siberian ginseng has no extensive historical use as a folk remedy; it is a recent discovery. Modern Chinese doctors have taken great interest in it and now prescribe it, usually as a single remedy, for many chronic illnesses. It is a reliable tonic with general restorative effects, especially useful for people who lack energy and vitality, and can be used safely over long periods of time. Take two capsules or tablets twice a day, unless the product you buy specifies otherwise.

GINSENG

Two species of *Panax* are the source of this most prized and famous tonic: *P. ginseng,* native to northeastern China, and *P. quinque-*

folium, native to northeastern North America. Both species are now widely cultivated for commerce, and both have similar restorative qualities, but Oriental ginseng is more of a stimulant and sexual energizer, while American ginseng may be more powerful as an adaptogen. The plants are very slow growing, and older roots are believed to have greater therapeutic benefit than younger ones. Ginseng fanciers pay dearly for old roots of wild plants, much less for young, cultivated roots. Many forms of ginseng are on the market, from whole dried roots to ginseng brandies, wines, teas, and candies, and a multitude of tableted and encapsulated extracts. Be warned: some of these products contain little or no ginseng. Whenever a medicinal plant is scarce and expensive, imitation and adulterated products will be sold. *Panax ginseng* owes its beneficial effects to an unusual group of compounds called ginsenosides that are not found in any other genus. If ginseng products are real, they must contain ginsenosides, the more the better, so unless you are buying whole roots (which are unmistakable once you have seen them), buy only products that are standardized for ginsenoside content.

Among Chinese and Koreans, ginseng is especially valued as a tonic for the elderly, because it can improve appetite and digestion, tone skin and muscles, and restore depleted sexual energy. Chinese men say that it is not for women, but it may be that men simply do not want to share a limited supply; however, ginseng may have estrogenic activity that would argue against its use by women with hormonal imbalances or those who have estrogen-dependent diseases like uterine fibroids, fibrocystic breast disease, and breast cancer. One Chinese man told me not to waste ginseng in my youth. Save it for old age, he advised. "Then you will see what it can do for you."

Ginseng is generally safe, but the Oriental variety can raise blood pressure in some individuals, as well as cause irritability. People who experience those side effects should lower the dose or switch to American ginseng (which is preferred by many Orientals). I recommend ginseng frequently to people who have low vitality or have been weakened by chronic illness or old age. Many people who take it tell me they are quite happy with its effects and plan to stay on it. Standardized ginseng extract, made by a Swiss method, is now available at drug stores throughout the world.

DONG QUAI (TANG KUEI)

The root of *Angelica sinensis,* a plant in the carrot family, dong quai is known in traditional Chinese medicine as a blood-building tonic that improves circulation. In this century it has come into common use in the West as a general tonic for women, and many Western herbalists and naturopaths prescribe it for disorders of the female reproductive system, especially for irregular or difficult menstruation. Chinese doctors recognize its ability to tone the uterus and balance female hormonal chemistry, but they think of it as beneficial to both sexes and often include it in tonic formulas for men, combining it with ginseng and ho shou wu (see below). In men it is supposed to help build muscle and blood.

Dong quai is nontoxic and does not have estrogenic activity, although many people think it does. I recommend it frequently to women experiencing menstrual problems or menopausal symptoms and women who lack energy, with good results. It is readily available in health food stores in tinctures and capsules, and since it is not a scarce or expensive herb, most products made from it are of good quality. If you want to experiment with it, try taking two capsules of the root twice a day or one dropperful of the tincture in a little water twice a day. Give it a six-to-eight-week trial to see what it does for you.

HO SHOU WU

The name of this tonic herb means "Mr. Ho has black hair," referring to its power as a rejuvenator and maintainer of youthfulness. The root of *Polygonum multiflorum,* ho shou wu is a very famous Chinese blood tonic, believed to clean the blood and increase energy, as well as to nourish the hair and teeth. It is widely believed to be a powerful sexual tonic when consumed regularly and to increase sperm production in men and fertility in women. Research in China has shown it to lower elevated cholesterol; there has been no research on it in the West, and it is usually available only from suppliers of Chinese herbal medicines.

One way to experience the benefits of this herb is to take it in a liquid formula known as shou wu chih, or Super Shou Wu, that combines it with other tonic herbs and flavors. This is a very dark liquid with a pleasant aromatic taste that should be diluted: two tablespoons to a cup of hot or cold water. Drink this amount once or twice a day for at least a month to see if it gives you increased energy and increased sexual energy. (To turn graying hair black, you would probably have to consume it every day for years, and I would like to see the before-and-after photographs.)

MAITAKE

Maitake is the Japanese name for an edible and delicious mushroom, *Grifola frondosa,* known to mushroom hunters in America as "hen-of-the-woods," because it grows in big clusters on the ground at the bases of trees or stumps, clusters that resemble the fluffed tailfeathers of a nesting hen. The Japanese name means "dancing mushroom," possibly because people danced with joy on finding this rare and prized species. Finding a big hen-of-the-woods—they can weigh up to a hundred pounds—can indeed be cause for celebration, not only because it is a huge quantity of a choice wild mushroom but also because it is an eminently salable commodity worth twenty dollars a pound or more. Italians love to cook it in sauces for pasta or pickle it in olive oil and vinegar marinades after parboiling. Unfortunately, maitake in the wild is uncommon, even though it will fruit in the same spot for many years.

In 1965 a master Japanese mushroom hunter wrote: "Top rank hunters are those who seek maitake. They go out to their own secret grounds to spend several days looking for maitake with a dream of fortune at a stroke. Maitake hunters are not supposed to let others know their secret spot. If he finds a spot where he can crop more than 10 kg (22 lbs) of maitake, he found a 'treasure island.' He would never tell anyone his secret location until he dies. He would only indicate the location in his will to his eldest son just before he dies. Some hunters are even willing to die without telling their own sons or families. . . ."

All this changed in the early 1980s, when Japanese scientists discovered how to cultivate maitake on sawdust; the cultivated form is now sold at reasonable prices in supermarkets throughout Japan.

Mushroom growers in this country are just beginning to experiment with it. In cultivation the mushroom looks like a floral bouquet in shades of gray and gray-brown, except, instead of flowers, it is made up of many overlapping, fan-shaped mushroom caps. The undersides are white, with tiny pores instead of gills. *Grifola* belongs to a family of mushrooms called polypores, distinguished by that kind of spore-bearing tissue. In general polypores are nontoxic, but only a few are edible; most are tough and woody, growing as brackets or shelves on dead or living trees. In the West, polypore mushrooms have mainly been of interest to forest pathologists, because they are important causes of heart rot in living trees and important decomposers of dead and dying trees; but in the Far East, many of them are highly esteemed as medicinal herbs, especially in the class of superior drugs, the tonics and panaceas that increase resistance and promote longevity.

Traditional Chinese doctors did not use maitake, but they did use many of its relatives, including a very close relative, *Polyporus umbellatus,* or zhu ling. Modern testing has shown zhu ling to have anticancer and immune-enhancing properties related to its content of polysaccharides. Now Japanese researchers have tested maitake for similar effects, with impressive results. In fact, extracts of maitake turn out to be more powerful anticancer and immune-enhancing agents than any of the other medicinal mushrooms tested so far. In combination with chemotherapy, they increase the effectiveness of lower doses of Western drugs, while protecting the immune system from toxic damage. Perhaps Chinese doctors will begin including this mushroom in their fu zheng therapy. Maitake extracts also show activity against HIV and hepatitis as well as an antihypertensive effect.

Until cultivated maitake turns up in supermarkets here—a likely prospect, because the mushroom is not difficult to grow, retains its freshness extremely well, and has a firm texture and good flavor—you will have to buy tablets and capsules of maitake extracts in health food stores. Several firms are now marketing these products, using material imported from Japan. Prices are high but should come down once cultivation catches on here.

I recommend supplements of maitake to people with cancer, AIDS, and other immune system problems as well as to those with chronic fatigue syndrome, chronic hepatitis, and environmental illnesses that may represent toxic overloads. As soon as fresh maitake becomes available, I will make it a regular addition to my diet.

CORDYCEPS

I will close this list of natural tonics with another mushroom, one that is stranger than maitake. *Cordyceps sinensis* grows not on trees but on the living bodies of certain moth larvae. The mushroom organism, in the form of fine threads, penetrates a larva, eventually killing and mummifying it. The mushroom then sends up its fruiting body: a slender stalk with a swollen end that will release spores. Cordyceps occurs in mountainous regions of China and Tibet and is now cultivated as well, because it is in great demand as a supertonic that builds physical stamina, mental energy, and sexual power. Chinese doctors say it is simultaneously invigorating and calming as well as life prolonging. Chinese people usually buy it in whole dried form, consisting of the mummified larva and attached fruiting body of the mushroom, which they add to soups and stews made from duck and chicken. In addition, extracts of cordyceps are included in many compound tonic formulas. Cordyceps is considered safe and gentle, indicated for both men and women of any age and state of health, even the most infirm.

This exotic remedy came to worldwide attention following the Chinese National Games of 1993, when a team of nine Chinese women runners broke nine world records, one by an unprecedented forty-two seconds. Charges of steroid use were leveled at the athletes, but their coach held a press conference to deny the accusations, holding up a box of the Chinese herbs he felt were responsible for his team's performance and a lab report stating that they were natural and safe. The main ingredient was cordyceps. The track world was unconvinced, with one American distance runner calling the broken records "tragic" and another saying the Chinese had set women's running back for years. In the words of one commentator:

> This suspicion was understandable. The improved performance of the Chinese distance runners had occurred suddenly and sensationally. The new 1,500-meter record-holder had been seventy-third at the same distance the previous year, and the forty-two-second improvement in the 10,000-meter race seemed impossible. And, as journalists and runners were aware, a number of East German coaches had moved to China after the fall of the Berlin Wall; their

former country had long been associated with steroid use. Further-more, the Chinese success was only among women runners, who are more apt to benefit from steroid use.

But there was strong evidence that the records were untainted. The Chinese runners had passed the drug tests. They also showed no outward signs of steroid use, such as acne, deepened voices, or highly defined musculature. And there is no doubt that—although they are not alone in this—the Chinese provide their runners with stringent training. . . .*

In any case, interest in and sales of cordyceps boomed. If you do not wish to add mummified, fungal-infected caterpillars to your chicken soup, cordyceps is also available in the form of tinctures and extracts, either singly or combined with other Chinese herbs. Ask for these products in health food stores. For general weakness, take it once a day, following dosage advice on the product. For health main-tenance, in the absence of specific problems, take it once a week.

MY INTENTION HAS not been to overwhelm you with information but rather to make you aware of substances that can help you resist the effects of toxins, stress, and aging on your healing system. Instead of despairing at the thought of all the harmful influences that exist, know that you can protect yourself and increase your healing poten-tial through the use of products that are safe and effective. Let me quickly recap the information in this chapter:

- Eat more garlic and ginger; they taste good, and the list of their beneficial effects keeps growing.

- If you use caffeine, switch to green tea all or some of the time, since it is the most healthful of the caffeinated beverages.

- If you worry about exposure to toxins or feel you have a toxic overload, take milk thistle to help your body recover.

- If you are generally weak or lacking in vitality, experiment with Siberian ginseng or cordyceps.

---

* This controversy is not settled. The Chinese runners may have been on steroids as well as cordyceps.

• If you have depressed immunity and find that you get every bug going around, do a course of astragalus or maitake.

• If you feel debilitated as a result of age and lack sexual energy, experiment with ginseng and ho shou wu. Ginseng is a good general tonic for men, while dong quai is a good general tonic for women.

Tonic herbs have always been immensely popular in many countries of the world. I predict that as medical researchers document their safety and effectiveness, doctors here will begin to prescribe them more.

12

ACTIVITY AND REST

YOU CAN INCREASE the chance of experiencing spontaneous healing by giving your body appropriate exercise and sufficient rest.

Physical exercise benefits the healing system in many different ways. It improves circulation, making the heart a more efficient pump and maintaining the elasticity of arteries. At the same time it tones the respiratory system, increasing exchanges of oxygen and carbon dioxide, which helps the body eliminate metabolic wastes. It further aids elimination by promoting the flow of perspiration and movement of the intestines. By stimulating release of endorphins in the brain, it fights depression and improves mood. It regulates metabolism and the body's economy of energy. It neutralizes stress, allowing greater relaxation and sounder sleep. It even enhances immune function. Any program intended to optimize the body's healing potential must include regular exercise.

But what is the best and simplest way to get these benefits? A great many people in our society, both young and old, do not like to exercise at all. Others exercise fanatically, spending hours in aerobics classes and on exercise machines, often in attempts to control weight. Some become addicted to strenuous exercise because it gives them a "buzz," probably the result of endorphin release. Exercise physiologists and sports medicine doctors have made the whole subject of exercise very complicated. It seems to me that many of these people—the couch potatoes, the fanatics and addicts, and the experts—are all missing something.

Whenever I come home after visiting traditional cultures in the Americas, Africa, or Asia, I am struck by the oddity of our habits of exercise. In nonindustrial societies the demands of daily life give bodies all the work they need. Muscles have good tone because people lift and carry burdens, and they walk constantly. They walk to gather water and wood, they walk to their fields, they walk to markets, they walk to visit friends and relatives. Of all the technological inventions that have changed our patterns of activity for the worse, the automobile gets the prize. I believe it has compromised health significantly, not only because it has darkened the air of our cities with exhaust emissions, but especially because it has deprived us of opportunities to walk.

Human beings are meant to walk. We are bipedal, upright organisms with bodies designed for locomotion. Walking is a complex behavior that requires functional integration of a great deal of sensory and motor experience; it exercises our brains as well as our musculoskeletal systems. Consider balance, which is merely one component of walking. In order to maintain the body's balance unconsciously and effortlessly as it changes position and moves over uneven surfaces in a gravitational field, the brain needs a lot of information. It relies in part on a mechanism in the inner ear responsible for sensing orientation in three-dimensional space; if this mechanism fails, people cannot maintain equilibrium. But in addition to data from the ear, the brain depends on visual input and information from other senses to keep us in balance: from touch receptors that let it know what part of the body is in contact with the earth and from proprioceptors in muscles, tendons, and joints that keep it continually informed of the exact position of each part of the body in space. Interference on any of these channels can lead to wobbling and falling. In the brain all of this information is processed by the cerebellum, which uses it to coordinate responses of muscles to the ever-changing requirements of locomotion.

When you walk, the movement of your limbs is cross-patterned: the right leg and the left arm move forward at the same time, then the left leg and the right arm. This type of movement generates electrical activity in the brain that has a harmonizing influence on the whole central nervous system—a special benefit of walking that you do not necessarily get from other kinds of exercise. Dr. Fulford, the old osteopath who first taught me the basic principles of healing, believed that cross-patterned movement was necessary for normal development and optimal functioning of the nervous system. When babies first start to crawl, this movement stimulates further brain development. I often heard Dr. Fulford instruct adult patients to crawl as a way of speeding recovery from injuries. "Go back to that simple movement, and you will help the nervous system move beyond any blocks," he would say. Dr. Fulford, a shining example of physical health in his nineties, does not go to aerobics classes or use exercise machines; he walks.

Many of the healthiest people I have met are dedicated walkers. Shin Terayama, the man who recovered completely from metastatic kidney cancer, takes a daily walk before breakfast whenever he can, always maintaining a brisk pace and always including uphill walking if possible. At a recent workshop I led in Montana, a seventy-six-year-old woman in the group greatly impressed me with her stamina on hikes in the mountains. She was in excellent health and looked much younger than her years. I was even more impressed when she told me that both of her parents had died in their fifties and that she had been in declining health in middle age until she started walking. She had also improved her diet, stopped taking medicines, and started using vitamins, but in her mind commitment to walking was the critical factor in her improvement. She walked at every opportunity and joined walking tours on vacations. "It's my life," she told me on top of a ridge along the Continental Divide, and I believed her.

So I am going to pare my advice and comments on exercise down to one word: Walk! In my opinion, walking is the most healthful form of physical activity, the one that has the greatest capacity to keep the healing system in good working order and increase the likelihood of spontaneous healing in case of illness.

The advantages of walking over all other forms of exercise are numerous. You do not have to learn how to do it. It does not require any equipment except a comfortable pair of shoes. It costs nothing, and you can do it anywhere: in cities, parks, even indoors in shopping malls if the weather is inclement. The chance of injuring yourself is small, in great contrast to running and competitive sports. It is much less boring than riding a stationary bike or running on a treadmill. You can walk outdoors and enjoy the beauty of nature. You can also walk with friends and enjoy their company.

Walking will satisfy all the body's needs for aerobic exercise if you do it in ways that increase heart rate and respiration sufficiently. For an ideal aerobic workout, your walks should last forty-five minutes, and you should be able to cover three miles in that time. If your heart and respiratory rate are not elevated at the end of a forty-five-minute walk, you should try walking faster part of the time or look for long, gradual hills to climb. But remember that you are not walking just to get aerobic exercise; you are also going for the neurological benefit of cross-patterned movement combined with visual, tactile, and proprioceptive stimulation. You can obtain this effect from short walks throughout the day as well as from long aerobic walks, and you can enhance it by accentuating your arm swing from time to time. Also try coordinating arm swing with breathing.

I have experimented with many forms of exercise in my life, and I keep coming back to walking as the best. As I get older, I think it will be the one I rely on to keep my body, mind, and healing system all in good shape.

ACTIVITY MUST BE balanced by rest. Everyone has experienced the adverse effects of fatigue and sleep deprivation; lack of good quality rest is one of the most common causes of susceptibility to illness, and a good night's rest is an effective healing technique that will abort many incipient illnesses. Therefore, improving the quality of rest and sleep should be another priority in a program aimed at enhancing your healing capacity.

Consider the common impediments to rest. Many people are unable to sleep because they are overstimulated, often by drugs they have ingested earlier in the day. Others cannot sleep because of noise or aches and pains. Others cannot turn off their minds. There are simple remedies for all of these problems.

Stimulant drugs that interfere with sleep include coffee, tea, cola, and other caffeinated beverages; ephedrine, the chief ingredient in many herbal diet and energy products sold over the counter in drug and health food stores; pseudoephedrine, a decongestant in over-the-counter cold remedies; and phenylpropanolamine, commonly used in appetite suppressants. Even when these drugs are taken early in the day, they can interfere with nighttime sleep patterns. If you have difficulty getting restful sleep, try to eliminate all of these substances from your life.

While we are on the subject of drugs, let me state my opinion that sedatives are not to be relied on except for short-term management of unusual stress. If you have a death in the family or have just lost a job, it may be appropriate to take sedative drugs for a few consecutive nights to help you sleep, but taking them every night is not wise. All sedatives depress function in the central nervous system, all are addictive, and all suppress rapid-eye-movement (REM) sleep, the phase of sleep in which dreaming occurs. Dreaming is necessary for the health and well-being of the brain and mind; if you are not doing it, you are not getting quality sleep, even though the quantity appears sufficient.

The safest sedative I know is valerian, a natural remedy obtained from the root of a European plant, *Valeriana officinalis*. You can buy tinctures of valerian root in health food stores—the dose is one teaspoon in a little warm water at bedtime. Still, this product is a depressant and should not be used long-term. Quite recently a nonaddictive, nondepressant regulator of sleep cycles has become available: melatonin, the hormone secreted by the pineal gland, which regulates the biological clock, especially in relation to day/night cycles. Melatonin comes in one- or three-milligram tablets and is sold in health food stores—the dose is one to two milligrams at bedtime. (Avoid animal-derived forms, which may contain dangerous contaminants; use only synthetic forms.) International travelers say melatonin is the first really effective treatment for jet lag, especially for west-to-east travel, which most people find harder. Melatonin also appears safe and effective for resetting wayward biological clocks. If you get bone tired at seven in the evening, then find yourself wide awake when you get into bed at ten or eleven, it might change your cycles of tiredness and wakefulness in just the right manner to allow you to enjoy full periods of restful sleep.

If you cannot get to sleep or stay asleep because of physical discomfort, I have several suggestions. One is to try a new mattress, since many different kinds are available, including futons and air mattresses whose firmness can be adjusted with the touch of a button. Another is to have a session or two of adjustment from an osteopathic physician who specializes in manipulation (or from a good chiropractor). This kind of therapy may allow you to find more comfortable positions to sleep in. You can also try soaking in a warm bath before bed and taking hops, an herbal muscle relaxant, which you will find in health food stores: two capsules at bedtime is the usual dose.

I find that noise is a major obstacle to sound sleep, everything from barking dogs in the country to the sounds of traffic in the city. A simple solution, better than ear plugs, is to buy a white-noise generator, an electronic device that produces restful sound. White noise contains a mixture of many different frequencies of sound waves, just as white light contains all frequencies of visible light. It sounds like water running from a shower head, and most units have variable controls that allow you to change the basic sound from that of a steady downpour to rhythmic ocean waves. White noise is soothing and masks offending sounds. A more exciting technology, soon to be on the market, actually eliminates noise by analyzing offending sound waves and producing mirror-image waves that cancel them out. Portable devices of this sort are already available as headsets to be worn on airplanes to eliminate engine noise.

No matter how comfortable my bed and how quiet the room, when my mind is overactive, I usually cannot fall asleep and may wake during the night. In the morning I am very aware that I have not had the rest I need. Learning to leave behind the worries of the day is not as easy as taking a pill or turning on a sound machine, but it is one of the most useful skills you can develop. I often read myself to sleep; there is no shortage of sleep-inducing books, and reading distracts me from pointless rumination. I also use a simple breathing exercise that I will describe in the next chapter, because I find that focusing attention on breathing is an effective way to withdraw attention from thoughts. Another possibility is to get out of the mind by attending to the body—for example, by tensing and relaxing groups of muscles. Here is a simple exercise that may help you get to sleep when your mind is racing: Lie on your back with your arms at your sides, close your eyes, and take five deep, slow breaths. Then squeeze your eyes shut and tense the muscles of your forehead for a few seconds. Relax for a few seconds. Then tense the muscles of your face and relax in the same way, then the chin and neck muscles, and so on, going down the arms and front of the body until you flex the feet and toes. Then go back to the head, pressing it against the bed for a few seconds and relaxing, and proceed down the back of the body, again reaching the feet, this time extending them. Finally, relax completely and take five deep, slow breaths. The whole exercise will take no more than a few minutes. It is an efficient relaxation technique, especially useful when mental turmoil threatens to keep you from falling asleep.

By the way, a major source of my own mental turmoil is the news. The percentage of stories in the news that make me feel good is very small; the percentage of stories that make me feel anxious or outraged is very large and increasing, as news media focus more and more on murder, mayhem, and misery. It is easy to forget that we have a choice as to whether we let this information into our minds and thoughts. I find it so useful to disengage myself from it that I recommend "news fasts" as part of the eight-week program to a more efficient healing system. I think you will find that these fasts will allow you to get better rest and sleep.

TO SUMMARIZE THIS chapter: Give your healing system a morning walk and a good night's rest, and it will be ready for whatever challenges may arise.

13

MIND AND SPIRIT

THE LOGO OF THE American Holistic Medical Association is a staff with a single snake coiled about it, on which are superimposed three interlocking circles. The staff with the snake is the staff of Asklepios, the symbol of the medical profession, while the circles are meant to symbolize body, mind, and spirit, the three components of the whole person. It is a common belief of holistic doctors that conventional medicine attends only to the physical body, neglecting mind and spirit. I have written that mind often holds the key to unlocking spontaneous healing, and I have alluded to cultural beliefs about spiritual causes of illness, but when it comes to the specifics of these interactions, our ignorance is vast. We know little about the mind and the ways it affects the physical body, less about spirit, if that is even knowable in the usual sense of the word. Science, with its present materialistic bias, is not of much help, because it denies the possibility of nonphysical causation of physical events. It is all very well to share a holistic philosophy of health and medicine, but what practical advice can a holistic doctor give to patients about optimizing healing potentials by mental and spiritual methods?

MIND

I would like you to consider four activities of the mind and ways they interact with the healing system. They are: belief, thought, mental imagery, and emotion.

Belief

Belief in healers, miracle shrines, and drugs is clearly the basis of placebo responses, which I regard as classic examples of spontaneous healing. Belief also strongly influences perception, determining what we see and what we do not see as we move through the world. Years ago I met a woman who was able to find four-leaf clovers in any clover patch. She liked to bet people that within a minute of being told to look, she could find a four-leaf clover, and she always won the bets. Never having found one, I was completely mystified by her ability. When I would look through patches of clover, I could search without success until my vision blurred, and whenever I thought I saw four leaves on one stem, they always turned out to belong to two different clovers. But after meeting this woman and watching her do it, something changed for me. I realized that the key to her success was her belief that in any clover patch there was a four-leaf clover waiting to be found. With that belief, there is a chance of finding it; without it there is none. After meeting her, I began to look again, and soon I started to find four-leaf clovers. Sometimes I found several in one patch, and sometimes I found five- and six-leaf clovers (though I do not know whether they bring any extra luck).

Recently I was teaching at a retreat center in Montana, an erstwhile hunting lodge with a large, clover-filled lawn. One afternoon when I had nothing to do I thought I would see what I could find. So I got down on the ground and began searching. A woman who was in the class came over and asked, "Did you lose something? Can I help you find it?"

"I'm looking for four-leaf clovers," I replied.

"Really?" she said. "I always thought they were just a story. Don't they just paste an extra leaf on the ones that come sealed in plastic?"

"No, they really exist," I told her. "I'm sure there's one here."

She joined me on the lawn, and we both started looking. "It takes some concentration," I explained, "but it's good training for the eyes and brain, and there are worse ways to spend time." Five minutes later, I found a six-leaf clover, then a four. My companion was amazed. "I've got a lot of clover on the lawn in front of my house," she said. "I'm going to look as soon as I get back home." She may start to find four-leaf clovers now that she believes they exist; before she would never even have looked.

Spontaneous healing is something like a four-leaf clover: lucky, mysterious, and sometimes elusive. If you do not believe it can occur, your chance of experiencing it will be small. I am interested in what people can do to increase belief in healing. One technique, recommended by many New Age therapists, is to repeat affirmations, such as "My body can heal itself," or "I am filled with healing energy," or "My gallstone is getting smaller and smaller." I do not recommend this technique, because I have no evidence that it works. It assumes that verbal repetition can produce a change in belief structure, but my experience is that the kind of belief that shapes perception and impacts the healing system—gut-level belief, if you will—is often at variance with what people say to themselves and others. I do not think I would have discovered my ability to find four-leaf clovers by repeating over and over, "I believe in four-leaf clovers." That discovery came about suddenly when I saw reality differently through the eyes of another person. Now I can provide that experience for others, as I did for the woman on the lawn in Montana. Therefore the strategy I recommend is to seek out people who have experienced healing so that their reality can become your reality.

I remember a patient who came to me with a large fibroid tumor of the uterus, almost the size of a grapefruit. She was forty-nine years old, the wife of a gynecologist. Her husband supported the opinion of her gynecologist (his colleague), who told her she had to have a hysterectomy. The fibroid was causing her considerable discomfort, painful periods, and heavy menstrual bleeding. She did not want to have her uterus removed and came to see me in the hope that I would alert her to an alternative to surgery. I told her that since she was near menopause, she could simply try to wait until her estrogen levels declined; uterine fibroids feed on estrogen and usually shrink at menopause, sometimes completely. I recommended an herbal remedy (blue cohosh, *Caulophyllum thallictroides*), dietary changes to minimize intake of foods with estrogenic activity, aerobic exercise to reduce estrogen levels, and visualization therapy to bring mental influence to bear on the tumor. She was willing to try this program, but I could tell that her belief in the possibility of the tumor's shrinking was not strong enough to counteract the message she got from the medical profession: that there was no way to avoid a hysterectomy.

Then I remembered that my next scheduled appointment was with a woman who had successfully dealt with an even larger—melon-sized—uterine fibroid a few years before. She had told me with great delight how she had proved her doctor wrong, avoided a hysterectomy, and now, having gone through menopause, was problem-free. I thought she would be willing to tell her story to the gynecologist's wife. With their permission, I introduced these two women to each other; but as it turned out, they already knew each other, since they were neighbors. My second patient, just by her presence, was able to do a much better job than I could to convince the first patient to refuse surgery. She did refuse the hysterectomy, followed the recommendations I gave her to control her symptoms, experienced menopause a year later, and now is symptom-free.

I can think of no better way to change belief in a manner that facilitates rather than obstructs healing than to seek out the company of persons who have experienced it. Four-leaf clovers did not exist in my reality until I met someone for whom they were an everyday occurrence. My world is now a bit richer for their presence. As more people come to believe in spontaneous healing, more people will experience it, and that will benefit everyone.

Thought

In Buddhist psychology, addiction to thought is seen as a major obstacle to enlightenment, because when our attention is focused on thought, we cannot experience reality. Thought takes us out of the here and now and into the past, into the future, and into fantasy—all unreal realms. On a practical level, thoughts are the major source of anxiety, guilt, fear, and sadness—emotions that probably obstruct healing and certainly cause us a great deal of anguish. It is not possible to stop thought, except perhaps in very advanced levels of mental training (hence the joke about a surefire way to make gold: put such-and-such ingredients into a pot, place it on a fire, and stir for thirty minutes while not thinking of the word "crocodile"), but it is possible to disengage attention from thought. One way to do that is to focus instead on sensations from the body. There is a great advantage to having bodies, according to Buddhist teaching, because they are anchored in the here and now while our minds are careering about the past and future. Whenever we pay attention to sensations in the body, attention is in present reality. In the last chapter I suggested a simple relaxation exercise before falling asleep based on alternately tensing and relaxing groups of muscles throughout the body. The reason it works to promote sleep when the mind is over-active is that it withdraws attention from thought and puts it into the here and now.

Another useful focus for attention is breath. I will have more to say about breathing in the latter part of this chapter. Here I will simply note that breath is the most natural object of meditation and gener-ally a much safer focus for attention than thought. If you find your-self having disturbing thoughts, instead of trying to stop them, try simply moving your attention to your breath.

Besides withdrawing attention from thought in general, there is another strategy for managing unwanted thoughts: putting atten-tion into their opposites. If you are plagued by recurrent, fearful thoughts of getting cancer, think about your immune system con-stantly weeding out abnormal cells, or when you eat broccoli or drink green tea or take antioxidant supplements, think about how you are strengthening your body's defenses against cancer. Contra-dictory thoughts will cancel each other out, much as mirror-image sound waves cancel each other out in the new technology of noise elimination.

Meditation is a technique to break addiction to thought; in essence it is directed concentration. By sitting and trying to maintain the focus of concentration on some object—the breath, body sensations, a visual image—you learn to control attention and keep it in one place. Meditation practice is both simple and difficult: simple because the method is nothing more than maintaining focused atten-tion, difficult because it requires changing lifelong habits of letting the mind wander where it will, especially into thoughts. Even when you learn to sit motionless for a half-hour and mostly keep your attention on your chosen object of meditation, you may not be able to extend that successful calming and focusing into the rest of your life. The real goal of meditation practice is to do it constantly, to practice meditation in action as you move through the world. Even if you are not ready to undertake that sort of training, you can begin by trying to move your attention to your body or your breath whenever you remember to do so, especially when you notice that your mind has been led away from the here and now by the endlessly fascinat-ing process of thought.

Mental Imagery

The mind's eye has a special relationship with the healing system. A great deal of the cerebral cortex is devoted to vision. Located at the back of the head, this part of the brain mostly occupies itself with processing of information from the retinas of the eyes, but when it disengages from that task and turns inward, one of the most important channels for mind/body communication becomes available.

All of us spend time watching images in the mind's eye, but few of us have had training in this process—for example, to make the images sharper, brighter, and more exact in detail—and society places no value on it. In daydreaming we mostly attend to internal visual imagery. Our outward-directed culture regards daydreaming as an escape: children caught daydreaming in school are ordered to pay attention. (They *are* paying attention—to inner visual reality instead of outer, consensus reality.) An elementary-school teacher once asked my advice about a problem child in her class, a boy who was the "worst" daydreamer she had ever encountered. "He's just not there much of the time," she told me. "But if I pester him too much to pay attention, he makes his temperature go up, and I have to send him to the school infirmary; from there he often gets sent home for the day even though nothing's wrong with him." She had not connected the facts that the worst daydreamer she had ever met was also the only child she knew who had voluntary control of body temperature and could create fever at will. My interpretation is that those talents go together, and I suggested she call the boy the "best" daydreamer she ever met, not the worst. When it is not occupied with processing information from the eyes, the visual cortex can connect mind and will with the controls of the autonomic nervous system. It can also elicit spontaneous healing.

Another occasion for focusing on mental imagery is sexual fantasy, also a powerful channel to the autonomic nervous system. Sexual fantasy involves an interplay of imagery, highly charged emotions, and body responses. If you have any doubts about the power of the mind to affect the body, pay attention to what happens to your body when you indulge in this experience! For most people, the pictorial content of sexual fantasy is intensely private; even longtime lovers may keep the details of this experience to themselves. Another quality is that it is quite fixed and resistant to change: the same movies play over and over, and it is very difficult to alter the content. I am sure that if we could take more control of this process and bring the same intensity of emotional charge to images of healing, we could activate the healing system at will and maybe access regenerative capacities that are latent in our genes.

Because most of the time we view mental images unconsciously and without purpose, I think it is useful to work with a therapist when trying to draw on their great potential power to elicit spontaneous healing, at least initially. Hypnotherapists, visualization therapists, and guided imagery therapists can help you learn methods to take advantage of the mind/body connection through the medium of visual imagination. Once you master a technique, you can then practice on your own. My experience is that images with emotional charge work best, as is the case in sexual fantasy. A good visualization therapist will explore with a client a range of possible images to discover which ones elicit the strongest emotional responses.

I have known many people to rid themselves of warts by visualizing their disappearance in one way or another. (Children are better at this than adults, and warts have high rates of spontaneous remission in children.) One man came to me with a large wart on his left hand. Doctors had burned it off more than once, but it had always regrown. I told him to try surrounding it with white light for a few minutes each day, once on falling asleep and again on waking. He did this faithfully for a month without any change in the wart. Then I sent him to a visualization therapist, who discovered in the initial interview that he had a great fascination with steam shovels. Steam shovels and other earth-moving equipment had thrilled him ever since he was a small child. She suggested that he visualize a steam shovel scraping away at the wart each morning and night, and when he made that change he got results in a week. After two weeks the wart had shrunk to almost nothing, and a short time later it was gone, never to return.

Earlier in this book (see page 99) I described the case of a young man whose immune system was destroying his red blood cells and platelets. He had been through years of suppressive therapy with prednisone and other immunosuppressive drugs and had undergone splenectomy as a method of symptomatic management, all without success. I was able to help him design a healthy lifestyle and guide him toward natural interventions that eventually allowed his autoimmunity to subside. One of the interventions was visualization therapy with a trained professional, but he had no success in working with her at first. "I like her," he told me when he called in from another city, "but she keeps giving me violent images that I have problems with, like asking me to use laser beams against the white cells that are causing the reactions. I feel I've had enough medical violence done to my body, and I need a more peaceful image." Eventually he came up with one that worked for him: he imagined other white cells (the suppressor T cells) as motorcycle policemen who escorted his red cells and platelets in sidecars to protect them from aggressive white cells as they moved through his bloodstream. This visualization exercise worked brilliantly for him and became a central part of a program that put his disease into long-term remission.

You can practice using mental imagery to influence your body by daydreaming more consciously and purposefully and by paying attention to the emotional responses that particular images elicit. Try using visualizations to speed up the healing of wounds, sore throats, and other common ailments. Then if you ever have to mobilize your healing resources to manage a serious illness, you will have a good headstart.

Emotions

Many counselors and advocates of meditation advise people to gain control of their emotions—to even out the ups and downs of mood swings and cultivate evenness of temperament. That advice may be useful for some people. When I see patients whose lives seem out of balance, whose energy levels fluctuate wildly, who eat erratically and have unstable relationships, I usually recommend breathing exercises and meditation as methods to restore balance. But when I look at the role of emotions in facilitating spontaneous healing, I think it may be more useful to encourage sick people to cultivate passion. I have mentioned healing responses that occur after falling in love or expressing anger. Whether the emotion felt is positive or negative seems not to matter; rather it is the intensity of the feeling that gives it power to affect body function. More than negative feelings, apathy may be the major emotional obstacle to spontaneous healing.

What about depression, which is now epidemic in our culture? I experience depression as a state of high potential energy, wound up and turned inward on itself. If that energy can be accessed and moved, it can be a catalyst for spontaneous healing. The psychiatric profession treats depression almost exclusively by prescribing drugs, especially a new class of antidepressants called serotonin reuptake inhibitors, of which Prozac is a prototype. The pharmaceutical industry markets these drugs aggressively and successfully, partly by convincing people that they cannot know their full human potential unless they use them. Recently a woman friend of mine in her early fifties went for a routine checkup to her gynecologist, also a woman. After the examination was over, the gynecologist asked her, "Well, do you want me to write you a prescription for Prozac?" "Why should I want to take Prozac?" my friend replied. "I'm not depressed." "How would you know?" asked the doctor.

People who take Prozac and its relatives often say they simply feel everything less intensely, including their depression. Drug treatment has its place as one option for treating severe mood disturbances, but I worry about such enthusiasm for drugs that damp down passion, because I see intensity of feeling as a key to activating the healing system. Moreover, our capacity to feel joy may be the same as our capacity to feel despair, so that a depressed person may be more capable of experiencing ecstasy than someone who is always on an even keel or someone on Prozac. One technique for managing the down periods is to pretend to feel otherwise. Rabbi Nachman of Bratislav, a great Jewish mystic of the late eighteenth and early nineteenth century, who regularly experienced ecstasy on solitary wanderings through forests, recommended it to his followers:

"Always be joyful, no matter what you are," he taught. "With happiness, you can give a person life." Every day, he further stressed, we must deliberately induce in ourselves a buoyant, exuberant attitude toward life; in this manner, we will gradually become receptive to the subtle mysteries around us. And, if no inspired moments seem to come, we should act as though we have them anyway, he advised. "If you have no enthusiasm, put on a front. Act enthusiastic, and the feeling will become genuine."

SPIRIT

Have you ever wondered why distilled alcoholic beverages are called "spirits"? The original usage was in the phrase "spirits of wine," an old name for brandy. ("Brandy"—a short form of "brandywine"—comes from a Dutch word meaning burnt or heated wine; it was the first distilled liquor.) In brandy, the alcoholic essence that gives fermented grape juice its intoxicating power has been concentrated, resulting in a much stronger drink. The original idea of Dutch distillers was to reduce the volume of wine to make it more easily transportable to colonies on other continents: you could seal brandy in barrels, then dilute it with water at the end of an ocean voyage to re-expand its volume. Of course, when people tasted the contents of the barrels, few bothered to add water, and a new, more powerful form of alcohol flooded the world. In the old name for this product and in the persistent use of the term "spirits" to describe all strong liquors is a clue to the nature of spiritual reality and its relationship to matter.

What is concentrated in brandy is the vital essence of wine, that which gives it power to alter consciousness. If you warm a snifter of brandy and hold it in your hand, you can inhale (and sometimes feel the effect of) the volatile fumes that rise from the glass. In this concentrated form the essence of wine behaves like a gas as well as a liquid; that is, it is less dense and more active than it was in the form of wine, as well as more powerful. Spirit is the source of life and power, without which material forms are nonliving husks. It interpenetrates matter but is itself nonmaterial.

Many mystics have looked within themselves and identified breath as the evidence of spirit in the body. Breath is nonmaterial, or, at least, it straddles the border between material and nonmaterial reality. It has inherent movement and rhythm and is the source of life and vitality. In many languages the words for spirit and breath are the same: Sanskrit, *prana;* Greek, *pneuma;* Hebrew, *ruach;* Latin, *spiritus.* And in many cultures life is thought to begin with the first breath and end with the last. Until the breath cycle begins, spirit and body are not connected; the fetus and the newborn baby have a vegetative life but are not invested with spirit. Some cultures believe that God allots each person a certain number of breaths and that one's lifetime ends when that number is used up—an argument for learning to breathe more slowly.

A few years ago, I wrote:

At the very center of our being is rhythmic movement, a cyclic expansion and contraction that is both in our body and outside it, that is both in our mind and in our body, that is both in our consciousness and not in it. Breath is the essence of being, and in all aspects of the universe we can see the same rhythmic pattern of expansion and contraction, whether in the cycles of day and night, waking and sleeping, high and low tides, or seasonal growth and decay. Oscillation between two phases exists at every level of reality, even up to the scale of the observable universe itself, which is presently in expansion but will surely at some point contract back to the original, unimaginable point that is everything and nothing, completing one cosmic breath.

If breath is the movement of spirit in the body—a central mystery that connects us to all creation—then working with breath is a form of spiritual practice. It is also one that impacts health and healing, because how we breathe both reflects the state of the nervous system and influences the state of the nervous system. You can learn to regulate heart rate, blood pressure, circulation, and digestion by consciously changing the rhythm and depth of breathing. You can tone the healing system in the same way. I am going to suggest some simple techniques for doing this kind of work. Although you can do each one in a very few minutes, you will not realize their potential power unless you practice them regularly, preferably every day.

1. *Observe the breath*. Sit in a comfortable position with your eyes closed, loosening any tight clothing. Focus your attention on your breathing without trying to influence it in any way. Follow the contours of the cycle through inhalation and exhalation and see if you can perceive the points at which one phase changes into the other. Do this for at least a few minutes. Your goal is simply to keep your attention on the breath cycle and observe. No matter how the breath changes, even if the excursions become very small, just continue to follow them. This is a basic form of meditation, a relaxation method, and a way to harmonize body, mind, and spirit.

2. *Start with exhalation*. Breathing is continuous, with no beginning or end, but we tend to think of one breath as beginning with an inhalation and ending with an exhalation. I want you to try to reverse this perception in the next exercise, which you can do either sitting or lying down. Again,

focus attention on the breath and let it come of its own accord without trying to change it, but now experience exhalation as the beginning of each new cycle. The reason for doing this is that you have more control over exhalation, because you can use the voluntary muscles between your ribs (the intercostal muscles) to squeeze air out of your lungs, and this musculature is much more powerful than that used for drawing air in. When you move more air out, you will automatically take more air in. It is desirable to deepen respiration; the easiest way to do that is to think of exhalation as the first part of the cycle and not worry at all about inhalation.

3. *Let yourself be breathed.* This exercise is best done while lying on your back, so you might want to try it while falling asleep or on waking. Close the eyes, let your arms rest alongside your body, and focus attention on the breath without trying to influence it. Now imagine that with each inhalation the universe is blowing breath into you and with each exhalation withdrawing it. You are the passive recipient of breath. As the universe breathes into you, let yourself feel the breath penetrating to every part of your body, even to the tips of your fingers and toes. Try to hold this perception for ten cycles of exhalation and inhalation.

You may do these first three exercises as often as you like, for as long as you like, up to a maximum of ten minutes, but do them every day.

The next two exercises are formal breathing techniques from *pranayama*, the ancient Indian science of breath control that forms a part of yoga. *Prana* is a term for universal energy, of which breath is the bodily expression, and *pranayama* practice is intended to harmonize body energies and attune them with cosmic energy. These two exercises are safe and very useful. They also take little time; but, again, to determine what they can do for you and your healing capacity, you must practice them regularly.

4. *Take a stimulating breath.* Sit comfortably with the back straight, eyes closed. Place the tongue in the yogic position: touch the tip of the tongue to the backs of the upper front teeth, then slide it just above the teeth until it rests on the

alveolar ridge, the soft tissue between the teeth and the roof of the mouth. Keep it there during the whole exercise. (Yoga philosophy says this contact closes an energy circuit in the body, preventing dissipation of *prana* during breathing practice.) Now breathe in and out rapidly through the nose, keeping the mouth lightly closed. Inhalation and exhalation should be equal and short, and you should feel muscular effort at the base of the neck just above the collarbones and at the diaphragm. (Try putting your hands on these spots to get a sense of the movement.) The action of the chest should be rapid and mechanical, like a bellows pumping air; in fact, the Sanskrit name of this exercise means "bellows breath." Breath should be audible on both inhalation and exhalation, as rapid as three cycles per second if you can do that comfortably.

The first time you try this exercise, do it for just fifteen seconds, then breathe normally. Each time you do it, increase the duration by five seconds until you get up to a full minute. This is real exercise, and you can expect to feel fatigue of the muscles you are using. You will also begin to feel something else: a subtle but definite movement of energy through the body when you return to normal breathing. I feel it as a vibration or tingling, especially in my arms, along with greater alertness and disappearance of fatigue. This is not hyperventilation (which produces physiological changes as a result of blowing off excess carbon dioxide) but a way of activating the central nervous system. Once you can do the bellows breath for a full minute, try using it instead of caffeine as a pick-me-up in the afternoon. I find it particularly useful if I start to feel sleepy while driving on a highway. The more you do it, the more you will become aware of the energy it creates.

5. *Take a relaxing breath.* You may do this sitting with the back straight, lying on the back, or even standing or walking. Place the tongue in the yogic position and keep it there during the whole exercise. Exhale completely through the mouth, making an audible sound. Then close the mouth and inhale quietly through the nose to a (silent) count of four. Then hold the

breath for a count of seven. Then exhale audibly through the mouth to a count of eight. Repeat for a total of four cycles, then breathe normally. If you have difficulty exhaling with your tongue in place, try pursing your lips; you will soon get the knack of how to do it. Note that the speed with which you do the exercise is unimportant. What is important is the ratio of four : seven : eight for inhalation, hold, and exhalation. You will be limited by how long you can comfortably hold the breath, so adjust your counting accordingly. As you practice this breath, you will be able to slow it down, which is desirable. Do it twice a day. After one month, if it agrees with you, increase to eight cycles twice a day.

I do these relaxing breaths in the morning before I meditate and in the evening when I am lying in bed just before falling asleep. I also try to remember to do it whenever I feel anxious or experience an emotional upset. I teach it to almost all patients I see, and I receive reports of remarkable benefits. It cures digestive problems, allows cardiac arrhythmias to subside, lowers high blood pressure, combats anxiety and insomnia, and more. I think of it as a tonic for the nervous system—a spiritual tonic rather than a material one—and cannot recommend it too highly.

These five exercises will get you started on a program of using breath to optimize your healing system. As I said earlier, this is genuine spiritual practice, not just a method of improving health. The science of conscious breathing is not taught in medical schools. Throughout history it has been an esoteric subject, mostly passed on as oral tradition, and even today remarkably few books about it are available.

The energy that you can feel in your body after doing the bellows breath is the energy that Chinese doctors call qi (chi), their term for universal life energy. Most people experience it as warmth or tingling or subtle vibration. With practice you can learn to feel it more, move it about the body, and even transmit it to another person. Many healing systems from both East and West make use of energy transmission, usually through the hands, with or without touch contact between giver and recipient. From China and Japan come systems like reiki, jin shin jyutsu, and johrei; from our own culture comes therapeutic touch, a form of energy healing mostly taught and practiced by nurses. It is useful to try to feel, send, and receive this subtle energy. Not only can this practice relieve pain and accelerate healing; it directs attention toward the spiritual pole of existence, away from the material pole. The more you can experience yourself as energy, the easier it is not to identify yourself with your physical body.

Mystics and spiritual adepts teach that it is possible to raise spiritual energy, to increase its rate of vibration. One way to do this is to put yourself in the vicinity of persons, places, or things that have high spiritual energy. Throughout the world millions of people make pilgrimages to sacred sites—mountains, groves, shrines, and temples— where they feel uplifted, renewed, recharged. You can join them or look in your own territory for places that make you feel good, turn your thoughts to higher purposes, and take you out of yourself. You can also read the writings or life stories of men and women of high spiritual attainment, and you can view great art or objects of special beauty or listen to great music, because beauty in any form has a salutary effect on spirit. A simple way to get this benefit is to have flowers in your living space, since most people find their natural beauty inspiring.

Finally, you can pay attention to how you feel in the presence of various friends and acquaintances. Do some people always make you feel happier and better and more positive? If so, spend more time in their company and less in the company of those with an opposite effect on you. In some way, our spiritual selves resonate with others; if the interaction is positive, human connectedness is a most powerful healer, capable of neutralizing many harmful influences on the material plane.

A much-publicized example is the story of the Italian-Americans of Roseto, Pennsylvania, with their lower-than-expected incidence of coronary heart disease. The town was populated by immigrants from two villages in northern Italy, who came to America in the 1930s seeking better lives. They were a very close-knit community comprising large extended families with strong social bonds. They also ate a lot of calories, meat, and fat, and many smoked tobacco; nonetheless, they had few heart attacks. But their children, now in their fifties and sixties and eating the same diets, have the same incidence of coronary heart disease as other Americans. What changed from the first to the second generation? Researchers who studied these people felt the most significant difference was the loss of extended family and community; the younger generation lives in typical nuclear families with all of the social isolation characteristic of modern life. Somehow the high level of connectedness in the first generation of immigrants protected them from the expected ill effects of high-fat diets and smoking. I classify that kind of beneficial interaction between human beings as a spiritual phenomenon, one that is lacking in the lives of many sick people I see as patients.

14

AN EIGHT-WEEK PROGRAM FOR OPTIMAL HEALING POWER

I HAVE TAKEN the information in the previous chapters and arranged it in the form of week-by-week suggestions to help you change your lifestyle in a way that favors spontaneous healing. Each week's suggestions build on what you have done in the previous week; after two months, you will have created the foundation of a healing lifestyle. Read over the program, then try to set a date when you can begin. When you finish, you can decide how many of the changes you want to incorporate into your lifestyle on a regular basis. If the program seems to move along too fast for you, do not hesitate to slow it down and go at your own pace.

WEEK ONE

Projects

• Go through your pantry and refrigerator and remove all oils other than olive oil. Get rid of any margarine, solid vegetable shortenings, and products made with them. Read labels of all food products so that you can dispose of any containing partially hydrogenated oils. If you do not have any extra-virgin olive oil on hand, buy a bottle and start using it. You might also want to buy a small bottle of organic, expeller-pressed canola oil.

Diet

• Start eating some fresh broccoli this week. If you do not have a favorite way of preparing it, try one of the recipes on pages 151–52.

• Eat salmon, sardines, or kippers at least once this week. If you do not like fish, buy some flax seeds at a health food store, grind them, and sprinkle them over your food.

Supplements

• Start taking vitamin C if you do not do so already: 1,000 to 2,000 milligrams with breakfast, another dose with dinner, and a third at bedtime, if convenient.

Exercise

• Try to walk ten minutes a day for five days of this week. If you are already on a program of aerobic exercise other than walking, do the walk in addition.

Mental/Spiritual

• Think about your own experiences of healing. Make a list of illnesses or injuries or problems you have recovered from in the past two years. Note down anything you did to speed the healing process.

• Practice breath observation (see page 204) for five minutes every day.

• Buy some flowers to keep in your home where you can enjoy them.

WEEK TWO

Projects

• Find out where your drinking water comes from if you do not know and what impurities it might contain. Stop drinking chlorinated water. Get information on a water purifying system for your home, if you do not have one. In the meantime, buy bottled water.

Diet

• Eat fish at least once this week.

• Go to a health food store and look through the frozen and refrigerated sections to familiarize yourself with the many different products made from soybeans. Select one to try.

• Buy some Japanese green tea and try it. If you drink coffee or black tea, try to substitute green tea for some or all of your usual beverage.

Supplements

• Start taking beta carotene, 25,000 IU a day with breakfast.

Exercise

• Increase your daily walk to fifteen minutes and try to do it five days of the week.

Mental/Spiritual

• Pay attention to your mental imagery and make a few notes on kinds of images that have strong emotional impact for you. Think about how you might adapt them to use in healing visualizations.

• Visit a park or some other favorite place in nature. Spend as much time as you can there, doing nothing in particular, just feeling the energy of the place.

• Try a one-day "news fast." Do not read, watch, or listen to any news for a day and see how you feel.

• Begin doing all of the breathing exercises described on pages 204–7.

WEEK THREE

Projects

• Find out where you can buy organic produce. Inquire in grocery stores, health food stores, or use the resource guide at the end of this book. Make a commitment to buy organically produced fruits and vegetables, especially the ones mentioned on page 165.

• If you use an electric blanket, stop. Pack it up and give it away. Remove electric clock radios from the vicinity of your bed. Buy a radiation shield for the video display of your computer. Buy a pair of UV-protective sunglasses if you do not have any.

Diet

• Make a conscious effort to eat an extra serving of fruits and vegetables with at least one meal this week.

• Start eating fish at least twice this week.

• Replace at least one serving of meat with a soy food of your choice.

Supplements

• With lunch or your largest meal take 400 to 800 IU of vitamin E and 200 to 300 micrograms of selenium.

Exercise

• Increase the daily walk to twenty minutes, five days of the week. If you do other aerobic exercise, consider cutting it down to two to three days and substituting an aerobic walk on the other days.

Mental/Spiritual

• Make a list of inspirational books you would like to read in the areas of spirituality, religion, self-help, poetry, biography, or any other category, and select one that you will begin this week.

• Make a list of friends and acquaintances in whose company you feel more alive, happier, more optimistic. Pick one whom you will spend some time with this week.

• Buy more flowers.

WEEK FOUR

Projects

• Check on your bed, mattress, and sleeping location. Is an uncomfortable bed or noisy bedroom interfering with restful sleep? If so, consider making changes, as suggested on pages 191–92.

• Find out about getting an air filter for your home or bedroom if you live in a polluted area.

Diet

• Begin eating some more garlic this week in any form that appeals to you.

• Try to replace another meal of animal protein with soy protein.

Exercise

• Increase your aerobic walk to twenty-five minutes, five days of the week.

Mental/Spiritual

• Try to do two days of news fasting this week.

• Continue to practice the breathing exercises. Make sure that you do the relaxing breath twice a day.

• Contact someone you know to have experienced healing or recovery from illness or injury. Ask for details of the experience.

WEEK FIVE

Projects

• Locate a steam bath or sauna that you can use. Use it for up to twenty minutes one day. It should be hot enough to make you sweat freely; be sure to drink plenty of pure water to replace lost fluid.

Diet

• Try a one-day fruit fast, eating as much fresh fruit as you like but nothing else except water and herbal tea. Take vitamin C but skip the other supplements on this day.

• Buy a piece of fresh ginger root and make yourself some ginger tea, as described on page 175. Also try some crystallized ginger to see if you like it.

Exercise

• Increase your aerobic walk to thirty minutes, five days of the week.

Mental/Spiritual

• See if you can extend your news fast to three days this week.
• Practice the breathing exercises every day.
• Listen to a piece of music that you find inspirational and uplifting.
• Bring more flowers into your home this week.

WEEK SIX

Projects

• Look over the information on tonics on pages 171–85. Decide which one is most appropriate for you and find out where to get it.

• See if you can uncover any other stories of healing in your circle of friends, acquaintances, and business associates.

• Take a steam bath or sauna twice this week.

Diet

• Try a one-day juice fast today: any amount of fruit and vegetable juices you care to drink, plus water and herbal tea. Take vitamin C but skip the other supplements on this day.

• Continue to eat fish twice this week and soy foods twice this week.

• Continue to eat broccoli at least twice.

Exercise

• Increase your aerobic walk to thirty-five minutes, five days this week.

Mental/Spiritual

• Extend your news fast to four days.

• Visit an art museum or try to view some work of art, sculpture, or architecture that you find beautiful and inspiring.

• Continue the breathing exercises every day.

WEEK SEVEN

Projects

• Think about some kind of service work that you could do this week, such as volunteering for a few hours at a hospital or charitable organization or helping someone you know who is disabled or shut in—any activity in which you give some of your time and energy to help others.

• Continue the steam baths or saunas, three times a week if possible.

Diet

• For your fast day this week, drink only fruit juice, water, and herbal tea. Take vitamin C but skip the other supplements on this day.

• On the other days, continue eating as above: at least two meals of fish and two of soy protein, generous servings of fruits, vegetables, whole grains, ginger, and garlic.

Exercise

• Increase the aerobic walk to forty minutes, five days of the week.

Mental/Spiritual

• Reach out to resume connection with someone from whom you are estranged.

• Make time for flowers, music, and art.

• Increase the relaxing breath to eight cycles, twice a day.

WEEK EIGHT

Projects

• Review the changes you have made in your lifestyle in the past eight weeks and think about how many of them you wish to make permanent. Develop a realistic plan that you can stick to over the next eight weeks.

Diet

• Try a one-day water fast this week. You can have herbal tea with lemon if you like, but nothing caloric. If this proves too difficult, drink some diluted fruit juice. Take vitamin C but skip the other supplements.

• Think about how you can continue the dietary changes of this program in coming weeks.

Supplements

• Start taking your tonic. Make a commitment to give it a two-month trial to see what it does for your energy level, resistance, and outlook.

Exercise

• Reach your goal of a forty-five-minute walk, five days of the week.

Mental/Spiritual

• Continue the breathing exercises. Start using the relaxing breath whenever you feel anxious or upset, and be sure to do it at least twice a day.

• Try to maintain your news fast for the whole week. At the end of the week, think about how much news you want to let back into your life in coming weeks.

• Think of people who have hurt you or made you angry. Try to bring yourself to understand their actions and forgive them. Can you express forgiveness to at least one of them?

• Reward yourself with especially beautiful flowers for completing this program, and buy some flowers for someone else.

Congratulations! I have asked you to do a lot in the past two months, some of it unfamiliar and challenging. Know that you have been very good to yourself and your healing system. As a result of the changes you have made, you have a greater chance of experiencing spontaneous healing if the need for it arises. Try to incorporate into your life as many of these steps as you can from now on.

PART THREE

IF YOU GET SICK

15

MAKING THE RIGHT DECISIONS

WHEN YOU GET sick, you must decide what course of action to take in order to recover your health. If you do not accept this responsibility, others will decide for you and will not necessarily make the best choices. The most important decision is whether visits to health professionals will help or hinder your own healing system. You will need to understand the nature of your illness and to know whether conventional medicine can do anything for it without reducing the possibility of spontaneous healing. You will also want to know whether any alternative treatments exist that might be of benefit.

A good place to start is with a review of what conventional medicine can do effectively and what it cannot. For example, it is very effective at managing trauma, so that if I were in a serious automobile accident, I would want to go directly to an urgent care facility in a modern hospital, not to a shaman, guided imagery therapist, or acupuncturist. (Once out of danger, I might use those other resources to speed up the natural healing process.) Conventional medicine is also very good at diagnosing and managing crises of all sorts: hemorrhages, heart attacks, pulmonary edema, acute congestive heart failure, acute bacterial infections, diabetic comas, bowel obstructions, acute appendicitis, and so forth. You must be able to recognize symptoms of potentially serious conditions, so that you will not waste time before getting needed treatment. In general, *symptoms that are unusually severe, persistent, or out of the range of your normal experience warrant immediate investigation.*

CASE EXAMPLE 1: A MEDICAL EMERGENCY

Frederick R., a sixty-five-year-old minister with a fairly healthy lifestyle and a strong commitment to natural medicine, came to me with the complaint of "worsening digestive pain of a year's duration." He said he wanted natural remedies for it, because he did not believe in allopathic medicine. The pain was episodic, beginning in the pit of the stomach, spreading upward to the chest and into the left arm, both sides of the jaw, and into his back. The episodes were becoming more frequent and recently had begun to wake him from sleep. Unable to control the pain himself, Frederick had gone to a gastroenterologist, who did various tests, including endoscopy—putting a tube into the stomach to visualize its lining. The tests revealed a hiatal hernia and a small gallstone that was probably causing no problems. The doctor prescribed a drug to suppress acid production in the stomach; Frederick took it for several months but got no relief. Then he consulted a naturopath who prescribed herbs and dietary changes, also to no avail. Now he was seeing a homeopathic doctor; but after trying several homeopathic remedies, he was no better. He told me the pain was made worse by exertion and by lying flat, made better by sitting up. It had no relation to what he ate or drank.

Burning pain in the chest that is worse lying down and better sitting up is typical of hiatal hernia (in which a portion of the stomach protrudes through the muscular ring at the esophageal junction and may become inflamed as a result of excess acidity), but hiatal hernia pain and digestive pain in general are not made worse by exertion. I questioned Frederick carefully about that association and got a very clear story from him of exertional chest pain, which suggested coronary heart disease, not a problem with his stomach. I asked him if the gastroenterologist or anyone else had taken a cardiogram; no one had. I was convinced from the history alone that this patient was experiencing unstable angina, a medical emergency, and I told him I would work with him only if he went immediately to a cardiologist for a treadmill stress test. I gave him the name of a nearby cardiologist, and he made an appointment for the next day. During the treadmill test, Frederick's heart went into a dangerously irregular rhythm, confirming the suspicion that it was seriously deprived of blood. The cardiologist stopped the test and told Frederick he would not be legally responsible for him if he left the office; he sent him directly to a hospital for emergency coronary artery bypass surgery. Frederick came through the operation well, is now in good health, and carefully follows a heart-healthy lifestyle.

Comment: Frederick's story illustrates the danger of paying insufficient attention to an unusual and persistent symptom that should have alarmed him and the health providers he saw. Any chest pain that wakes a person from sleep or occurs on exertion should be investigated allopathically. Both patients and doctors should know that exertional chest pain is more likely to be coming from the heart than from the digestive system. Without correct medical and surgical intervention Frederick would probably have had a heart attack, possibly a fatal one.

Common sense and intuition can help you analyze symptoms and decide whether they are serious or not. If you are suffering from headaches, for example, you should seek help if you have never before had headaches, if the headaches are more intense than any you have had before, if they last longer than any you have had before, if you have them regularly for a longer period of time than you have ever experienced, or if they are accompanied by other, novel symptoms (like vomiting or visual disturbance). The greater the sense you have of your body's normal range of changes, the more likely you are to pay attention to and seek professional help in diagnosing a symptom that is outside that range and may indicate a problem requiring conventional medical treatment.

Taking advantage of the diagnostic capability of standard medicine does not commit you to accepting its treatments. It is up to you to find out the success rates of conventional treatments as well as to determine their risks. If the treatments are suppressive and toxic, or if medicine has nothing to offer, then it is appropriate to look elsewhere for help. Remember also that whenever you visit conventional doctors—even if it is for diagnostic evaluation only—you must be on guard against their pessimism about healing.

CASE EXAMPLE 2: THE DOCTORS HAD NO IDEAS

Mary K., a forty-year-old intensive care nurse at a university hospital, thought she was in good health until she volunteered for a drug study and had to undergo a preliminary physical examination and blood tests. The blood tests showed elevated liver enzymes and high levels of iron and ferritin, the protein associated with iron storage in the body. She agreed to have a liver biopsy, which showed early cirrhosis and increased iron, but doctors were unable to determine a diagnosis. She told them she had had hepatitis twenty years before, following a period of intravenous drug use. Since then she had used no drugs, had had no recurrences of hepatitis, and had taken good care of herself.

Because she worked in a university medical center, Mary had access to outstanding allopathic specialists, several of whom became interested in her as a puzzling case. They ran further tests, pondered the results, and concluded that her cirrhosis was of unknown origin. They could find no reason for her elevated iron and had no treatments to suggest.

An intelligent person with medical training, Mary had some ideas of her own. She wondered, for example, whether phlebotomy—drawing off blood from a vein—might be a useful way to reduce the excessive iron in her system; but the doctors saw no merit in it. "Of the four specialists I saw initially, not one gave me any option for action or treatment," she wrote. "They did not even tell me there were dietary manipulations that could help reduce the iron load in my body. So where was any cause for hope?" Yet they certainly gave her cause for concern and fear. " 'I know you're thinking cancer,' one of them said to me during a consultation, and I remember saying to myself: 'The thought of cancer never entered my head until you just put it there.' At best, the doctors were tolerant of my ideas but not supportive. They displayed lack of common sense, no willingness to trust intuition, and no ability to be creative. In the end I felt disrespected."

Mary came to see me two years after the first abnormal blood tests. In that time she had avoided red meat and other iron-rich foods and kept up her good health habits. She still felt well but continued to worry about her liver and her iron metabolism. I began by reminding her that the liver has a remarkable capacity for regeneration, especially in a young, otherwise healthy person. I encouraged her to experiment and told her I thought phlebotomy would be worth a try. I also gave her additional suggestions about diet and vitamins and two herbal remedies for her liver: milk thistle (see page 177) and schizandra (the fruit of *Schisandra chinensis*), a Chinese medicine that helps the body heal chronic hepatitis. My impression was that Mary's primary problem was low-grade, chronic hepatitis that rendered her liver susceptible to damage from iron accumulation. Mary told me she knew a family-practice doctor at the university who was willing to supervise the bleeding. Over the next few weeks, she gave a number of units of blood and was delighted to see her iron levels drop and stay within the normal range. Over the next year her liver function gradually returned to normal and has stayed there, so that now she not only looks and feels as healthy as before but is also certified healthy by her medical test results. She no longer worries about cancer or other dire possibilities.

She wrote me recently:

> You and the other doctors who were helpful listened to me, supported me in my desire to experiment, used common sense, and were open to other therapies. You understood that I wanted/needed to heal myself rather than be healed. I don't believe my healing began until I was able to follow my own instincts and act on them. You gave me permission to do that. That's when my faith that I could improve my health began to grow, and instead of just waiting passively I was able to act. I want to tell other patients to search until they find practitioners they can trust, who respect them, listen to them, care about them, *and are competent.*

Comment: Faced with pessimistic doctors who had absolutely nothing to offer her, this patient sought out other professionals who empowered her to experiment with measures that solved her problem. Although she knew intuitively that healing was possible, she needed permission from a doctor to act.

Let me summarize for you what allopathic medicine can and cannot do for you:

CAN:

- Manage trauma better than any other system of medicine.
- Diagnose and treat many medical and surgical emergencies.
- Treat acute bacterial infections with antibiotics.
- Treat some parasitic and fungal infections.

- Prevent many infectious diseases by immunization.
- Diagnose complex medical problems.
- Replace damaged hips and knees.
- Get good results with cosmetic and reconstructive surgery.
- Diagnose and correct hormonal deficiencies.

CANNOT:

- Treat viral infections.
- Cure most chronic degenerative diseases.
- Effectively manage most kinds of mental illness.
- Cure most forms of allergy or autoimmune disease.
- Effectively manage psychosomatic illnesses.
- Cure most forms of cancer.

Here is another good rule to follow: *Do not seek help from a conventional doctor for a condition that conventional medicine cannot treat, and do not rely on an alternative provider for a condition that conventional medicine can manage well.*

LET'S LOOK AT some more case examples of people who made the right decisions about how to resolve illness. I have chosen cases from my practice that are representative of broad classes of disease and that illustrate successful strategies for controlling them.

CASE EXAMPLE 3: NATURAL MEDICINE RELIEVES RHEUMATOID ARTHRITIS

Joyce N., a seventy-year-old retired teacher, has had rheumatoid arthritis for almost forty years. Despite pain and deformity in her hands and neck, she is a cheerful, positive woman, who, to my surprise, told me she had never taken any medication stronger than aspirin for her symptoms. "Many doctors over the years tried to talk me into taking gold, prednisone, and other strong drugs," she told me at our first meeting, "but I knew intuitively that they would not be good for me, and I always refused. I have a high tolerance for pain and have been able to manage using aspirin alone." Joyce came to see me at the beginning of one November, saying that her pain had increased recently, which worried her, because it was the beginning of the winter season, usually her worst time. "Is there anything you can suggest that might help me live with this condition more comfortably?" she asked.

I had never before met anyone with severe rheumatoid arthritis who had been able to avoid the strong suppressive drugs that allopathic doctors prescribe for it. Although Joyce was a quiet, retiring woman with significant deformity from her disease, she radiated a glow of emotional contentment. The glow increased when she described her marriage and family life, making me feel that this was the source of the inner strength that enabled her to live so well with chronic pain. I discovered also that she knew little about options for moderating rheumatoid arthritis without prescription drugs and told her I thought she could expect great improvement if she would make changes in her diet and activity, take a few supplements, and explore the mind/body connection. I asked her to eliminate all dairy products, eat less meat, add fish sources of omega-3 fatty acids, and eliminate all polyunsaturated and partially hydrogenated fats. I recommended an antioxidant formula (see pages 159–61) and an herbal remedy, feverfew (*Tanacetum parthenium*), which is nontoxic and known to alleviate rheumatoid arthritis. I recommended that she begin to swim regularly and to practice the relaxing breath (pages 206–7). Finally, I sent her to a hypnotherapist, who is skilled at working with chronically ill people. The patient reported back six weeks later that she had followed this program faithfully and was amazed at the degree of improvement she had experienced, all the more remarkable because it was now the coldest, wettest time of year, when she expected to suffer the most.

Comment: Rheumatoid arthritis is a prototypical autoimmune disease. (Others in this class are lupus, scleroderma, and multiple sclerosis.) Autoimmunity has an inherent tendency to wax and wane, with the ups and downs often mirroring emotional highs and lows. Conventional medicine has only immunosuppressive drugs to offer, which may be necessary for getting through periods of severe exacerbation of symptoms but are inappropriate for long-term treatment. The chronic inflammation of autoimmunity often causes pain and eventual damage to body structures, but inflammation can be moderated by a variety of nontoxic methods, especially dietary change and herbal remedies. Hypnotherapy and guided imagery therapy are often very effective at nudging the disease in the direction of remission. This patient's rapid and dramatic response to natural medicine, despite her age and the chronicity of her disease, may be due to two factors: her never having used suppressive medication and her psychospiritual good health, rooted in positive relationships and high self-esteem.

CASE EXAMPLE 4: TURNING AROUND CHRONIC DERMATITIS

Nancy S., the forty-five-year-old wife of a successful surgeon, developed an itching, red rash on both hands that gradually spread to much of her body. The skin became thickened, cracked, and raw, causing her great discomfort. She saw several dermatologists, who told her the problem was dermatitis of unknown origin and prescribed steroid creams and oral prednisone. Prednisone made the rash disappear; but knowing its toxicity with long-term use, Nancy stopped it, whereupon the condition returned worse than before. This experience, repeated several times, made her wary of using steroids in any form. Eventually she went to a leading dermatologist in another city who biopsied the skin and told her that she might have a rare form of lymphoma, a cancer with a bad prognosis. This made her quite upset, although a subsequent biopsy by yet another dermatologist failed to support this possibility. The doctors had no treatments to offer other than steroids and antihistamines to control the itching. As the condition progressed, Nancy became fatigued, and her awareness of disfigurement led her to retreat from social contact into depression and isolation. She spent most of her time lying in bed or soaking her body in soothing baths.

When she came to see me, she had had the dermatitis for two years. One month before, she had consulted a homeopath, who gave her remedies that did not work, but she still felt there must be some way to solve the problem. In listening to her history, I thought it was significant that her children had left home about the time of the onset of her problem. Her husband's profession left him little time for home life, and she generally felt uprooted and isolated since they moved from another part of the country some years before. I assured her that her body could heal itself if given a chance, outlined a low-protein diet that excluded milk, and recommended supplementation with black currant oil, a source of an unusual fatty acid (GLA, gamma-linolenic acid), good for the health of the skin. I also taught her to make a tea of a desert shrub (chaparral, *Larrea divaricata*) for application to affected areas; recommended calendula lotion, another herbal product available in health food stores; and sent her to a hypnotherapist. This last suggestion frightened her, because she did not like the idea of "anyone taking over my mind," but she implemented the other recommendations, and her husband supported her in following them. He even bought her a little stove to brew the strong-smelling chaparral tea out of doors. She came to love this ritual and found the tea very soothing. After six weeks she began to experience some improvement but still had not made an appointment with the hypnotherapist. It took much urging to get her to overcome her reluctance; when she did, she was pleasantly surprised. The hypnotherapist taught her relaxation methods, which she now practices faithfully. Her improvement accelerated and has continued steadily; she has been able to dispense with the antihistamines and steroids and resume her social life.

Comment: Dermatitis is an allergic and psychosomatic condition, for which conventional medicine can offer only suppressive therapies. Diseases of the skin (and gastrointestinal tract) should be assumed to have an emotional basis until proved otherwise, because these systems are the most frequent sites of expression of stress-induced imbalances. Mind/body interventions combined with lifestyle change and nontoxic symptomatic management will often allow the body to heal itself completely from these conditions.

CASE EXAMPLE 5: CHILDREN WHO ARE ALWAYS SICK

Terry, age six, and Ryan, age four, were spending more of their time on antibiotics than off. Their frustrated parents brought them to me in the hope that I could suggest a way to change their pattern of continual ear infections, colds, and bronchitis. "We'll try anything," they told me, adding that they liked their pediatrician but felt he knew how to do only one thing: prescribe drugs. Both boys were active and well developed, apparently healthy except for the susceptibility to upper respiratory and ear infections. I explained to the parents that frequent use of antibiotics can worsen the very problem it is meant to alleviate, both by weakening immunity and by increasing the number and virulence of resistant germs. I suggested they try to reserve antibiotics for very severe infections after other remedies had failed. I taught them how to use echinacea, an herbal immune enhancer and antibiotic substitute made from the root of a native American plant (*Echinacea purpurea*, purple coneflower) that is nontoxic and readily available in health food stores. As general preventive measures I recommended excluding milk and milk products from the boys' diet, giving them daily doses of vitamin C, and taking them to an osteopath specializing in cranial therapy in order to relieve any restrictions in their breathing. The parents implemented all of these suggestions, and within three months the children's pattern of illness changed. Now episodes of infection are infrequent, and use of antibiotics in this household is unusual.

Comment: Antibiotics are powerful tools for containing susceptible infections but must be reserved for instances where they are really needed. The frequent use of antibiotics is not wise. In case of recurrent or chronic infections, it is important to increase natural resistance. Disease-causing germs are always present, but by enhancing immunity and natural healing capacity it is possible to reduce the chance that they can harm us. Doctors must bear much of the responsibility for getting us into our growing predicament with aggressive bacteria; by overprescribing and misprescribing antibiotics, they have brought on the coming catastrophe.

CASE EXAMPLE 6: REVERSING CHRONIC DISEASE BY CHANGING LIFESTYLE

When Henry D. was diagnosed with adult-onset diabetes at age sixty, his doctor started him on an oral hypoglycemic drug and advised him to exercise and lose weight. At about the same time Henry's blood pressure, which had long been in the high normal range, climbed to levels requiring treatment, so his doctor also prescribed an antihypertensive drug. Henry did not like its side effects and stopped taking it, but his doctor scared him into starting again by saying he would probably have a stroke without it. Henry took it but complained constantly. Shortly afterward, his wife, who was also overweight and hypertensive, read an article about a center that offered residential programs of lifestyle modification to treat cardiovascular diseases. The program emphasized a very low-fat diet (ten percent of total calories from fat), exercise, relaxation training, group discussion, and lectures aimed at helping people incorporate the program's changes into their lives upon returning home. Henry and his wife signed up for a ten-day program and loved it. On returning home they began cooking food according to the program's guidelines and exercising regularly. Henry's wife eventually lost twenty pounds, while Henry lost thirty-two. Both of them saw their blood pressure return to normal without medication, and Henry's diabetes disappeared as well. They say they feel much better now; both have more energy and greater confidence in their own healing abilities.

Comment: Lifestyle modification is a proven method for reversing a number of common, debilitating, chronic diseases, including hypertension, non-insulin-dependent diabetes, and coronary heart disease. The only requirement for patients is motivation.

CASE EXAMPLE 7: STOMACH PAIN

Ben K., a thirty-eight-year-old environmental consultant, suffered from chronic upper gastrointestinal pain and discomfort that he had lived with for several years. Eventually the episodes forced him to seek help from a family-practice doctor, who prescribed a course of antibiotics and a strong acid-suppressive drug. The doctor told Ben that he probably had an infection with *Helicobacter pylori,* the germ now believed to cause many cases of peptic ulcer and gastritis; hence the antibiotics. He did not give Ben any advice about changing his lifestyle or diet. On his own, Ben cut out coffee, which he had been drinking regularly, and started practicing relaxation techniques. When I saw him, three weeks into the treatment, the pain had lessened but was not entirely gone. I advised him to discontinue the acid-

suppressive drug and to substitute a licorice extract called DGL,*
which strengthens the mucus coating in the stomach, making it more
resistant to acid. I encouraged him to eliminate caffeine entirely and
to practice the relaxing breath. One month later, he was free of pain.

Comment: The doctor prescribed antibiotics without conducting
a test to determine if *Helicobacter* was present. Antigen testing for
this bacterium is very simple and should be done in all cases of persistent upper GI pain. If the test is positive, a course of antibiotic
treatment (two different drugs) plus a course of bismuth subsalicy-
late (the active ingredient in Pepto Bismol) is definitely indicated. In
this case, the doctor did not prescribe the correct antibiotic regimen
and left out the bismuth. Of course, he did not know about DGL,
since few conventional doctors are familiar with botanical remedies.
This is a case where selective allopathic diagnostic work and treatment combined with alternative treatment was in the patient's best
interest.

CASE EXAMPLE 8: IRREGULAR HEARTBEAT

Marjorie O., a sixty-two-year-old widow, was bothered by irregular
heartbeats: frequent "skipped beats" and runs of rapid beats. Her
internist examined her and took an electrocardiogram, which
showed premature ventricular contractions, a common, usually
benign arrhythmia that people perceive as skipped beats. He recommended an antiarrhythmic drug, but Marjorie declined to take it,
because she was afraid of toxicity. When I saw her, I determined that
her habits of diet and exercise were good. I advised her to avoid caffeine, to practice the relaxing breath twice a day, and to take supplemental magnesium, which helps stabilize irritable muscle tissue in the
heart. With this regimen, her irregular heartbeats disappeared and
have not returned.

Comment: Marjorie's use of conventional medicine to rule out a
serious heart condition was appropriate, as was her refusal to take a
strong chemical drug before exploring safer alternatives.

---

* Deglycyrrhizinated licorice is an extract of licorice root (*Glycyrrhiza glabra*) with
a fraction removed that can cause sodium retention and elevated blood pressure. It
is available in health food stores.

CASE EXAMPLE 9: ULCERATIVE COLITIS AND CHINESE MEDICINE

Susan K. was diagnosed with ulcerative colitis in her mid-twenties. The disease had gone in and out of remission; but now, at age thirty-five, she required much suppressive medication, including prednisone, to keep the symptoms under control. She had frequent episodes of abdominal pain and diarrhea, and her doctor told her that if the condition worsened, the only remedy would be surgery to remove a length of affected colon. Although Susan hated being so dependent on doctors and drugs, she had been unable to find other ways to manage the colitis. She had been through psychotherapy, biofeedback, and several forms of relaxation training, and felt she had explored the mental/emotional roots of her illness without discovering practical solutions. I taught her the relaxing breath and urged her to keep exploring. Then on a trip away from home she suffered a severe exacerbation of symptoms and feared she might have to check in to a hospital. Instead she was able to find a Chinese doctor who practiced traditional Chinese medicine. He gave her instructions for making rice gruel, which he prescribed as her sole nourishment during the crisis, and treated her with acupuncture and herbal teas. After a few days the symptoms subsided without the need for allopathic intervention. With continued acupuncture and herbal treatment, the colitis went into remission, and Susan was able to eliminate most of the suppressive drugs.

Comment: Ulcerative colitis (and its relative, Crohn's disease) is a complex problem with genetic, autoimmune, and psychosomatic components. Suppressive medication is often required during periods of exacerbation but is never curative. Traditional Chinese medicine, with its unique therapies, may be able to manage illnesses of this sort with much less risk and expense.

CASE EXAMPLE 10: ASTHMA AND AYURVEDIC MEDICINE

Michael B., a twenty-seven-year-old university student, had a long history of allergic asthma, controlled imperfectly with an array of allopathic drugs. He used a bronchodilator inhaler, a steroid inhaler, and oral theophylline, another bronchodilator; previously he had gone through several series of desensitization shots for some of the allergens that he reacted to most strongly. Nevertheless, his asthma attacks gradually became more frequent, forcing him to restrict his activities. When I saw him, he had just moved, because he felt the carpeting in his old apartment was a problem, and he now found it difficult to exercise because of breathing difficulties. Michael ate a healthy diet, took vitamins, and had experimented with a number of alternative treatments, including homeopathy, dietary change, and herbs. Nothing had given him substantial improvement. He worried that he was becoming more dependent on medication and might soon have to start taking oral prednisone, which he wanted to avoid at all costs.

I recommended further modifications in his diet, suggested he buy an air filter for his bedroom, and told him to take a natural product called quercetin, which reduces allergic responsiveness. I also sent him to an osteopath for manipulative treatment to free up restrictions in his chest. These measures helped some. Later, Michael called to tell me he had consulted a practitioner of Ayurvedic medicine in New Mexico, with wonderful results. Ayurveda is the traditional healing system of India, based on classifying people into constitutional types, then recommending appropriate dietary and herbal therapy. The practitioner had given Michael a list of foods to eat and a list of foods to avoid, along with herbal remedies and instructions for a detoxifying regimen. After two months on this program, Michael's asthma subsided to such an extent that he was able to dispense with most of his medication. He now uses his bronchodilator inhaler only occasionally, mainly before starting exercise, and finds that he can tolerate exposure to many allergens that he could not tolerate previously. This is the first time in his adult life that he has had long periods free of any breathing difficulties.

Comment: Bronchial asthma is not one disease but several. Some forms respond more easily to treatment than others. Allopathic measures are toxic and addictive, yet it is often impossible to do without them. The potential for spontaneous healing of asthma is significant, especially with major lifestyle change or application of alternative medical methods. The Ayurvedic approach, with its emphasis on the right diet for each person and its wealth of medicinal plants upon which to draw, might be worth exploring if you have a stubborn, chronic disease that conventional medicine cannot cure.

CASE EXAMPLE 11: LONG-TERM HIV INFECTION

Mark M. knows exactly when he got infected with the AIDS virus and from whom he got it. It was in 1983 from a male sexual partner; the man's previous partner died shortly afterward. One month after this contact Mark became very sick with a skin rash and a mysterious pneumonia that was never identified. He remained very sick for three months, then recovered and has been healthy ever since. In 1985 he tested positive for HIV. At that time his helper T cell count was over 1,000. (Helper T cells are the targets of HIV; as their numbers decline, people become more susceptible to opportunistic infections.) In 1989 his T cell count had dropped to 700.

Since his recovery from the initial infection, Mark has been very conscientious about his health, especially about his diet and mental state. He eats a lot of raw garlic—one head a day, chopped and mixed with food—because he read about garlic's beneficial effects on the immune system. He also eats a lot of hot chile peppers and buys only organically produced food, including some meat and chicken and a substantial quantity of fruits, fruit juice, and vegetables. He takes vitamins, drinks purified water, and walks, swims, and gardens regularly. He lives in a monogamous relationship, works as director of a program that provides counseling for persons with HIV, and creates art objects that he uses in healing rituals. In 1991, Mark's T cell count was up to 1,300; and when he was last tested, in 1994, it was still 1,300, which is in the normal range.

"The medical professionals gave me six to eighteen months to live when I was first diagnosed," Mark told me when I met him. "Since 1985 I can't tell you how many doctors have shown me the Curve— that is, the graph showing the percentage of people per year who develop AIDS after infection. They all try to tell me I'm somewhere along it, headed for destruction. This is really Western medicine's fascination with illness. Here I am with normal T cells, in great health, and they have the audacity to tell me I'm on this curve heading for death. When I see doctors now, I tell them right at the start:

'Look, I don't even want to hear about your curve. Just check me out, answer my questions, and keep your opinions to yourself!' They have also all tried to get me to take AZT [the antiviral drug that is conventional medicine's current treatment of choice for HIV], but all of the people I've known who have used it are dead, so I've refused. And none of them have been interested to hear what I'm doing to stay healthy. They pat me on the head and say, 'Whatever you're doing, just keep it up!'

"I have developed an ability not to buy into the medical system and a willingness to accept that I have control over what happens to me with HIV. I am also committed to not being afraid. I use visualization every day to neutralize fear; I've been doing it since I was a kid, because I came from a disastrous family and was subjected to incest and a lot of verbal and physical abuse. Things come up every day—like a funny spot on my arm recently. I visualized it going away, and it did. It was nothing. I'm also in ongoing psychotherapy. For the past seven years I've used it to keep centered. In my work I act as a healthy role model for persons newly diagnosed with HIV. I counsel them and don't reveal that I'm HIV-positive till later. It's an effective technique. Many of these people, especially as a result of their interactions with doctors, think they'll die within two years. I'm here to show them it doesn't have to be that way."

I did not have much to tell Mark except to make him aware of some of the Chinese herbal tonics that look promising for keeping HIV in remission.

Comment: With a life-threatening illness for which conventional medicine has no effective treatment, it takes conscious effort to get needed services from doctors (like monitoring of T cell counts) without taking on their pessimism. One of the most interesting and encouraging features of HIV infection is its tendency to go into a long latent period before it begins to compromise immunity. Conventional therapy centers on chemical weapons against the virus, but these drugs are all toxic and may select for strains of HIV that are less inclined to live in balance with their human hosts. For many years, medical doctors paid no attention to long-term survivors of HIV infection like Mark. Now enough cases have surfaced that researchers are beginning to study them. One possibility is that some of these people are infected with less virulent strains of HIV and may have developed immunity to them (which could help scientists develop an effective vaccine). Many long-term survivors have relied on healthy lifestyles and therapies to support the healing system, such as Chinese herbal remedies. If the latent period of HIV infection could be extended to twenty-five or thirty years, people with the virus might live out relatively normal lives. (They could, of course, still infect others.)

THESE CASE EXAMPLES show how correct decisions about treatment, particularly about whether and how to use conventional medicine, can allow the healing system to resolve a variety of serious health problems. Once you establish the right relationship with the conventional system, your next task is to make wise choices from among the great variety of alternative therapies now available.

16

CONSIDERING THE ALTERNATIVES

WHEN YOU VENTURE out of the world of standard medicine to look for alternative treatments, it is even more important to be an informed consumer. Alternative medical practices range from those that are grounded in long traditions of careful work to those that are nonsensical. In general, alternative treatments are less risky than allopathic drugs and surgery, but they can be expensive and wasteful of time and effort. I have written at length elsewhere about the history and philosophy of major systems of alternative medicine; what I will do here is give capsule summaries of a number of popular therapies, along with indications for their use. You will find a guide to locating practitioners in the Appendix to this book.

ACUPUNCTURE

Insertion of needles into particular points of the body is a unique therapeutic intervention of traditional Chinese medicine (TCM); Western doctors have taken the technique out of context, using it mostly to treat acute and chronic pain. As a symptomatic treatment for pain, acupuncture has the advantage of being free of the side effects of analgesic drugs, although relief is usually temporary, necessitating frequent visits to the therapist. I have known acupuncture to cure the pain, pressure, and congestion of acute sinus infections as well as to speed the healing of joint injuries. Some dentists use it as the sole form of anesthesia for dental work, including drilling and extraction of teeth. Another interesting use is in addiction treatment: placement of needles in points in the ear has helped some people quit smoking, withdraw from heroin and cocaine, and moderate addictive eating. In TCM acupuncture is used to manipulate energy flows around the body, not primarily to relieve pain or change behavior.

AYURVEDIC MEDICINE

One of the oldest medical systems in the world, Ayurveda has only recently become widely available in the West. Practitioners diagnose by observing patients, questioning them, touching them, and taking pulses. With this information the practitioner is able to assign patients to one of three major constitutional types and then to various subtypes. This classification dictates dietary modifications and selection of remedies. Ayurvedic remedies are primarily herbal, drawing on the vast botanical wealth of the Indian subcontinent, but may include animal and mineral ingredients, even powdered gemstones. Other treatments include steam baths and oil massages.

Although Ayurvedic herbs are little known outside India and few have been studied by modern methods, many may have great therapeutic value. For example, guggul (*Commiphora mukul*), a plant indicated traditionally for control of obesity, has been shown to lower cholesterol in a manner similar to pharmaceutical drugs used for that purpose, but with much less risk. An extract of it called gugulipid is now available in health food stores. Another Ayurvedic preparation, called triphala, is the best bowel regulator I have come across, much better than Western herbal remedies for constipation. It is a mixture of three fruits and can be found in capsule form in health food stores.

Finding a good Ayurvedic doctor takes some effort. Many practitioners in the West are members of the international religious organization of Maharishi Mahesh Yogi, the Holland-based billionaire, whose promotion of Ayurveda is definitely a for-profit endeavor. (In India Ayurveda is medicine of the people, an inexpensive alternative to allopathic treatment. Maharishi Ayurveda is anything but inexpensive.) This group offers training programs for physicians that certify them to be Ayurvedic practitioners after minimal exposure to the philosophy and methods of the system. I recommend seeking out practitioners who are independent of this organization. One way to find them is by inquiring in Indian communities, even in Indian restaurants and grocery stores.

BIOFEEDBACK

Training in biofeedback, a relaxation technique employing electronic equipment to amplify body responses until they become perceptible, is offered by certified therapists, many of them clinical psychologists. In the most common version, patients learn to raise the temperature of their hands and by so doing relax the whole sympathetic nervous system, which controls many involuntary functions. Biofeedback training is enjoyable, and almost everyone succeeds at it. It is especially useful for alleviating Raynaud's disease (see page 15), migraine, hypertension, bruxism (involuntary grinding of the teeth, especially during sleep), temporomandibular joint (TMJ) syndrome, and other ailments with a prominent stress component. Brainwave biofeedback, requiring more complex technology, may be helpful for people with seizure disorders, narcolepsy, and other central nervous system problems.

It is easy to find biofeedback therapists—they are usually listed in the yellow pages of the telephone book—but harder to find ones who are creative and do not use the technology in a mechanical fashion. A typical training program consists of ten one-hour sessions as well as daily practice on your own. Biofeedback teaches you what it feels like to be relaxed internally. It is then up to you to recreate the feeling and make it part of your way of being.

BODY WORK

In addition to prescribing massage therapy as a form of stress reduction, I often recommend specific kinds of body work. Here are the four I most prefer:

- *Feldenkrais work* is a system of movements, floor exercises, and body work designed to retrain the central nervous system, particularly to help it find new pathways around any areas of blockage or damage. Feldenkrais work is innovative, gentle, and often strikingly effective at rehabilitating victims of trauma, cerebral palsy, stroke, and other serious disabilities. I find it to be much more useful than standard physical therapy.

• *Rolfing,* a more invasive form of body work, aims at restructuring the musculoskeletal system by working on patterns of tension held in deep tissue. The therapist applies firm pressure to different areas of the body, which can be painful while it is administered. "Getting Rolfed" means going through a basic series of ten sessions, each focusing on a different part of the body. Rolfing can release repressed emotions as well as dissipate habitual muscle tension.

• *Shiatsu,* a traditional healing art from Japan, makes use of firm finger pressure applied to specified points on the body and is intended to increase the circulation of vital energy. The client lies on the floor with the therapist seated alongside. Japanese practitioners use much firmer pressure than many Westerners find comfortable, but it is worth tolerating because shiatsu can be remarkably effective at dissipating muscle tension and recharging the body. Western practitioners generally use a lighter touch.

• *Trager work* is one of the least invasive forms of body work, using gentle rocking and bouncing motions to induce states of deep, pleasant relaxation. In addition to its relaxing effects, Trager work can also help facilitate the nervous system's communication with muscles, so that it can be helpful as a rehabilitation method, especially for people suffering from traumatic injuries, disabilities, post-polio syndrome, and other chronic neuromuscular problems.

TRADITIONAL CHINESE MEDICINE (TCM)

Traditional Chinese medicine is a comprehensive system of diagnosis and treatment that has now established itself throughout the world. Practitioners include Chinese immigrants and Westerners trained in China or in numerous schools in other countries. Diagnosis in TCM is based on history, on observation of the body (especially the

tongue), on palpation, and on pulse diagnosis, an elaborate procedure requiring considerable skill and experience. Treatment involves
dietary change, massage, medicinal teas and other preparations made
primarily from herbs but also including animal ingredients, and
acupuncture. The Chinese herbal pharmacopeia is vast, with many
plants now under serious scrutiny by Western pharmacologists.
Many Chinese remedies appear to have significant therapeutic value,
and some work on conditions for which Western doctors have no
pharmaceutical drugs.

In my experience, TCM is worth trying for a wide range of allergic,
autoimmune, infectious, and chronic degenerative conditions, including asthma, ulcerative colitis, Crohn's disease, chronic bronchitis,
chronic sinusitis, osteoarthritis, chronic fatigue syndrome, HIV infection and other states of immune deficiency, sexual deficiency, and general debility.

CHIROPRACTIC

Chiropractic has come a long way since the days of its invention a century ago. Today's chiropractors have had basic scientific education and
are not likely to claim that spinal adjustment alone can cure cancer,
diabetes, or any other serious disease. In my experience chiropractors
still take too many X-rays and are too likely to have patients commit
to long and costly treatment packages. (Some people see their chiropractors once or twice a week just to get adjusted, whether or not they
have anything wrong with them.) Chiropractic treatment can be helpful in cases of acute musculoskeletal pain, tension headaches, and
recovery from trauma; it is less effective with chronic pain syndromes.

GUIDED IMAGERY AND VISUALIZATION THERAPY

At several points in this book (see pages 93–7 and 199–201) I have
indicated my enthusiasm for these methods of employing the
mind/body connection to modify illness. Here I will simply repeat my
assertion that no disease process is beyond the reach of these therapies
and that it is best to work with a trained professional, at least initially,
to ensure you are using them correctly. Guided imagery and visualiza-

tion can enhance the effectiveness of other treatments, including allopathic drugs and surgery. Certainly try them for all autoimmune disorders and for any illness in which healing seems blocked or stalled.

HERBAL MEDICINE

As a physician with botanical training, I recommend herbal treatments for a wide range of diseases. Unfortunately, few allopathic physicians have the knowledge or experience to do this. You are more likely to find knowledgeable practitioners in the fields of Ayurvedic medicine, traditional Chinese medicine, and naturopathy. There are also professional herbalists, persons who do not have degrees in any of the major systems of medicine but who have studied on their own or with experienced preceptors.

To be a wise consumer of the great variety of herbal remedies available in health food stores, you must buy reliable preparations and brands. Tinctures (alcoholic extracts), freeze-dried extracts, and standardized extracts are recommended. Herbal medicines tend to be milder than chemical drugs and produce their effects more slowly; they are also much less likely to cause toxicity, because they are dilute forms of drugs rather than concentrated ones.

HOLISTIC MEDICINE

Holistic doctors subscribe to the principles that human beings are more than their physical bodies and that good medicine should embrace the whole spectrum of available treatments, not just the drugs and surgery of conventional medicine. Although holistic doctors share a common general philosophy, there is little uniformity of practice from one to the next, nor is there any assurance that a doctor is good just because he or she is a member of a holistic medical association.

HOMEOPATHY

Homeopathic medicine, a system of diagnosis and treatment based on the use of highly diluted remedies made from natural substances, has a distinguished two-hundred-year history and is now enjoying new popularity. Its main virtue is that it cannot possibly cause harm, because the medicines it employs are so diluted. Homeopaths say that the diluted substances work on the body's energy field, catalyzing natural healing responses; critics charge that homeopathic remedies are nothing but placebos.

It is confusing to seek homeopathic treatment today, because it is practiced in many different forms by people with very different training. Classical homeopathy—the kind taught by the founder of the system—specifies the administration of one dose of one remedy selected on the basis of information gained during a lengthy interview with the patient. Nonclassical homeopathy prescribes multiple or regular doses of formulas combining several remedies. Homeopathic practitioners may be M.D.'s, osteopaths, naturopaths, chiropractors, or lay persons without formal training as health professionals. My own preference would be to seek out classical homeopathy from an M.D., but I have met a few highly accomplished lay homeopaths. Homeopathic remedies are now widely sold in both drugstores and health food stores, another deviation from the classical system, which requires the expertise of a doctor to pick the proper remedy for each individual.

Although I cannot explain how homeopathy works in scientific terms, I have known it to be effective for a diversity of health problems, including allergies, skin and digestive ailments, rheumatoid arthritis, ear and upper respiratory infections in children, gynecological problems, and headaches. Homeopaths often object to combining their treatment with other types of treatment, especially allopathic drugs, herbal medicines, and vitamins and supplements. They also believe that coffee, camphor, mint, and a few other substances act as antidotes to the remedies and must be avoided once you begin treatment with this system.

HYPNOTHERAPY

Hypnotherapy takes advantage of the mind/body connection by encouraging patients to enter a trance, a state of heightened suggestibility. In this state, verbal suggestions are often able to pass from the mind to the nervous system, influencing the body in ways that seem impossible in ordinary states of awareness. I frequently refer patients to hypnotherapists because I have seen it produce excellent results in many illnesses that are managed poorly by conventional medicine, among them a wide range of skin and gastrointestinal ailments, allergy and autoimmune disease, and chronic pain. Some people fear hypnotherapy, seeing it as mind control; but, in fact, hypnotherapists simply arrange circumstances to allow patients to move on their own into natural states of focused concentration, similar to daydreaming or watching a movie. Patients then learn to re-create the experience on their own. It is important to shop around for a therapist you trust and feel comfortable with. One problem I encounter as a referring physician is that many hypnotherapists lack imagination and limit their work to relaxation, pain control, and overcoming bad habits. If I send them patients with challenging physical diseases like multiple sclerosis or ulcerative colitis, they are likely to regard these problems as beyond their expertise and are reluctant to take them on. So as well as being someone you can trust, a good hypnotherapist should be inventive and willing to try new strategies to access spontaneous healing.

NATUROPATHY

Many people think of naturopathic physicians as being "New Age." In fact, naturopathy comes from the old tradition of European health spas with their emphasis on hydrotherapy, massage, and nutritional and herbal treatment. Older naturopaths may actually be chiropractors with mail-order degrees in naturopathy. Younger naturopaths are well trained in basic sciences and have had exposure to subjects omitted from the conventional medical curriculum, such as nutritional and herbal medicine. Except for their adherence to a general philosophy of taking advantage of the body's natural healing capacity and avoiding the drugs and surgery of conventional medicine, naturopaths show a great deal of individuality in their styles of practice. Some use acupuncture, some use body work, some practice herbalism, others practice homeopathy.

As a profession, naturopathy is smaller than the other major systems of alternative medicine, licensed in only a few states in the United States, mostly in the West. Good naturopaths are worth consulting for childhood illnesses, recurrent upper respiratory infections and sinusitis, gynecological problems, and all ailments for which conventional doctors have only suppressive treatments. Naturopaths can be valuable as advisors to help people design healthy lifestyles.

OSTEOPATHIC MANIPULATIVE THERAPY (OMT)

Most osteopaths (D.O.'s) today are indistinguishable from M.D.'s in their reliance on drugs and surgery; only a small percentage of them still use manipulation as a primary therapeutic modality. Unlike chiropractic, osteopathic manipulation does not focus solely on the spine but works on all parts of the body, often with gentler techniques than the high-velocity adjustments favored by chiropractors. Since osteopaths have the same educational background as M.D.'s, they are much more competent than chiropractors in assessing general health problems. Skilled practitioners of OMT can relieve a variety of acute and chronic musculoskeletal problems, undo effects of past traumas (like automobile accidents), and help treat headaches and TMJ syndrome. Cranial therapy, a specialized form of OMT, may benefit asthma, recurrent ear infections in children, sleep disorders, and other conditions rooted in nervous system imbalances. I frequently refer patients to D.O.'s for OMT and often encourage medical students to learn the technique, because I have found it to be safe and highly effective.

RELIGIOUS HEALING

A considerable body of research data supports the beneficial effects of prayer on health. Good documentation also exists for the efficacy of Christian Science healing. It is reasonable to think that belief on the part of patients is the crucial factor here; however, some research shows prayer to be effective even when sick people are unaware that they are the objects of prayer, suggesting that unknown mechanisms might also be at work. Since religious practices can clearly activate healing responses and cannot cause direct harm, there is no reason not to use them as adjunctive or primary treatments in cases of medically hopeless disease.

THERAPEUTIC TOUCH

Therapeutic touch, a form of energy healing taught and practiced mostly by nurses, is a learnable skill of great utility. It can relieve pain without the side effects of drugs, can speed healing from injury, and can identify and dissipate energy blockages that may be impeding the healing system. As with prayer, therapeutic touch cannot harm, so there is no reason not to try it. Many healers outside the therapeutic touch movement also work by the laying on of hands and achieve good results. In addition, you can learn to use this therapy on yourself. Put yourself in a relaxed state and begin by trying to sense and transmit energy with the palms of the hands; then direct it to a part of the body that is hurting.

17

SEVEN STRATEGIES
OF SUCCESSFUL PATIENTS

IN ADDITION TO the case reports already recounted, I have known and interviewed many other patients who have experienced spontaneous healing. Reflecting on their stories, I have identified a few common strategies they used, strategies that would benefit anyone who is sick and struggling with difficult decisions. If more patients adopted them, I believe, the incidence of spontaneous healing would rise dramatically.

I observe that successful patients:

1. DO NOT TAKE "NO" FOR AN ANSWER

Most of the people whose experiences I have related heard discouraging words from health professionals, especially from medical doctors who told them there was no hope, nothing more to be done, and no possibility of getting better. They did not buy it. Instead they never gave up hope that there was help to be found somewhere.

The young man with chronic autoimmune disease, described on page 99, had been told for years by hematologists that nothing could be done for him but to maintain him on the high doses of steroids that were destroying his health. For years he accepted that view, but as the toxicity of suppressive treatment became more and more obvious, he acted on his intuitive belief that other methods had to exist and began a search that led him to me. I told him I thought he could alter the behavior of his immune system by making significant changes in his lifestyle, exploring alternative therapies, and working with mind/body approaches. He was interested but skeptical. I gave him reading assignments about psychoneuroimmunology, and he followed up on these by going to the University of Arizona medical library to look up more articles on the subject. After reading this material, he was excited and motivated to begin the work. He told me he wanted his hematologist on his team as well, in order to monitor his blood counts and be there in case of a crisis. I agreed and said I would be happy to review a treatment plan with his doctor.

A few days later he came back to see me. The hematologist had told him his ideas were crazy; that if he tried to discontinue his medication, he would land in the hospital in a matter of days. He had tried to give the hematologist copies of the articles he had found on mind/body approaches to autoimmunity, but the doctor had laughed at him and said he would not waste his time "reading garbage." This remark so infuriated the patient that he worked up his courage to fire his doctor, the first time in his life that he had defied a medical authority and taken into his own hands responsibility for treatment. With some effort he found another hematologist, who, despite some discomfort, was willing to watch over him and let him experiment. The patient made the recommended changes in his life and weaned himself from prednisone. His blood counts fluctuated for a period, then stabilized at better levels than when he was on the drug. This convinced him he was on the right track and bolstered his motivation to proceed.

2. ACTIVELY SEARCH FOR HELP

Successful patients search out possibilities for treatments and cures and follow up every lead they come across. They ask questions, read books and articles, go to libraries, write to authors, ask friends and neighbors for ideas, and travel to meet with practitioners who seem promising. Such behavior leads some doctors to label these patients difficult, noncompliant, or simply obnoxious, but there is reason to think that difficult patients are more likely to get better while nice ones finish last.

Remember the words of Kristin, the young woman who was healed from aplastic anemia (page 20): "There may be different ways to healing for different people but there is always a way. Keep searching!"

3. SEEK OUT OTHERS WHO HAVE BEEN HEALED

One of the most effective ways to neutralize medical pessimism is to find someone who had the same problem you do and is now healed. Whenever I come across people who have solved serious health problems, I ask them if they will allow me from time to time to send similarly affected patients for advice and guidance. For example, I know a man in his late thirties who developed rheumatoid arthritis fifteen years ago. For years he took larger and larger doses of suppressive medication, and he required several surgeries to correct worsening deformity of one hand. Then he began to notice that the fluctuating course of the disease followed his emotional ups and downs. He made a conscientious effort to develop a healthy lifestyle and cultivate evenness of mood; as a result, he has been able to stop the progression of the arthritis and eliminate the medication. I have sent him several patients with rheumatoid arthritis—young people who knew only the perspective of conventional rheumatologists and had no reason to believe they could take charge of their health. He helped convince them that they could modify their disease without depending on drugs and then got them started on the road to healing.

4. FORM CONSTRUCTIVE PARTNERSHIPS WITH HEALTH PROFESSIONALS

Successful patients often ally themselves with health professionals who support them in their search for answers. An ally can simply be a doctor who says, "I don't know what you're doing, but whatever it is, keep it up!" Or it can be a practitioner who takes an active hand in suggesting experiments. What you want is a professional who believes in you and in your ability to heal yourself, someone who empowers you in your search and makes you feel that you are not alone. Good doctors are willing to say "I don't know," and they will take the greatest pleasure in seeing you heal, whatever methods you decide to use.

5. DO NOT HESITATE TO MAKE RADICAL LIFE CHANGES

Many of the successful patients I have known are not the same people they were at the onset of illness. Their search for healing made them aware that they had to make significant changes in their lives: changes in relationships, jobs, places of residence, diet, habits, and so forth. In retrospect they see these changes as steps that were necessary to personal growth, but at the time the process was wrenching. Change is always difficult; major change can be very painful. Illness often forces us to look at issues and conflicts in our lives that we have ignored in the hope that they would disappear. Continuing to ignore them may block any possibility of spontaneous healing, while willingness to change may be a strong predictor of success.

6. REGARD ILLNESS AS A GIFT

Because illness can be such a powerful stimulus to change, perhaps the only thing that can force some people to resolve their deepest conflicts, successful patients often come to regard it as the greatest opportunity they have ever had for personal growth and development—truly a gift. Seeing illness as a misfortune, especially one that is undeserved, may obstruct the healing system. Coming to see illness as a gift that allows you to grow may unlock it.

7. CULTIVATE SELF-ACCEPTANCE

To accept oneself, with all of the imperfections, limitations, and defects that characterize every human being, represents a surrender to a higher will. Change seems more likely to occur in this climate of surrender than in a climate of confrontation with the universe. When you are sick, surrender does not mean giving up hope of renewed health. Rather it means accepting all the circumstances of your life, including present sickness, in order to move beyond them. Recall the stages of the process of grieving (see page 83): only with acceptance of loss does it become possible to move on to completion and healing. Recall also the words of one man who experienced spontaneous healing: "The trick is to get your ego out of the way, get your concepts out of the way, and just let the body heal itself. It knows how to do it."

18

MANAGING GENERAL
CATEGORIES OF ILLNESS: SECRETS
OF A HYGEIAN PRACTITIONER

IF YOU GET SICK, it is useful to know about therapeutic approaches that can give the healing system a boost, especially dietary modifications, specific supplements, herbal medicines, and alternative methods unknown to most conventional doctors. It is not my purpose to go through an exhaustive list of diseases with complete treatment plans, particularly since I believe that treatment must be customized for each individual, but I can offer you advice about the management of general categories of illness. Bear in mind that the suggestions in this chapter are not meant to be total replacements for standard medicine. Remember also that people react in different ways to substances they ingest. Although the treatments outlined below are safe and effective in my experience, idiosyncratic adverse reactions can occur in response to taking any herb or supplement. Stop using any remedy that causes problems. Also be patient with natural treatments; they usually take longer to work than strong, suppressive drugs. If you change your diet and begin a regimen of natural therapies, it may be six to eight weeks before you notice improvement. The improvement will be gradual, steady, and solid, because it represents lasting activity of the healing system rather than suppression of symptoms.

ALLERGY

Allergy is a learned response of the immune system to environmental agents that are not intrinsically harmful. The goal of good treatment should be to calm an overreactive immune system so that you can live with allergens and not sneeze, cough, or itch. Conventional treatments are more or less toxic and, because they are purely suppressive, may increase immune reactivity over time. The fact that allergies can suddenly come and suddenly go is encouraging; it indicates that the learned patterns of response are not fixed, that what the immune system has learned, it can unlearn. Spontaneous healing of allergy is not an infrequent occurrence. To increase its likelihood, it is a good idea to work on several fronts:

Dietary modification can reduce allergic responsiveness. The most important suggestions I can give are to follow a low-protein diet, to cut down on animal protein in general and, specifically, to eliminate cow's milk and products made from it, since milk protein acts as an irritant of the immune system in many people. Additionally, I recommend eating organically grown foods as much as possible, because I think residues of agricultural chemicals frequently contribute to immune system reactivity.

Supplement the diet with quercetin, a natural product obtained from buckwheat and citrus fruits. Quercetin stabilizes the membranes of cells that release histamine, the mediator of many allergic reactions. You can buy quercetin tablets in health food stores (some brands contain vitamin C and other related compounds). The recommended dose is 400 milligrams twice a day between meals. Quercetin is a preventive, not a symptomatic, treatment, so it is best to use it regularly. If allergies are seasonal, start taking it several weeks before you expect the onset of symptoms. Otherwise try it for two to three months, then gradually reduce the dose to determine if the improvements are maintained.

A good *herbal treatment* for hay fever, especially for allergic sneezing and itching eyes, ears, and throats, is stinging nettles (*Urtica dioica*), especially a freeze-dried extract of the leaves of this plant. (See Appendix for a source.) One to two capsules every two to four hours as needed will control symptoms with none of the toxicity of antihistamines and steroids. The safest standard drug for this problem is cromolyn sodium in the form of a nasal spray (Nasalcrom nasal solution), which works by a mechanism similar to that of quercetin.

Environmental modifications, such as installing air filters in the home, can reduce the allergenic load on the immune system and give it a better chance to calm down.

Mind/body interventions are important. Some people strongly allergic to roses will have allergic reactions on being shown plastic roses, indicating that learning at the level of the higher brain is involved in these misdirected responses of the immune system. Interactive guided imagery therapy may be especially helpful for allergic skin conditions like chronic hives and eczema.

AUTOIMMUNE DISEASE

In autoimmune disease, immune responses are directed against the body's own tissues, causing inflammatory changes and eventual damage to body structures. Predisposition to autoimmune disease may be inherited, and the disease may be triggered by infection or other physical stress or by emotional trauma. Any number of tissues and organs can become targets for the abnormal immune responses: nerves (multiple sclerosis), joints (rheumatoid arthritis), endocrine glands (myasthenia gravis and forms of thyroiditis), muscles (polymyositis), connective tissues throughout the body (systemic lupus erythematosus), kidneys (glomerulonephritis), and so on. The natural history of all of these diseases is marked by alternating periods of exacerbation and remission—a welcome pattern because it demonstrates the potential of the healing system to curb autoimmune disease. The conventional medical approach to this type of illness is unsatisfactory, relying as it does on suppressive drugs that are highly toxic.

Because autoimmune disease has multiple roots (among them heredity, stress, and environmental interactions), good treatment should address the total lifestyle of each patient. In addition to helping the healing system modulate immunity, it is useful to make adjustments in the diet that aim to reduce inflammation, since inflammatory changes mediate the tissue damage in these diseases.

Dietary modification would be the same as it is for allergy: a low-protein diet with minimal intake of foods of animal origin, especially milk and milk products; plenty of organically grown fruits, vegetables, and grains; elimination of polyunsaturated vegetable oils and artificially hydrogenated fats; inclusion of fish or other sources of omega-3 fatty acids, such as flax seeds.

Supplement the diet with antioxidant vitamins and minerals.

Herbal treatments include ginger for its anti-inflammatory effect (capsules of powdered, dried ginger are best; start with one twice a day) and feverfew, which shows efficacy in the treatment of autoimmune arthritis. (I recommend one to two capsules of freeze-dried feverfew leaves twice a day; see the Appendix for a source.) Another possibility is turmeric (*Curcuma longa*), the spice that makes curry and much prepared mustard yellow. Obtained from the rhizome of a ginger relative, turmeric has significant anti-inflammatory properties and can simply be added to food; however, it is more efficient to take curcumin, the yellow pigment that is the active component, in doses of 400 to 600 milligrams three times a day. Health food stores sell products that combine curcumin with bromelain, an enzyme from pineapple that enhances curcumin's absorption and has anti-inflammatory effects of its own.

Alternative medical treatments may be of great benefit, especially traditional Chinese medicine and Ayurvedic medicine. I have also seen cases of autoimmune disease respond to homeopathic treatment. (See Appendix for information on finding practitioners.)

Mind/body interventions are key in autoimmune disease, because the ups and downs of these diseases often correlate with emotional ups and downs, and because we know that mental factors influence immune responses. Psychotherapy, hypnotherapy, and guided imagery therapy are all useful and worth exploring.

CARDIOVASCULAR DISEASE

Most diseases of the heart and blood vessels are diseases of lifestyle that can be prevented by following a heart-healthy diet, by not smoking, by getting proper exercise, and by working at building nurturing emotional relationships and neutralizing anger and stress. Even when these diseases appear, their progress can be slowed, halted, or even reversed by changing lifestyle in the proper manner. Here are some additional suggestions:

Dietary modification should stress reduction of fat, especially saturated fat, and substitution of olive oil for other kinds of fat in the diet. A high-fiber, low-fat, vegetarian or semivegetarian diet with fish or other sources of omega-3 fatty acids is probably most protective of the heart. Garlic, onions, chili peppers, green tea, and turmeric all have protective effects on the cardiovascular system.

Supplement the diet with antioxidant vitamins and minerals, especially vitamin E. Also take folic acid, 400 micrograms a day, to lower blood levels of homocysteine, which appears to be another cause of atherosclerosis. Two other natural products that I recommend are coenzyme Q (also known as Co-Q-10) and L carnitine. The former improves the use of oxygen at the cellular level, especially in heart muscle cells. I recommend taking 60 milligrams once a day, more if you can afford it, up to 200 milligrams a day. (It is not worth buying Co-Q-10 in dosage forms less than 60 milligrams per capsule.) L carnitine is an amino acid that also improves the metabolism of heart muscle cells (it, too, is not cheap). The recommended dose is 250–500 milligrams twice a day. Both products are available in health food stores and from vitamin suppliers. For cardiac arrhythmias, supplementation with magnesium may be very helpful. Try 1,000 milligrams of magnesium (citrate, gluconate, or chelate) at bedtime plus another 500 milligrams in the morning, along with equal amounts of calcium (citrate). I recommend the same doses of calcium and magnesium for help in managing high blood pressure.

Herbal treatments for the cardiovascular system include hawthorn (*Crataegus oxycantha*), a natural diuretic and heart tonic, useful in persons with coronary heart disease and heart failure, and tree ear mushrooms (*Auricularia polytricha*), an ingredient in Chinese cuisine that has an anticoagulant effect similar to that of aspirin. Encapsulated, freeze-dried extract of hawthorn is available (see Appendix); the dose is one to two capsules two to four times a day. You can buy dried tree ears in Oriental grocery stores. Reconstitute them by soaking in hot water until they expand and become soft; then discard any hard bits and add the mushrooms to soups or stir-fries. A reasonable dose is one tablespoon of the soaked mushrooms a day. Horse chestnut (*Aesculus hippocastanum*) provides a topical treatment for varicose veins. Creams containing horse chestnut extract, sometimes called "escin," are available in health food stores.

Regular aerobic exercise is one of the best influences on the heart, as are all techniques of relaxation and stress reduction.

DIGESTIVE DISORDERS

Here is another large category of diseases that are mostly related to lifestyle, especially to poor habits of eating and managing stress. Conventional medicine controls them poorly. Alternative medicine offers many safe and effective treatments, probably because the healing system, if given a chance, is often able to resolve these conditions completely. A common root cause of many digestive disorders, from esophageal reflux to constipation, is an imbalance between the intrinsic motility of the gastrointestinal musculature and the regulating influence of involuntary nerves that coordinate the whole system. There is so much nervous input to the GI tract that it is very susceptible to stress-induced distortions. In fact, along with the skin, the digestive system is the most common site of expression of stress-related illness.

Dietary modification should always be employed to improve digestive health and function. As a start, eliminate caffeine (especially coffee), tobacco, and other stimulant drugs. Alcohol can be a major irritant of the esophagus and stomach. Pay attention to which foods and combinations of foods cause distress, and change eating habits accordingly. Sometimes eating smaller amounts more frequently will make your digestive system function more smoothly.

Herbal treatment for digestive disorders is often quite effective. Chamomile and peppermint teas both work for simple heartburn and nausea; but peppermint, because it relaxes the sphincter muscle where the esophagus joins the stomach, may make esophageal reflux worse. Ginger in any form works for nausea. For severe gastritis, reflux, or peptic ulcer, try the licorice preparation DGL (see footnote on page 232), which increases the natural, protective mucus that coats the stomach lining. Peppermint oil in enteric-coated capsules, available at health food stores, is an excellent treatment for irritable bowel syndrome, diverticulitis, and other intestinal ailments. A good natural remedy for diarrhea and intestinal inflammation is carob powder, available at health food stores. Start with one tablespoon, mixed with some applesauce and honey to make it palatable. Take it with acidophilus (liquid or capsules from the health food store) on an empty stomach (at least an hour and a half before or three hours after eating). For constipation, the Ayurvedic preparation triphala is excellent; follow dosage recommendations on the product.

Relaxation is all-important. The breathing exercise described on pages 206–7 has especially beneficial effects on the GI system, but it must be practiced regularly. Biofeedback and yoga can be helpful, and I cannot recommend hypnotherapy and guided imagery therapy too highly.

Alternative medical approaches to digestive disorders that give the best results are naturopathy, homeopathy, traditional Chinese medicine, and Ayurvedic medicine. I would try these systems before resorting to allopathic drugs and surgery.

INFECTION

I have noted more than once in this book that the effectiveness of antibiotics for bacterial infections is rapidly declining as organisms develop resistance to them. Infections that are severe, fast moving, or involve vital organs are emergencies requiring allopathic supervision, but even in those cases it is worth using complementary methods to stimulate healing responses. For less severe infections and for chronic or recurrent infections that resist allopathic treatments, the primary focus should be to rouse the healing system to action. For accessible, localized infections, one of the best ways to accomplish this is to increase blood flow to affected areas by applying heat—for example, by using hot, wet compresses or soaks. You can also help the healing system fight infection by giving the body more rest, eating less, increasing fluid intake, and sweating in a steam room or sauna.

Dietary modification can reduce susceptibility to some kinds of infection. For example, cutting down on sugar of all sorts may decrease the frequency of urinary tract infections in women, and increasing intake of fresh fruits and vegetables will help build immunity.

Supplement the diet with antioxidant vitamins and minerals, especially with vitamin C, 2,000 milligrams two to three times a day for chronic or recurrent infections.

Herbal treatments abound for infections, from the familiar (garlic) to the exotic (Oriental mushrooms). Add raw garlic to the diet as a general measure and experiment with echinacea (*Echinacea purpurea* and related species), a native American herb with antibiotic and immune-enhancing properties. Echinacea preparations are readily available in health food stores and some drugstores. Taste them to make sure they cause a distinct numbing sensation on the tongue after a minute; otherwise they are not effective. Follow dosage recommendations on the product or use one dropperful of the tincture in a little warm water four times a day. For topical infections, try tea tree oil, obtained from an Australian tree (*Melaleuca alternifolia*).

Buy only one hundred percent pure tea tree oil from a health food store; it is an excellent disinfectant, useful in first-aid kits for the home and when traveling. For chronic or recurrent viral infections, try astragalus (see pages 177–79).

Alternative medicine can sometimes succeed with infectious illnesses when conventional medicine cannot. My first choice would be traditional Chinese medicine, which has a vast array of medicinal plants with antiviral, antibacterial, and immunomodulating properties.

Mind/body approaches should always be tried. At the least, they can enhance the efficacy of conventional drugs. At best, they can change the balance between the immune system and pathogenic germs in a way that favors resolution of the infection.

MEN'S HEALTH PROBLEMS

The prostate gland is a vulnerable point of male anatomy, often harboring stubborn infections in youth and enlarging in age to the point of interfering with urination. The main irritants of the prostate are coffee and other forms of caffeine, decaffeinated coffee, alcohol, tobacco, red pepper, dehydration, and either too frequent or too infrequent ejaculation. Prolonged sitting and repetitive jarring motion (as from riding a horse, bicycle, or motorcycle) also stress the gland.

Supplement the diet with zinc, 30 milligrams a day of the picolinate form. Also increase intake of soy foods; their phytoestrogens might protect the prostate from the unbalanced influence of male sex hormones.

Herbal treatment for prostatic enlargement relies on two plants: saw palmetto (*Serenoa repens*) and pygeum (*Pygeum africanum*). Use one or both, following dosage recommendations on the products. You can continue taking them indefinitely.

For sexual deficiency, traditional Chinese medicine offers many treatments, including ginseng (see pages 179–80), the preeminent male sexual tonic. Ayurvedic medicine contributes ashwaganda (*Withania somnifera*), newly available in health food stores. Follow dosages recommended on the product.

Mind/body methods are worth exploring in all sexual and genital problems, hypnotherapy and guided imagery therapy being especially useful.

MENTAL, EMOTIONAL, AND NERVOUS DISORDERS

For anxiety, even the most severe forms of anxiety, the best treatment I know is the breathing exercise on pages 206–7. By gradually changing the tone of the involuntary system, it allows deep, internal relaxation that promotes emotional healing. If you start practicing it now, you will have it ready to use in case of need. Regular exercise is also important, and, obviously, relaxation training can be very helpful. Two herbal treatments that I recommend frequently are passion flower (*Passiflora incarnata*) and valerian (*Valeriana officinalis*). The former, which is quite mild, can be taken as a tincture: one dropperful in a little warm water as needed, up to four times a day. The latter is a strong enough sedative to be used for insomnia, but small doses—say, ten drops of the tincture in a little warm water—can be used for daytime calming.

For depression, the best single treatment is vigorous, regular aerobic exercise, at least thirty minutes a day, five days a week. Avoidance of alcohol, sedatives, antihistamines, and other depressant drugs is advisable. Dietary modification—less protein and fat, more starches, fruits, and vegetables—may also make a difference. Try this regimen of supplements as well: In the morning, on arising, take 1,500 milligrams of DL-phenylalanine (DLPA, an amino acid), 100 milligrams of vitamin B-6, 500 milligrams of vitamin C, and a piece of fruit or a small glass of juice. Do not eat breakfast for at least an hour. (Use this formula cautiously if you have high blood pressure, as DLPA may worsen that condition temporarily. Start with a lower dose of the amino acid and monitor blood pressure frequently.)

MUSCULOSKELETAL DISORDERS

Acute and chronic musculoskeletal pain brings more patients to doctors' offices than many other categories of illness combined. Conventional drugs and surgery should be regarded as last resorts to be used only after aggressive experimentation with natural and alternative methods has failed to provide relief.

Dietary modification is less important here, except that it is useful to manipulate dietary fats to reduce any inflammatory processes.

That means eliminating polyunsaturated and artificially saturated fats and increasing intake of omega-3 fatty acids in any form.

Supplementation with the B-vitamin niacinamide can be very helpful for osteoarthritis. Start with 500 milligrams twice a day, increasing by 500 milligrams at three-week intervals if necessary to a maximum daily dose of 2,000 milligrams.

Herbal treatments for musculoskeletal pain include ginger, especially in dried form, and the Ayurvedic herb *Boswellia,* or the extract made from it, boswellin. Health food stores sell it; follow dosage recommendations on the products. Ginger and boswellin may provide relief in fibromyalgia and other conditions in which people complain that "it hurts all over." Also consider using curcumin, the anti-inflammatory agent from turmeric, as described under "Autoimmune Disease." For extensive bruises and hematomas resulting from trauma, an excellent treatment is bromelain, the pineapple enzyme you can find in capsules at health food stores. Take 200 to 400 milligrams three times a day on an empty stomach. Bromelain promotes healing of tissue injuries, but occasional individuals may develop an allergic rash from it; discontinue it if you develop any itching.

Mind/body interventions, again, are critical. Hypnotherapy can teach people how to distance themselves from chronic pain, which can help the pain to resolve more quickly. Other forms of stress reduction, including guided meditation, have worked for chronic pain syndromes after all conventional approaches have failed.

Alternative treatment is always worth trying for these maladies, especially osteopathic manipulation, chiropractic, therapeutic massages, and other forms of body work. Acupuncture can provide dramatic temporary relief of musculoskeletal pain and may promote healing of some conditions. In combination with Chinese herbal treatment, it may do wonders for individuals with arthritis and other chronically painful musculoskeletal ailments.

PAIN

Pain has two aspects: the physical sensation arising from some disturbance of body structure or function and the psychic perception of it. The latter aspect can be modified in several ways. My preference is for hypnotherapy, guided imagery, meditation, and acupuncture. Review the story of Ethan's back pain on pages 118–22, which describes the healing of chronic pain through purely psychic intervention.

To the extent that pain is the result of inflammation at the tissue level, it can be approached through all of the dietary changes, herbal treatments, and alternative medical approaches listed under "Auto-immune Disease" and "Musculoskeletal Disorders."

Therapeutic touch and other forms of energy healing can be dramatically effective in relieving pain.

SKIN DISORDERS

Because the skin has so many nerve endings, it is another very frequent site for stress-related problems. Again, conventional treatments for many skin diseases, especially topical steroid preparations, are suppressive in nature and potentially toxic.

Lifestyle changes can make a huge difference to the health of the skin, particularly protection from the damaging effects of sun exposure; decrease in frequency of washing with soap, which removes natural protective oils; assiduous use of moisturizers immediately after a bath or shower; and elimination of cosmetic products containing dyes and other harsh chemicals.

Dietary modification is also important in order to eliminate foods that may promote allergic and inflammatory changes and to provide nutrients needed for healthy development of skin, hair, and nails. In general, make the changes recommended under "Autoimmune Disease," being sure to provide adequate sources of omega-3 fatty acids.

Supplement the diet with antioxidant vitamins and minerals and with GLA (gamma-linolenic acid, an essential fatty acid of particular benefit to the skin); best sources are black currant oil and evening primrose oil, available in capsules at health food stores. The recommended dose of black currant oil is 500 milligrams twice a day. You will see changes in the skin, hair, and nails after six to eight weeks of continuous use.

Mind/body interventions should be tried in all cases of skin disease to take advantage of the high level of innervation of the skin. I usually send patients to skilled hypnotherapists and guided imagery therapists.

Alternative medicine can be more effective and less toxic than conventional medicine in managing skin disorders. In my experience the greatest chance for success is with homeopathy, Ayurvedic medicine, and traditional Chinese medicine, even for cases of psoriasis and other severe, chronic problems.

STRESS-RELATED DISORDERS

All illnesses should be assumed to be stress-related until proved otherwise. Even if stress is not the primary cause of illness, it is frequently an aggravating factor. To say that a bodily complaint is stress-related does not in any way mean that it is unreal or unimportant; it simply means that time spent at stress reduction and relaxation training may be very worthwhile in terms of obtaining relief. Some of the most common stress-related ailments are headache, insomnia, musculoskeletal pain (especially in the back and neck), gastrointestinal disorders of all sorts, skin disorders of all sorts, sexual deficiency, menstrual problems, and increased susceptibility to infection; that accounts for quite a few symptoms, visits to doctors, and prescriptions for suppressive drugs. In all of these conditions, regardless of what other interventions you try, I recommend working with the relaxing breath, using mind/body approaches, and all relaxation methods that appeal to you in order to give the healing system the best possible chance to solve any problems on the physical level.

URINARY SYSTEM DISORDERS

Lifestyle change is critical here, because the most common stressors of the kidneys are tobacco; high blood pressure; dehydration; alcohol, caffeine, and other stimulant drugs; and high-protein diets. The metabolism of protein puts a huge workload on the kidneys. If you know that you have abnormal kidneys or have had any kidney disease in the past, the most important preventive strategies you can employ are to adopt a very low-protein diet and never to allow yourself to become dehydrated.

Because the urinary system filters toxins from the blood and concentrates them in urine, it is susceptible to toxic injury that may initiate malignant transformation, especially in the bladder. Following the advice in Chapter 10 of this book on protecting yourself from toxins will help you, as will the regular use of antioxidant supplements.

Women are much more vulnerable than men to urinary tract infections. They can reduce susceptibility by eliminating or minimizing the use of tobacco, alcohol, and caffeine, by avoiding traumatic or excessive sexual activity, and by always maintaining good urinary output by drinking plenty of water. Also, cranberries contain a substance that makes it harder for bacteria to stick to the bladder wall. If you are experiencing frequent urinary tract infections, try drinking cranberry juice often or use unsweetened cranberry concentrate from the health food store that you can dilute to your own taste with water or sparkling water. Taking acidophilus in liquid or capsule form after meals can also help increase resistance to bladder infections.

An *herbal treatment* that can help the urinary tract is bearberry, or uva ursi (*Arctostaphylos uva-ursi*). Tinctures and encapsulated extracts of the leaves can be found at health food stores and are useful for a variety of urinary problems. The dose is one dropperful of the tincture in a little water or one or two capsules of extract three to four times a day. This should be used as a short-term remedy only, since prolonged use may cause irritation.

Mind/body methods can be extremely valuable in managing urinary problems. Guided imagery with a trained therapist would be my first choice.

Alternative medicine can also be helpful, especially naturopathy, homeopathy, and traditional Chinese medicine.

WOMEN'S HEALTH PROBLEMS

Menstrual problems, including painful periods and premenstrual syndrome (PMS), can be moderated by eliminating caffeine and inflammation-promoting fats (see "Autoimmune Disease," pages 255–56) and by supplementing the diet with GLA (see "Skin Disorders," pages 263–64), vitamin E, and vitamin B-6 (100 milligrams twice a day). Dong quai (*Angelica sinensis*) is a useful tonic for a wide range of female problems (see page 181). Another useful herbal treatment is chaste tree (*Vitex agnus-castus*), which may be taken in tincture or capsule form (one dropperful of the tincture in water or one or two capsules twice a day); it helps regulate the female reproductive cycle. Regular, moderate aerobic exercise is also important.

To avoid imbalances of estrogen metabolism, it is essential to avoid consuming foods with added estrogen (commercially raised meats and poultry), to avoid exposure to pollutants that may have estrogenic activity, to minimize consumption of alcohol, to eat a low-fat diet, and to increase intake of soy foods for their protective phytoestrogens.

Menopausal symptoms can be managed without resorting to hormone replacement therapy, although women who are already losing bone density or are at high risk for coronary heart disease may choose hormone replacement for those reasons. An herbal formula that will reduce or eliminate hot flashes in most women consists of dong quai, chaste tree, and damiana (*Turnera diffusa*). Take one dropperful of the tinctures of each, or two capsules of each, once a day at noon.

Mind/body approaches are invaluable in all disorders of the female reproductive system. Results of hypnotherapy and guided imagery therapy can be rapid, dramatic, and surprisingly effective.

19

CANCER AS A SPECIAL CASE

CANCER HAS ALWAYS been with us. All living organisms are susceptible to it, and the more complex the organism, the higher the risk. A
great many pressures on cells push them toward malignant transformation; malignant cells are dangerous because they do not die when
they are supposed to, do not stay in place, and do not limit their
growth to conform to the general laws that regulate the economies of
whole organisms.

Nevertheless, there is a radical difference between a transformed
cell and a cancerous growth with power to kill its host. When cells
become malignant, they announce their new identity by displaying
abnormal antigens on their surface membranes. An ongoing job of
the immune system is to scan cells in order to recognize and eliminate those that are not-self, that do not belong in the body. Given
the number of cell divisions constantly occurring, and given all the
possibilities for malignant transformation, the seeds of cancers are
surely being created unceasingly, and just as surely the immune system eliminates them. Immune surveillance to weed out malignant
cells is a key function of the healing system, a defense against cancer
that our bodies developed in the course of evolution. Yet the incidence of cancer is rising sharply in the world today, because our
defenses are overwhelmed. In addition to the natural carcinogenic
agents that have always been with us, we have added to the environment a great number of manmade ones. By following the advice
in Part Two of this book on optimizing the healing system, you can
strengthen your defenses and reduce your risks of getting cancer.

Given the inadequacy of current treatments for this disease, prevention is all-important.

Once cancer becomes established in the body, and particularly when it has spread from its initial site (metastasis), it is very difficult to cure. We fear cancer because it develops insidiously from within, because it resists our best technological weaponry, and because it has great destructive potential. To understand why cancer presents such a difficult challenge, you need grasp only one basic fact: *The presence of cancer in the body, even in its earliest stages, already represents significant failure of the healing system.* In order for a transformed cell to give rise to a detectable tumor, it must have escaped immune destruction, undergone many divisions, and produced countless generations of daughter cells, all without interference. With most other diseases, even severe ones like coronary heart disease and multiple sclerosis, it is reasonable to expect much of the healing system. With cancer, by the time a lump is noticed, failure of healing mechanisms is already a fixed pattern.

Current therapies for cancer, both conventional and alternative, are far from satisfactory. Conventional medicine has three main treatments: surgery, radiation, and chemotherapy, of which only the first makes sense. If cancer is in one location only and accessible to a surgeon's knife, it can be excised and eliminated permanently. Unfortunately, only a small percentage of cancers meet those criteria, principally cancers of the skin and uterine cervix. In far too many cases cancer has already spread to more than one site by the time of its discovery or is somewhere in the body that is beyond the reach of a surgical cure.

Radiation and chemotherapy are crude treatments that will be obsolete before long. Both work by killing dividing cells; the assumption made by doctors who use them is that cancerous cells divide faster than normal ones. Unfortunately, that is true only for a small percentage of cancers, principally childhood cancers, leukemias, lymphomas, testicular cancer, and a few others. In most cases, cells of cancers have lower division rates than the most active normal tissues of the body: the skin, the lining of the gastrointestinal tract, the bone marrow, and other immune structures. The well-known side effects of radiation and chemotherapy—loss of hair, loss of appetite, nausea, and vomiting—represent damage to the skin and the GI tract. Damage to the immune system is less obvious and much more of a concern. If you have cancer and are faced with a decision about whether to use conventional therapies, the question you must try to answer is this: Will the damage done to the cancer justify the damage done to the immune system?

Ultimately, hopes for cures of cancer are equivalent to hopes for immune responses, because the immune system has the potential to recognize and eliminate malignant tissue. The future of cancer treatment is not in bigger and better cytotoxic weapons (which will never be capable of killing malignant cells without also killing fast-growing normal cells). Instead, the future will bring immunotherapy capable of rousing a slumbering immune system to action. Some forms of immunotherapy are now available, but most are still experimental.

Spontaneous remission of cancer—an all-too-rare event—appears to result from sudden immune activation, which demonstrates the potential of the immune system to react against malignant growth, sometimes with such vigor that large masses of tumor tissue dissolve in a matter of hours or days. Here is an account of that kind of cancer remission, sent to me by Robert Anderson, M.D., of Edmonds, Washington, a past president of the American Holistic Medical Association.

The patient, Helen B., was a sixty-seven-year-old hairdresser who came to him in 1985 for a routine checkup. Dr. Anderson felt a suggestion of a mass during the vaginal examination; he thought it might be scar tissue from a previous hysterectomy but worried when blood tests revealed the patient to be anemic with abnormal liver function. Dr. Anderson referred her to a gynecologist, but she procrastinated, believing that her previous physician had described these same findings several years before. Both of her former doctors had died, and her records could not be located. When Dr. Anderson re-examined her six weeks later, the mass was "significantly larger," and blood test results were significantly worse. He insisted that she see a gynecologist and undergo further tests, one of which, an ultrasound examination, revealed "a left pelvic mass consistent with ovarian origin."

One month later, Helen B. underwent exploratory surgery. The surgeon found a large tumor mass in the left and central pelvis, extensively involving the small and large bowel, and noted that "widespread 3–9 mm peritoneal lesions were studded throughout the pelvic and abdominal cavities, exceeding one hundred in number;

five of them were biopsied." The pathology report of the biopsies described "malignant tumor with moderate variation in cell size and shape. . . . The tumor appears as a poorly differentiated carcinoma, possibly of ovarian origin." Several days later, Helen underwent more surgery, for removal of the mass and attached portions of small and large bowel. She was left with a colostomy and obvious tumor still in her abdomen. The pathologist's final diagnosis was "poorly differentiated carcinoma of probable ovarian origin."

Poorly differentiated carcinoma of any origin is not a good kind of tumor to have. The primitive cells tend to be highly malignant and invasive; in Helen B.'s case, widespread metastasis had already occurred throughout the abdominal cavity, making for a poor prognosis. The surgeon wrote to Dr. Anderson: "I recommend oncological consultation and commencement of chemotherapy. The colostomy does not need to be considered permanent. After the first course of chemotherapy, probably within six months, we should re-explore her, and at that time we could close the colostomy." But Helen did not want to go to an oncologist or to take chemotherapy. She went to Dr. Anderson again and said, "I want you to tell me what I have to do to recover." He outlined for her a comprehensive program that included a low-fat, low-sugar, high-fiber vegetarian diet, supplementation with antioxidant vitamins and minerals, regular exercise when possible, regular meditation incorporating visualization of tumor shrinkage, and "modifying her attitude toward her husband, including forgiveness," since marital discord was a major source of stress in her life. He also insisted on a visit to an oncologist, and Helen went, albeit reluctantly. The oncologist, who was very concerned about the residual cancer, urged chemotherapy "now rather than later when the tumor is bulkier and our chances for a good outcome are much less," but Helen refused, saying that she and God would win the battle.

A month after the surgery her anemia resolved and her liver function returned to normal. She felt strong and confident. Dr. Anderson encouraged her, noting that "her belief in the divine was evangelistic; I reinforced her hope with every encouragement." Helen hated the colostomy and began to demand that the surgeon undo it. He was unwilling to operate until she had undergone chemotherapy, but her refusal was so adamant and so persistent that he finally relented and reoperated two and a half months after the removal of the tumor. He reported of this operation that "the surgery was long and tedious. The adhesions encountered merely entering the peritoneal cavity were among the worst I had ever seen. . . . The hundreds of 3–9 mm peritoneal tumors appeared as before. Seven of them from various locations were biopsied." But this time the pathology report on the biopsies was quite different; it showed "inflammatory tissue with moderate cell variation and no malignant characteristics." The surgeon's comment on receiving this news was, "She is a very interesting lady."

Helen B. quickly returned to normal life and health, continuing the program that Dr. Anderson had recommended to her. Two years later she was divorced from her husband, which seemed to provide emotional relief. Dr. Anderson wrote: "In 1987, approximately two years following her first visit with me, she developed an incisional hernia at the site of the previous surgical operation. It became problematic, and she underwent surgery for yet a fourth time to repair it. At the time of operation, the surgeon, with my assistance, took advantage of the opportunity to reexplore her abdomen briefly. The adhesions were totally gone; *there were no residual peritoneal tumors and no evidence of cancer anywhere.*" Helen B. died at seventy-five of unrelated causes, nearly eight years after her original diagnosis.

What happened in this woman's abdomen that eliminated widely disseminated cancer and restored her internal organs to good health? Her healing system, probably making use of immune mechanisms, was surely responsible; but why did it not act before? Did removal of the main mass of tumor tissue somehow activate a healing response? If so, why doesn't this happen more often? In most patients with metastatic cancer of this sort, tumors will regrow, often in spite of aggressive cytotoxic therapy and often with fatal results. If an immune response is the best hope for a total cure of cancer, then one must be cautious indeed about using cytotoxic treatments that can damage the immune system.

Cancer treatments abound in the world of alternative medicine, most of them much less toxic than radiation and chemotherapy, but none of them works reliably for large numbers of patients. Many of the therapies I have looked into appear to have induced remissions in some people; in many more they improve quality of life for a time, yet the cancers remain and continue to grow. If there were a reliably effective alternative treatment for cancer, we would all know about it soon enough.

Let me summarize the information in this chapter so far: Cells turn malignant constantly, and normally the healing system eliminates them. Given the increasing environmental pressures toward malignant transformation and the inadequacy of cancer treatments, it is imperative to maintain our healing systems in good working order and to know how to reduce cancer risks. Spontaneous healing of cancer occurs but is much less common than spontaneous healing of most other diseases because the healing system has already failed if a malignant cell is able to give rise to a detectable tumor. When remission does occur, the mechanism is immune activation; therefore, great care must be exercised in deciding whether or not to use cytotoxic treatments (radiation and chemotherapy), because damage to the immune system may reduce the long-term possibility of a curative healing response.

So how should you proceed if you or a loved one develops cancer? The first step must be to determine whether, and how, to use conventional treatments. Here are some guidelines:

• If surgical excision of a tumor is possible, have it done. Even partial removal of a large tumor mass ("debulking") may help the healing system contain cancerous growth.

• Find out whether any forms of immunotherapy are available for your particular type of cancer. If your oncologist does not know of any, call the National Cancer Institute or cancer research centers at universities.

• If radiation and chemotherapy are urged on you, obtain statistics on their success rates for the particular type and stage of cancer you have. You cannot always rely on oncologists here, since they have a vested interest in promoting these therapies and are usually unfamiliar with alternatives. I have known oncologists to represent a regimen of chemotherapy as producing an "eighty percent cure rate" when all the scientific literature showed was an eighty-percent five-year cancer-free survival. What happened to the patients after five years? If you are trying to place your bet wisely, you want to know the accurate odds. In a few cases, books exist to guide patients in making these difficult decisions. More often than not, the only way you will acquire the information you need is to visit a medical library and look up articles on the proposed treatment.

• Remember that radiation and chemotherapy are themselves mutagenic and carcinogenic. It is possible to calculate the percentage of patients exposed to these therapies who, if they survive long enough, will develop independent cancers that are direct results of treatment.

• Natural chemotherapeutic agents like vincristine from the Madagascar periwinkle and taxol from the Pacific yew tree are no safer than synthetic ones. All forms of chemotherapy—natural or chemical, old or new, singly or in combination—are cell-killing agents that damage DNA and injure actively dividing cells, including those of the immune system.

• In general, radiation is safer than chemotherapy because it can be directed to one part of the body. Still, it may cause severe scarring that can interfere with future organ function.

• If immunotherapy is not an option and if the success rates of conventional therapies are good for your type and stage of cancer, then avail yourself of them without worrying about the risks. Those therapies may give you time to explore other options; and by working to optimize your healing system, you can moderate their side effects.

• If you decide to proceed with radiation or chemotherapy, discontinue use of antioxidant supplements during treatment, since they may protect cancer cells along with normal cells. Resume the supplements as soon as treatment ends.

• If, after reviewing the statistical evidence for the usefulness of radiation and chemotherapy for your particular type and stage of cancer, you decide not to undergo those treatments, you should then investigate alternative therapies.

Here are a few suggestions regarding alternative cancer therapies:

• It is just as important to seek good statistical information on outcomes from the use of alternative treatments. Ask to see any published data supporting treatments that interest you. Published data may be scant or lacking here, so you may have to rely on the statements of providers.

• Try to determine whether there is any risk of toxicity or harm from the therapies in question.

• Ask for names of patients you might contact who have undergone the therapies. If providers will not give you this information, be wary.

Regardless of whether you choose conventional or alternative treatment, there are general recommendations that everyone with cancer should follow:

• Because it represents failure of the healing system, cancer, even in its early and localized stages, is a systemic disease. Patients must work to improve general health and resistance by making changes on all levels: physical, mental/emotional, and spiritual.

• As a minimum, I recommend changing diet according to the principles reviewed in Part Two, Chapter 2; maintaining a program of regular exercise; taking antioxidant supplements; using tonic herbs, especially those with immune-enhancing effects; learning visualization or guided imagery techniques to help the healing system contain the cancer; working to heal relationships (with parents, children, and spouses, for example); and making whatever changes in lifestyle are necessary to give yourself the best chance for healing to occur.

• In addition, try to find people who have experienced healing of cancer, preferably those who have had your particular kind of cancer. Read accounts of healing and books that increase your confidence in your own healing capacity.

• Seek out healers. Get all the help you can find.

If the healing system is not able to eliminate cancer completely, it may be able to do something else: slow or contain malignant growth to allow a period of relatively good health. Here is the story of one patient who did remarkably well even though cancer eventually caused her death.

Barbara S. came to me at the beginning of 1989, five and a half years after she was diagnosed with breast cancer and had undergone standard treatment: mastectomy and chemotherapy. She believed that if she made it through five years without a recurrence, she would be out of danger; but just at the fifth anniversary of her diagnosis, she fell and injured her right hip, which would not heal. Tests revealed the bone to be weakened by the presence of tumor. The cancer was not gone; it was now present as bone metastases throughout her skeleton—shocking news for Barbara and her family. Her doctor started her on tamoxifen, an estrogen antagonist, and told her he would order another course of chemotherapy if that did not shrink the tumors in her bones.

In the next few months Barbara made drastic changes in her life. She took a sabbatical from her job as a college dean, visited a number of counselors and psychotherapists, started yoga, began practicing visualization therapy, inaugurated a vitamin regimen, improved her diet, began swimming regularly, made arrangements to receive regular shiatsu treatments, took a Chinese herbal formula for cancer, and worked with healers. For the next three years, contrary to all the statistics for disseminated breast cancer, Barbara was in good health and looked so well that most people who met her could not believe she had cancer. During this period, I sent to Barbara several patients of mine newly diagnosed with breast cancer, who were frightened and confused about which steps to take. She was a great help to them. I also invited her to my classes to tell her story to groups of medical students. They found her to be an inspiring speaker who made a great case for taking charge of one's life and learning how to combine conventional and alternative therapies. Above all she demonstrated that recurrence of cancer does not automatically condemn a patient to sickness and rapid decline.

In the fall of 1992, Barbara's cancer advanced, with new metastases in her liver. She underwent chemotherapy and a trial of an experimental drug, investigated other alternative therapies, and continued most of the program she had developed to maintain her general health. She lived for another year and a half, during which she was very close to her family. Her doctors constantly expressed amazement at her longevity and vigor in the face of an overwhelming disease, and she continued to inspire many people with whom she came in contact. Barbara's healing system was unable to eradicate her cancer, but it held it in check for a long time, during which she accomplished a great deal.

CANCER WILL ALWAYS be with us. Prevention remains the best strategy for managing it, and that depends on the integrity of the healing system. As environmental pressures toward malignant transformation of cells increase, it will be ever more important to know how to optimize your healing potential. New and better cancer treatment is on the horizon in the form of immunotherapy, methods that will take advantage of natural healing mechanisms to recognize and destroy malignant cells without harming normal ones. In the meantime, a concerted effort to discover and study cases of spontaneous remission may help us understand that phenomenon and increase its incidence. To make wise decisions regarding the use of existing therapies for cancer you must have reliable information about their benefits and risks. Whatever specific treatments people decide to use, they must also work with all due diligence to improve general health in order to give the healing system the best chance to check cancer's spread.

AFTERWORD:
PRESCRIPTIONS FOR SOCIETY

IMAGINE A FUTURE world in which medicine was oriented toward healing rather than disease, where doctors believed in the natural healing capacity of human beings and emphasized prevention above treatment. Except for urgent care facilities, hospitals in such a world might more resemble spas, where patients could learn and practice the principles of healthy living, where they would learn to eat and prepare healthy food, learn to take care of the physical needs of their bodies, learn to use their minds in the service of healing, and become less rather than more dependent on health professionals. Even in urgent care facilities, technology would be used to help the healing system, as by stimulating regeneration of damaged organs. In these facilities the best ideas and methods of both conventional and alternative medicine would be available to all patients. In such a world doctors and patients would be partners working toward the same ends, with malpractice litigation a rare event rather than a commonplace. Insurance companies would happily reimburse for preventive education and natural treatments, knowing that these efforts were in their own best interests.

What stands in the way of moving health care in these directions? Here are the main obstacles that I see:

• Medical education is frozen in a disease-oriented mode. The clinical training of doctors remains a brutal initiation that makes it very difficult for students to maintain healthy lifestyles and develop the mental and spiritual qualities of healers.

• An atmosphere of distrust has poisoned doctor/patient relationships, so that every patient coming through the door is now seen as a potential plaintiff in a lawsuit. Doctors are more afraid than ever to deviate from conventional standards of practice.

• Insurance companies dictate how medicine is practiced by their policies of reimbursement. They will not pay for most of the interventions described in this book because they say they do not have research data to support their effectiveness or their cost-effectiveness compared to conventional treatments.

• Research on healing and on alternative medicine is primitive or nonexistent because the people who set research priorities and disburse research funds are not interested in these fields.

• The biomedical model from which medical scientists work stifles movement toward Hygeian medicine. From that model's materialistic perspective, doctors can easily dismiss most of the ideas in this book as unscientific and unworthy of investigation.

And what are the remedies for this situation?

I believe that the root problem is medical education. If future doctors were taught alternative models of science and health, were encouraged to study the healing power of nature, and were allowed to develop themselves into healthy role models for patients, all the obstacles listed above would begin to melt away. These new doctors would want to do the research that will eventually change standards of practice and lead insurance companies to spend their money in better ways. They would know how to take belief projected onto them by patients and reflect it back in ways that increase the occurrence of spontaneous healing. They would be able to design and staff new kinds of health care institutions that would be more like spas than hospitals, and they would recreate the trust between doctors and patients that makes lawsuits unthinkable.

Having said that, I must also say that I am cynical about the prospects for radical reform of medical education, even though I am committed to trying to bring it about. My cynicism goes back to my days as a first-year medical student in 1964 and has been reinforced by my experience on a medical school faculty. Many of my classmates at Harvard had majored in humanities rather than science as undergraduates, and many were not sure they wanted to be doctors. We were a restive group, and we were dismayed by the quality of instruction we received in our basic science courses. Instead of being taught how to think about science and health, instead of learning general principles of human biology, we were inundated with masses of detail that we were expected to regurgitate on frequent exams. Many of us had experienced much better teaching in college, and we complained bitterly. The faculty put us off by saying that a brand-new curriculum, the product of much work by committees and subcommittees, was to be unveiled in the second semester: an integrated curriculum that was to be a model for medical schools of the future. What you are getting now is the old stuff, they told us, so please stop complaining and be patient.

Came the first day of the new curriculum. Instead of studying traditional subjects like embryology, anatomy, physiology, and biochemistry, we were now going to study systems of the body, and the first unit was to focus on the heart. An embryologist delivered an incredibly detailed sixty-minute lecture on the embryology of the heart. Then an anatomist gave an equally detailed lecture on cardiac anatomy. And so on for physiology and biochemistry. At the end of four hours, we were dazed, confused, and angry. This was supposed to be integrated teaching? It was integration by juxtaposition, nothing more. And I am sorry to say that in all the years since, I have listened to committees and subcommittees proposing ideas for curriculum reform and there has been no progress whatsoever. It all amounts to reshuffling the deck and dealing out the same cards in a different order.

What I mean by radical reform of medical education is this:

• Basic instruction in the philosophy of science, with reference to new models based on quantum physics that replace old concepts of Newtonian mechanism and Cartesian dualism. Such instruction would include information on probability and gambling theory, would discuss possible interactions of the observer and the observed, and would present models that could account for the nonphysical causation of physical events.

• Instruction in the history of medicine with reference to the development of major systems like traditional Chinese medicine, homeopathy, and osteopathy.

• Emphasis on the healing power of nature and the body's healing system.

• Emphasis on mind/body interactions, including placebo responses, medical hexing, and psychoneuroimmunology.

• Instruction in psychology and spirituality in addition to information about the physical body.

• Reduction in the amount of factual knowledge students are now required to memorize to pass certifying examinations. If students learn how to learn and know the general structure of knowledge in the various medical sciences, they will be able to look up the details as they need them, especially as this information becomes available in computerized formats.

• Provision of practical experience in the areas of nutrition, exercise, relaxation, meditation, and visualization. Students should be evaluated not only on factual knowledge but on personal progress in developing healthy lifestyles.

• Practical experience with the basic techniques of alternative medicine, such as herbalism, nutritional medicine, manipulation, body work, breath work, acupuncture, and guided imagery, in addition to the basic techniques of allopathic medicine.

• Instruction on how to design and conduct research in medicine and how to evaluate published research.

• Instruction in the art of communication, including interviewing patients, taking medical histories, and presenting treatments in ways that are likely to activate the body's healing system.

In addition to these changes in the training of doctors, I would insist on the creation of a National Institute of Health and Healing within the National Institutes of Health. The mission of this institute would be to investigate all healing phenomena, including spontaneous remissions of cancer and other diseases, placebo responses, and faith healing. The present Office of Alternative Medicine should operate within this organization with a greatly expanded budget to conduct research on the efficacy of alternative treatments and their cost-effectiveness compared to conventional treatments. Another goal of the Institute of Health and Healing should be to develop a National Registry of Healing, classified by diseases and extensively cross-referenced. This information should be available to all health professionals and patients, so that if you develop scleroderma, for example, you can obtain a list of persons in your area of the country who have experienced healing of scleroderma, and you or your doctor can contact them to discover what steps they took. Not only will this information permit researchers to compile data on the most promising treatments for particular diseases, it will also, I predict, increase the incidence of spontaneous healing in our society.

You can help bring these changes about by adding your voice to the chorus demanding changes in health care. A powerful consumers' movement is responsible for the growth of alternative medicine around the world and for the growing openness to it within the medical profession. The fact that there is an Office of Alternative Medicine in the National Institutes of Health is testament to this change. In addition, conventional medicine is now caught in an economic crunch that is forcing hospitals, insurance companies, and doctors to consider ideas that would have been unthinkable a decade ago. The time is right for change. The direction in which medicine needs to move is clear.

ACKNOWLEDGMENTS

This book was written mostly during a summer of record heat and dryness in the Sonoran Desert of southern Arizona and in the midst of a major move my family made from one end of the Tucson valley to the other. Early in the move I lost my office and a comfortable place to write. Mel Zuckerman of Canyon Ranch came to the rescue by offering me a guest house to use as a writing studio. Without his help, this book would not have seen the light of day so soon. I am much indebted to him and to Enid Zuckerman, and to Gary Frost, Jerry Cohen, Jonah Liebrecht, and other personnel at Canyon Ranch for their generous hospitality. I also thank my wife Sabine for holding down the home fort during this time so that I was free to write.

My agent, Richard Pine of Arthur Pine Associates, was instrumental in finding the right publisher for the book and motivating me to get to work on it. He also contributed useful insights and facts. And I thank Marly Rusoff and Sara Davidson for introducing me to Richard. Jonathan Segal, my editor at Alfred A. Knopf, gave the manuscript great attention while it was in preparation, for which I am most grateful.

Persons who contributed information to the book include Dr. James Dalen and Dr. Jean Wilson of the University of Arizona Health Sciences Center; Dr. Robert Anderson, Dr. William Manahan, Dr. Amy Stine, Dr. Michael T. Murray, Dr. Gail L. Lamb, Mark Blumenthal, Stephen Foster, Deborah Coryell, Kay Swetnam, Paul Stamets, and all the patients who graciously consented to let me use their stories of healing in these pages. Pete Craig of the University of Arizona College of Medicine gave me excellent research assistance, and a number of readers of the manuscript made valuable suggestions: Melanie Anderson, Brian Becker, Sue Fleishman, Woody Wickham, and Sabine Kremp especially.

Kevin Barry, senior hydrotherapist at Canyon Ranch, kept me relaxed and in good spirits while I was writing, and Dr. Dean Ornish gave me pep talks when I was feeling overwhelmed.

Finally, I must express special thanks to my old friend and sometime coauthor, Winifred Rosen, who spent a great deal of time and energy helping me polish the writing to a point that satisfied both of us.

Andrew Weil
Tucson, Arizona
Spring 1995

Appendix:

Finding Practitioners, Supplies, and Information

Here is a listing of organizations that can help you find practitioners of therapies mentioned in this book:

Acupuncture

American Academy of Medical Acupuncture
5820 Wilshire Boulevard, Suite 500
Los Angeles, California 90036
213 937-5514

Biofeedback

Biofeedback Certification Institute of America
10200 West 44th Avenue, Suite 304
Wheat Ridge, Colorado 80033
303 420-2902

Cranial Therapy

Cranial Academy
8606 Allisonville Road, Suite 130
Indianapolis, Indiana 46250
317 594-0411

Feldenkrais Work

The Feldenkrais Guild
P.O. Box 489
Albany, Oregon 97321
800 775-2118

Guided Imagery™ Therapy

Academy for Guided Imagery
P.O. Box 2070
Mill Valley, California 94942
415 389-9324

Herbal Medicine

American Herbalists Guild
P.O. Box 1683
Soquel, California 95073
408 464-2441

Herb Research Foundation
1007 Pearl Street, Suite 200
Boulder, Colorado 80302
303 449-2265

Holistic Medicine

American Holistic Medical Association
4101 Lake Boone Trail, Suite 201
Raleigh, North Carolina 27607
919 787-5146

Homeopathy

National Center for Homeopathy
801 North Fairfax Street, Suite 306
Alexandria, Virginia 22314
703 548-7790

Hypnotherapy

American Society of Clinical Hypnosis
2250 East Devon Avenue, Suite 336
Des Plaines, Illinois 60018-4534
708 297-3317

Milton H. Erikson Society for Psychotherapy and Hypnosis
P.O. Box 1390
Madison Square Station
New York, New York 10159
212 628-0287

Naturopathy

American Association of Naturopathic Physicians
2366 Eastlake Avenue East, Suite 322
Seattle, Washington 98102
206 323-7610

Osteopathic Manipulative Therapy

American Academy of Osteopathy
3500 De Pauw Boulevard, Suite 1080
Indianapolis, Indiana 46268
317 879-1881

Rolfing

Rolf Institute
205 Canyon Boulevard
Boulder, Colorado 80306
303 449-5903

Traditional Chinese Medicine

The American Foundation of Traditional Chinese Medicine
505 Beach Street
San Francisco, California 94133
415 776-0502

Institute for Traditional Medicine
2017 Southeast Hawthorne
Portland, Oregon 97214
503 233-4907

Trager Work

The Trager Institute
33 Millwood
Mill Valley, California 94941
415 388-2688

The following companies sell products mentioned in this book:

Chinese Tonics and Medicinal Herbs

The Tea Garden Herbal Emporium
903 Colorado Boulevard, Suite 200
Santa Monica, California 90405
310 450-0188

Freeze-Dried Herbal Extracts and Tinctures

Eclectic Institute
14385 Southeast Lusted Road
Sandy, Oregon 97055
800 332-4372

Ginger Preparations

New Moon Extracts, Inc.
99 Main Street
Brattleboro, Vermont 05301
802 257-0018

Maitake Mushrooms

Maitake, Products, Inc.
P.O. Box 1354
Paramus, New Jersey 07653
800 747-7418

Fungi Perfecti
P.O. Box 7634
Olympia, Washington 98507
800 780-9126

Franklin Mushroom Farm
931 Rte 32
N. Franklin, CT 06254-0018
860 642-3000

Organic Produce

Eden Acres, Inc.
12100 Lima Center Road
Clinton, Michigan 49236
517 456-4288
(distributes directories of organic growers)

Mothers & Others for a Livable Planet
40 West 10th Street
New York, New York 10011
212 242-0010

Radiation Shields for Computer Displays

NoRad Corporations
1549 11th Street
Santa Monica, California 90401
800 262-3260

Vitamins and Supplements

L & H Vitamins
37-10 Crescent Street
Long Island City, New York 11101
800 221-1152

The Vitamin Shoppe
4700 Westside Avenure
North Bergen, New Jersey 07047
800 223-1216

Detailed instructions for management of common medical conditions with natural remedies that take advantage of the body's healing system will be found in my book *Natural Health, Natural Medicine: A Comprehensive Manual for Wellness and Self-Care* (Boston: Houghton Mifflin, revised edition, 1995).

If you would like information on my seminars, lectures, and informational products, including a monthly newsletter I write on health and healing, please send a postcard to:

Andrew Weil, M.D.
P.O. Box 697
Vail, Arizona 85641

NOTES

Introduction

4 Quotation from René Dubos: *Mirage of Health: Utopias, Progress, and Biological Change* (New York: Harper & Brothers, 1959), 110–11.

5 Resistance to antimicrobial agents: Michael D. Katz in *Clinical Research News for Arizona Physicians* 5 (September 1994):9 (published by the University of Arizona Health Sciences Center, Office of Public Affairs). For further information on this subject, see A. Tomascz, "Multiple-Antibiotic-Resistant Pathogenic Bacteria: A Report on the Rockefeller University Workshop," *New England Journal of Medicine* 330 (1994):1247–51; and J. A. Fisher, *The Plague Makers: How We Are Creating Catastrophic New Epidemics—and What We Must Do to Avert Them* (New York: Simon & Schuster, 1994).

PART ONE: THE HEALING SYSTEM

1. Prologue in the Rain Forest

15 Hahnemann on disease suppression: Samuel Hahnemann, *The Chronic Diseases: Theoretical Part* (New Delhi: B. Jain, 1993). This was originally published in German in 1835.

19 The fate of the Kofán: See Joe Kane, "Letter from the Amazon," *New Yorker,* September 27, 1993.

2. Right in My Own Backyard

31 Confirmation of cranial motion: V. M. Frymann, "A Study of the Rhythmic Motions of the Living Cranium," *Journal of the American Osteo-*

pathic Association 70 (1971):928–45; D. K. Michael and E. W. Retzlaff, "A Preliminary Study of Cranial Bone Movement in the Squirrel Monkey," *Journal of the American Osteopathic Association* 74 (1975):866–9; E. W. Retzlaff et al., "Cranial Bone Mobility," *Journal of the American Osteopathic Association* 74 (1975):869–73.

36 Documentary film of Dr. Fulford: *Robert Fulford: An Osteopathic Alternative,* available from Biomedical Communications, University of Arizona Health Sciences Center, Tucson, Arizona 85724.

3. Testimonials

51 Effects of *Ginkgo biloba:* J. Kleijnen and P. Knipschild, "*Ginkgo biloba* for Cerebral Insufficiency," *British Journal of Clinical Pharmacology* 34 (1992):352–8.

4. Medical Pessimism

60 People who go to alternative practitioners: D. M. Eisenberg et al., "Unconventional Medicine in the United States: Prevalence, Costs, and Patterns of Use," *New England Journal of Medicine* 328 (1993):246–52.

61 Voodoo death: See W. B. Cannon, "Voodoo Death," *Psychosomatic Medicine* 19 (1957):182–90.

Hexing in exotic cultures: See, for example, R. A. Kirkpatrick, "Witchcraft and Lupus Erythematosus," *Journal of the American Medical Association* 245 (1981):1937.

66 Bibliography of spontaneous remission: Brendan O'Regan and Carlyle Hirshberg, *Spontaneous Remission: An Annotated Bibliography* (Sausalito, California: Institute of Noetic Sciences, 1993).

Quotation on remission and cancer: O'Regan and Hirshberg, *Spontaneous Remission,* 13.

Wart cures: See "Why Warts Fall Off," Chapter 18 of my book *Health and Healing* (Boston: Houghton Mifflin, 1988).

5. The Healing System

73 Enzymes: See Donald Voet and Judith G. Voet, *Biochemistry* (New York: John Wiley & Sons, 1990), Chapter 12, "Introduction to Enzymes," 316–28, and Chapter 14, "Enzymatic Catalysis," 355–90.

74 DNA repair enzymes: See E. C. Friedberg, *DNA Repair* (New York: Freeman, 1985). Also, A. Sancar and G. B. Sancar, "DNA Repair Enzymes," *Annual Review of Biochemistry* 57 (1988):29–67.

75 Many different enzymes available for the healing of DNA: See Voet and Voet, *Biochemistry,* Chapter 31, "DNA Replication, Repair, and Recombination," 948–86.

77 Recycling of LDL receptors: J. L. Goldstein et al., "Receptor-mediated Endocytosis," *Annual Review of Cell Biology* 1 (1985):1–39.

79 Growth factors in wound healing: Ramzi S. Cotran, Vinay Kumar, and Stanley L. Robbins, *Robbins Pathologic Basis of Disease*, 4th ed. (Philadelphia: W. B. Saunders, 1989), 74–77.

80 Bone healing: Cotran, Kumar, and Robbins, *Robbins Pathologic Basis*, 1322–33.
Becker on bone healing and regeneration: Robert O. Becker and Gary Selden, *The Body Electric: Electromagnetism and the Foundation of Life* (New York: William Morrow, 1985).
Regeneration of the liver: Cotran, Kumar, and Robbins, *Robbins Pathologic Basis*, 72, 913.

81 Absence of regeneration in heart and nerve cells: Cotran, Kumar, and Robbins, *Robbins Pathologic Basis*, 72–73.

82 Reversibility of atherosclerosis: Dean Ornish, *Dr. Dean Ornish's Program for Reversing Heart Disease Without Drugs or Surgery* (New York: Ballantine, 1992).

84 Case report from Lourdes: J. Garner, "Spontaneous Regressions: Scientific Documentation as a Basis for the Declaration of Miracles," *Canadian Medical Association Journal* 111 (1974):1254–64.

85 Case of Vittorio Micheli: J. Garner, "Spontaneous Regressions," quoted in Brendan O'Regan and Carlyle Hirshberg, *Spontaneous Remission: An Annotated Bibliography* (Sausalito, California: Institute of Noetic Sciences, 1993), 548.

6. The Role of the Mind in Healing

90 Article on ulcerative colitis and smoking: E. J. Boyko et al., "Risk of Ulcerative Colitis Among Former and Current Cigarette Smokers," *New England Journal of Medicine* 316 (1987):707–10.

91 Ulcer as an infectious disease: See Terence Monmaney, "Annals of Medicine," *New Yorker*, September 20, 1993.

92 Candace Pert on neuropeptides: C. B. Pert et al., "Neuropeptides and Their Receptors: A Psychosomatic Network," *Journal of Immunology* 135 (1985):820s–826s.

93 Quotation from Pert: C. B. Pert et al., "Neuropeptides," 824s.

103 Quotation from Lao-tzu: *The Way of Life According to Lao Tzu*, translated by Witter Bynner (New York: Perigee Books, 1972), verses 43 and 55.

7. The Tao of Healing

110 The art of dying: See, for example, Mary Catharine O'Connor, *Art of Dying Well: Development of the* Ars Moriendi (New York: Columbia University Press, 1967).

113 Cancer seems almost to be an occupational hazard of sainthood: Larry Dossey, *Meaning in Medicine* (New York: Bantam, 1991), 208–9.

119 Book by John Sarno: John E. Sarno, *Healing Back Pain: The Mind-Body Connection* (New York: Warner Books, 1991).

120 Lack of correlation between subjective experience of back pain and objective measures: M. C. Jensen et al., "Magnetic Resonance Imaging of the Lumbar Spine in People Without Back Pain," *New England Journal of Medicine* 331 (1994):69–73.

PART TWO: OPTIMIZING THE HEALING SYSTEM

8. Optimizing Your Healing System: An Overview

133 Lupus in Nogales, Arizona: K. Bagwell, "Lupus Is Found at Highest Rate in Nogales, Ariz.," *Arizona Daily Star,* November 7, 1993.

9. A Healing Diet

136 Low-fat diet and longevity: S. A. Grover et al., "Life Expectancy Following Dietary Modification or Smoking Cessation," *Archives of Internal Medicine* 154 (1994):1697–704.

137 Animals live longer with less disease on fewer calories: E. J. Masoro, "Assessment of Nutritional Components in Prolongation of Life and Health by Diet," *Proceedings of the Society for Experimental Biology and Medicine* 193 (1990):31–34.

142 Olive oil and better health: M. Aviram and K. Eias, "Dietary Olive Oil Reduces Low-Density Lipoprotein Uptake by Macrophages and Decreases the Susceptibility of the Lipoprotein to Undergo Lipid Peroxidation," *Annals of Nutrition and Metabolism* 37 (1995):75–84.

143 Omega-3 fatty acids and health: For example, see A. Leaf, "Cardiovascular Effects of Omega-3 Fatty Acids," *New England Journal of Medicine* 318 (1988):549–57; W. Hermann, "The Influence of Dietary Supplementation with Omega-3 Fatty Acids on Serum Lipids, Apolipoproteins, Coagulation, and Fibrinolytic Parameters," *Zeitschrift für Klinische Medizin* 46 (1991):1363–69; R. A. Karmali, "Omega-3 Fatty Acids and Cancer," *Journal of Internal Medicine* 225 (suppl. 1, 1989):197–200; J. M. Kremer, "Clinical Studies of Omega-3 Fatty Acid Supplementation in Patients Who Have Rheumatoid Arthritis," *Rheumatic Disease Clinics of North America* 17 (1991):391–402; and H. R. Knapp, "Omega-3 Fatty Acids, Endogenous Prostaglandins, and Blood Pressure Regulation in Humans," *Nutrition Reviews* 47 (1989):301–13.

149 Soy phytoestrogens: A. Cassidy et al., "Biological Effects of a Diet of Soy Protein Rich in Isoflavones on the Menstrual Cycle of Premenopausal Women," *American Journal of Clinical Nutrition* 60 (1994):333–40.

10. Protecting Yourself from Toxins

154 Quotation on pesticides on food crops: T. H. Jukes, "Organic Food," *CRC Critical Reviews in Food Science & Nutrition* 9 (1977):395–418.
155 Quotation on aldicarb in watermelon: A. M. Fan and R. J. Jackson, "Pesticides and Food Safety," *Regulatory Toxicology and Pharmacology* 9 (1989): 158–74, 168.
163 Quotation on DDT in fish: Fan and Jackson, "Pesticides," 169.
165 Most heavily contaminated vegetable crops: R. Wiles et al., *Washed, Peeled, Contaminated* (Washington, D.C.: Environmental Working Group, 1994).
169 Biological hazards of energy: Robert O. Becker, *Cross Currents: The Perils of Electropollution, The Promise of Electromedicine* (Los Angeles: Tarcher, 1991).

11. Using Tonics

173 Garlic lowers blood pressure: J. E. Brody, "Personal Health: Modern Doctors Confirm the Ancient Wisdom That Garlic Has Many Benefits," *New York Times,* July 27, 1994.
Effects of garlic on cholesterol and blood clotting: "Garlic," *Lawrence Review of Natural Products* (St. Louis, Missouri: Facts and Comparisons), April 1994. See also S. Warshafsky et al., "Effect of Garlic on Total Serum Cholesterol: A Meta-analysis," *Annals of Internal Medicine* 119 (1993): 599–605.
Garlic as an anticancer agent: Brody, "Modern Doctors Confirm."
174 Effects of ginger on the digestive system: Paul Schulick, *Ginger: Common Spice & Wonder Drug* (Brattleboro, Vermont: Herbal Free Press, rev. ed., 1994), passim. This book contains an excellent list of references to the scientific literature.
175 Anti-inflammatory effect of ginger: Schulick, *Ginger.*
176 Health benefits of green tea: Jean Carper, *Food—Your Miracle Medicine* (New York: HarperCollins, 1993), 212–3. See also H. N. Graham, "Green Tea Composition, Consumption, and Polyphenol Chemistry," *Preventive Medicine* 21 (1992) 334–50; Y. Sagesaka-Mitane et al., "Platelet Aggregation Inhibitors in Hot Water Extract of Green Tea," *Chemical and Pharmacological Bulletin* (Tokyo) 38 (1990):790–93.
177 Protective effect of milk thistle on liver: V. Fintelmann and A. Albert, *Therapiewoche* 30 (1980):5589–94; H. Hikino and Y. Kiso, "Natural Products for Liver Disease," in H. Wagner, H. Hikino, and N. R. Farnsworth, *Eco-*

nomic and Medicinal Plant Research, Vol. 2 (New York: Academic Press, 1988), 39–72.

178 Fu zheng therapy: Subhuti Dharmananda, *Chinese Herbal Therapies* (Portland, Oregon: Institute for Traditional Medicine, 1988), Chapter 2. Astragalus enhances immune function: See "Astragalus" in A. Y. Leung and S. Foster, *Encyclopedia of Common Natural Ingredients* (New York: John Wiley & Sons, 1995).

179 Protective effects of Siberian ginseng: N. R. Farnsworth et al., "Siberian Ginseng (*Eleutherococcus senticosus*): Current Status as an Adaptogen," in H. Wagner, H. Hikino, and N. R. Farnsworth (eds.), *Economic and Medicinal Plant Research,* Vol. 1 (Orlando, Florida: Academic Press, 1985), 155–215; and B. W. Halstead and L. L. Hood, *Eleutherococcus senticosus, Siberian Ginseng: An Introduction to the Concept of Adaptogenic Medicine* (Long Beach, California: Oriental Healing Arts Institutre, 1984).

182 Quotation on maitake: From H. Namba, "Maitake Mushroom: Promising Immune Therapy for Cancer Treatment," *New Editions Health World,* October 1994, 20–24.

183 Anticancer and immune-enhancing effects of maitake: N. Ohno et al., "Structural Characterization and Antitumor Activity of the Extracts from Matted Mycelium of Cultured *Grifola frondosa*," *Chemical and Pharmacological Bulletin* (Tokyo) 33 (1985):3395–401; also, I. Suzuki, "Antitumor and Immunomodulating Activities of a β-Glucan Obtained from Liquid-cultured *Grifola frondosa*," *Chemical and Pharmacological Bulletin* (Tokyo) 37 (1989):410–13.

184 Quotation on Chinese distance runners: Cameron Smith, "Gold Medal Herbs," *Natural Health,* May/June 1994, 85–7.

13. Mind and Spirit

202 Quotation from Rabbi Nachman of Bratislav: Edward Hoffman, *The Way of Splendor: Jewish Mysticism and Modern Psychology* (Northvale, New Jersey: Jason Aronson, 1992), 124.

203 Quotation on breath: Andrew Weil, *Natural Health, Natural Medicine* (Boston: Houghton Mifflin, 2nd rev. ed., 1995), 89.

207 Few books about breathing are available: An excellent one of recent publication is *Conscious Breathing* by Gay Hendricks, Ph.D. (New York: Bantam, 1995). It has detailed instructions for working with breath to improve physical, mental, and spiritual health.

208 Italian-Americans of Roseto, Pennsylvania: C. Stout et al., "Unusually Low Incidence of Death from Myocardial Infarction: Study of an Italian American Community in Pennsylvania," *Journal of the American Medical Association* 188 (1964):845–49; A. Keys, "Arteriosclerotic Heart Disease in Roseto, Pennsylvania," *Journal of the American Medical Association*

195 (1966):137–39. The conclusions of these papers are questioned in a more recent article by S. Wolf et al., "Roseto Revisited: Further Data on the Incidence of Myocardial Infarction in Roseto and Neighboring Pennsylvania Communities," *Transactions of the American Clinical and Climatological Association* 85 (1973):100–08.

PART THREE: IF YOU GET SICK

15. *Making the Right Decisions*

224 Schizandra and chronic hepatitis: L. Geng-tao, "Pharmacological Actions and Clinical Use of Fructus Schizandrae," *Chinese Medical Journal* 102 (1989):740–49.

227 Feverfew and rheumatoid arthritis: H. O. Collier et al., "Extract of Feverfew Inhibits Prostaglandin Biosynthesis," *Lancet* 11 (1981):1054; M. I. Berry, "Feverfew Faces the Future," *Pharmacy Journal* 232 (1984):611–14.

229 GLA for eczema: V. A. Ziboh, "Implications of Dietary Oils and Polyunsaturated Fatty Acids in the Management of Cutaneous Disorders," *Archives of Dermatology* 125 (1989):241–5.

230 Echinacea as an immune enhancer: B. Bräunig et al., "Echinacea purpureae Radix for Strengthening the Immune Response in Flu-like Infections," *Zeitschrift für Phytotherapie* 13 (1992):7–13.

232 DGL (licorice extract): See Bardhan et al., "Clinical Trial of Deglycyrrhizinated Liquorice in Gastric Ulcer," *Gut* 19 (1978):779–82; A. G. Morgan et al., "Comparison Between Cimetidine and Caved-S in the Treatment of Gastric Ulceration, and Subsequent Maintenance Therapy," *Gut* 23 (1982):545–51.

234 Quercetin reduces allergic responsiveness: E. Middleton and G. Drzewieki, "Naturally Occurring Flavonoids and Human Basophil Histamine Release," *International Archives of Allergy and Applied Immunology* 77 (1985): 155–77; M. Amelia et al., "Inhibition of Mast Cell Histamine Release by Flavonoids and Bioflavonoids," *Planta Medica* 51 (1985):16–20; E. Middleton and C. Kundaswami, "Effects of Flavonoids on Immune and Inflammatory Cell Functions," *Biochemical Pharmacology* 43 (1992):1167–79.

16. *Considering the Alternatives*

238 I have written elsewhere about alternative medicine: See Andrew Weil, *Health and Healing* (Boston: Houghton Mifflin, rev. ed., 1988).

239 Guggul lowers cholesterol: G. V. Satyavati, "Gum *Guggul (Commiphora mukul)*—the Success Story of an Ancient Insight Leading to a Modern Discovery," *Indian Journal of Medical Research* 87 (1988):327–35; S. Nityanand et al., "Clinical Trials with Gugulipid, a New Hypolipi-

daemic Agent," *Journal of the Association of Physicians of India* 37 (1989):323–28.

246 Beneficial effects of prayer on health: Larry Dossey, *Healing Words: The Power of Prayer and the Practice of Medicine* (San Francisco: Harper San Francisco, 1993).

18. *Managing General Categories of Illness: Secrets of a Hygeian Practitioner*

254 Stinging nettles for hay fever: P. Mittman, "Randomized, Double-Blind Study of Freeze-Dried *Urtica dioica* in the Treatment of Allergic Rhinitis," *Planta Medica* 56 (1990):44–46.

256 Anti-Inflammatory effect of feverfew: See "Feverfew," *Lawrence Review of Natural Products* (St. Louis, Missouri: Facts and Comparisons), September 1994.

Turmeric and curcumin: M. Murray, "Curcumin: A Potent Anti-inflammatory Agent," *American Journal of Natural Medicine* 1 (1994):10–13.

257 Coenzyme Q: T. Kawasaki, "Antioxidant Function of Coenzyme Q," *Journal of Nutritional Science and Vitaminology* 38 (1992), special number, 552–55.

L carnitine improves the metabolism of heart muscle cells: C. J. Pepine, "The Therapeutic Potential of Carnitine in Cardiovascular Disorders," *Clinical Therapeutics* 13 (1991):2–21.

Tree ear mushrooms have an anticoagulant effect: D. E. Hammerschmidt, "Szechuan Purpura," *New England Journal of Medicine* 302 (1980): 1191–93.

259 Antibiotic and immune-enhancing properties of echinacea: B. Bräunig et al., "Echinacea purpureae Radix for Strengthening the Immune Response in Flu-like Infections," *Zeitschrift für Phytotherapie* 13 (1992):7–13.

260 Saw palmetto and *Pygeum* for prostatic enlargement: G. Champault et al., "A Double-blind Trial of an Extract of the Plant *Serenoa repens* in Benign Prostatic Hyperplasia," *British Journal of Clinical Pharmacology* 18 (1984):461–62; A. Barlet et al., "Efficacy of *Pygeum africanum* Extract in the Medical Therapy of Urination Disorders Due to Benign Prostatic Hyperplasia: Evaluation of Objective and Subjective Parameters: A Placebo-controlled Double-blind Multicenter Study," *Wiener Klinische Wochenschrifte* 102 (1990):667–73.

262 Niacinamide can be very helpful for osteoarthritis: W. Kaufman, "The Use of Vitamin Therapy to Reverse Certain Concomitants of Aging," *Journal of the American Geriatric Society* 3 (1955):927–36.

Boswellia for musculoskeletal pain: C. K. Reddy et al., "Studies on the Metabolism of Glycosaminoglycans Under the Influence of New Herbal Anti-inflammatory Agents," *Biochemical Pharmacology* 20 (1989): 3527–34.

19. Cancer as a Special Case

269 Account of Helen B.: Dr. R. A. Anderson, "Carcinoma of the Ovary: A Case Report," December 1992.

271 Alternative treatment for cancer: For a review of this subject with detailed information on the nature and availability of therapies, see Michael Lerner, *Choices in Healing* (Boston: MIT Press, 1994).

272 It is imperative to maintain our healing systems in good working order: In addition to the information in Part Two of this book, see my previous book, *Natural Health, Natural Medicine* (Boston: Houghton Mifflin, 2nd rev. ed., 1995), especially Chapter 11, "How Not to Get Cancer," and Chapter 12, "How to Protect Your Immune System."

Books exist to guide patients in making these difficult decisions: For example, S. Austin and C. Hitchcock, *Breast Cancer: What You Should Know (But May Not Be Told) About Prevention, Diagnosis, and Treatment* (Rocklin, California: Prima Publishing, 1994), which includes an excellent analysis of the choices facing women with breast cancer.

INDEX

About the Author

ANDREW WEIL, M.D., a graduate of Harvard Medical School, has worked for the National Institute of Mental Health and for fifteen years was a research associate in ethnopharmacology at the Harvard Botanical Museum. As a fellow of the Institute of Current World Affairs, he traveled extensively throughout the world collecting information about the medicinal properties of plants, altered states of consciousness, and healing. He is currently Associate Director of the Division of Social Perspectives in Medicine and Director of the Program in Integrative Medicine at the University of Arizona in Tucson, where he practices natural and preventive medicine. This is Dr. Weil's sixth book.

You can reach Dr. Weil via HotWired on the WorldWide Web at http://www.drweil.com/

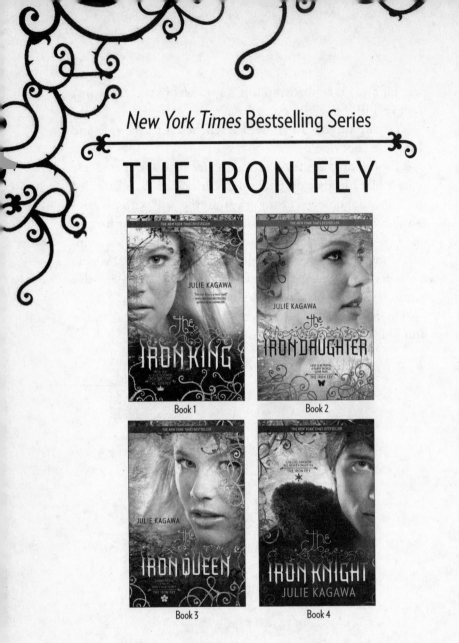
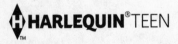

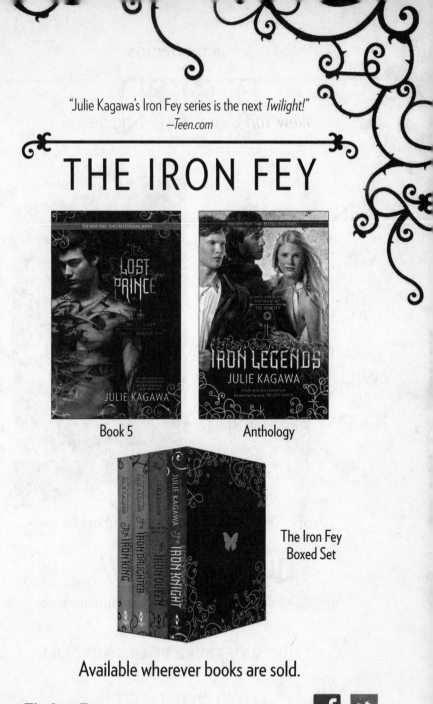

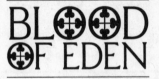
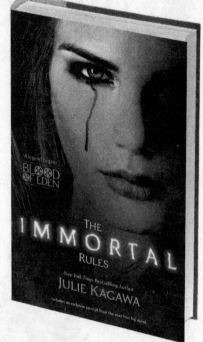
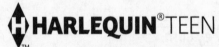

THE GODDESS TEST NOVELS

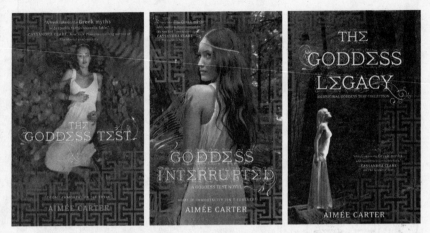

Available wherever books are sold!

A modern saga inspired by the Persephone myth.

Kate Winters's life hasn't been easy. She's battling with the upcoming death of her mother, and only a mysterious stranger called Henry is giving her hope. But he must be crazy, right? Because there is no way the god of the Underworld—Hades himself—is going to choose Kate to take the seven tests that might make her an immortal...and his wife. And even if she passes the tests, is there any hope for happiness with a war brewing between the gods?

Also available:
The Goddess Hunt, a digital-only novella.

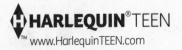

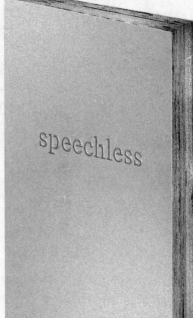
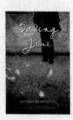
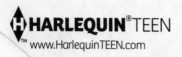

CHAPTER ONE
NEW KID

My name is Ethan Chase.

And I doubt I'll live to see my eighteenth birthday.

That's not me being dramatic; it just is. I just wish I hadn't pulled so many people into this mess. They shouldn't have to suffer because of me. Especially...her. God, if I could take back anything in my life, I would never have shown her my world, the hidden world all around us. I *knew* better than to let her in. Once you see Them, they'll never leave you alone. They'll never let you go. Maybe if I'd been strong, she wouldn't be here with me as our seconds tick away, waiting to die.

It all started the day I transferred to a new school. Again.

The alarm clock went off at 6:00 a.m., but I had been awake for an hour, getting ready for another day in my weird, screwed-up life. I wish I was one of those guys who roll out of bed, throw on a shirt and are ready to go, but sadly, my life isn't that normal. For instance, today I'd filled the side pockets of my backpack with dried Saint-John's-wort and stuffed a canister of salt in with my pens and notebook. I'd also driven three nails into the heels of the new boots Mom had bought me for the semester. I wore an iron cross on a chain beneath my shirt, and just last summer I'd gotten my ears pierced with metal studs. Originally, I'd gotten a lip ring and an eyebrow bar, too, but Dad had thrown a roof-shaking fit when I came home like that, and the studs were the only things I'd been allowed to keep.

Sighing, I spared a quick glance at myself in the mirror, making sure I looked as unapproachable as possible. Sometimes, I catch Mom looking at me sadly, as if she wonders where her little boy went. I used to have curly brown hair like Dad, until I took a pair of scissors and hacked it into jagged, uneven spikes. I used to have bright blue eyes like Mom and, apparently, like my sister. But over the years, my eyes have become darker, changing to a smoky-blue-gray—from constant glaring, Dad jokes. I never used to sleep with a knife under my mattress, salt around my windows, and a horseshoe over my door. I never used to be "brooding" and "hostile" and "impossible." I used to smile more, and laugh. I rarely do any of that now.

I know Mom worries about me. Dad says it's normal teenage rebellion, that I'm going through a "phase," and that I'll grow out of it. Sorry, Dad. But my life is far from normal. And I'm dealing with it the only way I know how.

"Ethan?" Mom's voice drifted into the room from beyond the door, soft and hesitant. "It's past six. Are you up?"

"I'm up." I grabbed my backpack and swung it over my white shirt, which was inside out, the tag poking up from the collar. Another small quirk my parents have gotten used to. "I'll be right out."

Grabbing my keys, I left my room with that familiar sense of resignation and dread stealing over me. *Okay, then. Let's get this day over with.*

I have a weird family.

You'd never know it by looking at us. We seem perfectly normal; a nice American family living in a nice suburban neighborhood, with nice clean streets and nice neighbors on either side. Ten years ago we lived in the swamps, raising pigs. Ten years ago we were poor, backwater folk, and we were happy. That was before we moved into the city, before we joined civilization again. My dad didn't like it at first; he'd spent his whole life as a farmer. It was hard for him to adjust, but he did, eventually. Mom finally convinced him that we needed to be closer to people, that *I* needed to be closer to people, that the constant isolation was bad for me. That was what she told Dad, of course, but I knew the real reason. She was afraid. She was afraid of Them, that They would take me away again, that I would be kidnapped by faeries and taken into the Nevernever.

Yeah, I told you, my family is weird. And that's not even the worst of it.

Somewhere out there, I have a sister. A half sister I haven't seen in years, and not because she's busy or married or across the ocean in some other country.

No, it's because she's a queen. A faery queen, one of Them, and she can't ever come home.

Tell me *that's* not messed up.

Of course, I can't ever tell anyone. To normal humans, the fey world is hidden—glamoured and invisible. Most people wouldn't see a goblin if it sauntered up and bit them on the nose. There are very few mortals cursed with the Sight, who can see faeries lurking in dark corners and under beds. Who know that the creepy feeling of being watched isn't just their imagination, and that the noises in the cellar or the attic aren't really the house settling.

Lucky me. I happen to be one of them.

My parents worry, of course, Mom especially. People already think I'm weird, dangerous, maybe a little crazy. Seeing faeries everywhere will do that to you. Because if the fey *know* you can see them, they tend to make your life a living hell. Last year, I was kicked out of school for setting fire to the library. What could I tell them? I was innocent because I was trying to escape a redcap motley that followed me in from the street? And that wasn't the first time the fey had gotten me into trouble. I was the "bad kid," the one the teachers spoke about in hushed voices, the quiet, dangerous kid whom everyone expected would end up on the evening news for some awful, shocking crime. Sometimes, it was infuriating. I didn't really care what they thought of me, but it was hard on Mom, so I tried to be good, futile as it was.

This semester, I'd be going to a new school, a new location. A place I could "start clean," but it wouldn't matter. As long as I could see the fey, they would never leave me alone. All I could do was protect myself and my family, and hope I wouldn't end up hurting anyone else.

Mom was at the kitchen table when I came out, waiting for me. Dad wasn't around. He worked the graveyard shift at UPS and often slept till the middle of the afternoon. Usually, I'd see him only at dinner and on weekends. That's not to say he was happily oblivious when it came to my life; Mom might know me better, but Dad had no problem doling out punishments if he thought I was slacking, or if Mom complained. I'd gotten one D in science two years ago, and it was the last bad grade I'd ever received.

"Big day," Mom greeted me as I tossed the backpack on the counter and opened the fridge, reaching for the orange juice. "Are you sure you know the way to your new school?"

I nodded. "I've got it set to my phone's GPS. It's not that far. I'll be fine."

She hesitated. I knew she didn't want me driving there alone, even though I'd worked my butt off saving up for a car. The rusty, gray-green pickup sitting next to Dad's truck in the driveway represented an entire summer of work—flipping burgers, washing dishes, mopping up spilled drinks and food and vomit. It represented weekends spent working late, watching other kids my age hanging out, kissing girlfriends, tossing away money like it fell from the sky. I'd *earned* that truck, and I certainly wasn't going to take the freaking bus to school.

But because Mom was watching me with that sad, almost fearful look on her face, I sighed and muttered, "Do you want me to call you when I get there?"

"No, honey." Mom straightened, waving it off. "It's all right, you don't have to do that. Just…please be careful."

I heard the unspoken words in her voice. *Be careful of* Them. *Don't attract their attention. Don't let Them get you into trouble. Try to stay in school this time.*

"I will."

She hovered a moment longer, then placed a quick peck on my cheek and wandered into the living room, pretending to be busy. I drained my juice, poured another glass, and opened the fridge to put the container back.

As I closed the door, a magnet slipped loose and pinged to the floor, and the note it was holding fluttered to the ground. *Kali demonstration, Sat.*, it read. I picked it up, and I let myself feel a tiny bit nervous. I'd started taking kali, a Filipino martial art, several years ago, to better protect myself from the things I knew were out there. I was drawn to kali because not only did it teach how to defend yourself empty-handed, it also taught stick, knife and sword work. And in a world of dagger-toting goblins and sword-wielding gentry, I wanted to be ready for anything. This weekend, our class was putting on a demonstration at a martial arts tournament, and I was part of the show.

If I could stay out of trouble that long, anyway. With me, it was always harder than it looked.

★ ★ ★

Starting a new school in the middle of the fall semester sucks.

I should know. I've done all this before. The struggle to find your locker, the curious stares in the hallway, the walk of shame to your desk in your new classroom, twenty or so pairs of eyes following you down the aisle.

Maybe third time's the charm, I thought morosely, slumping into my seat, which, thankfully, was in the far corner. I felt the heat from two dozen stares on the top of my head and ignored them all. *Maybe this time I can make it through a semester without getting expelled. One more year—just give me one more year and then I'm free.* At least the teacher didn't stand me up at the front of the room and introduce me to everyone; that would've been awkward. For the life of me, I couldn't understand why they thought such humiliation was necessary. It was hard enough to fit in without having a spotlight turned on you the first day.

Not that I'd be doing any "fitting in."

I continued to feel curious glances directed at my corner, and I concentrated on not looking up, not making eye contact with anyone. I heard people whispering and hunched down even more, studying the cover of my English book.

Something landed on my desk: a half sheet of notebook paper, folded into a square. I didn't look up, not wanting to know who'd lobbed it at me. Slipping it beneath the desk, I opened it in my lap and looked down.

U the guy who burned down his school? it read in messy handwriting.

Sighing, I crumpled the note in my fist. So they'd already heard the rumors. Perfect. Apparently, I'd been in the local paper: a juvenile thug who was seen fleeing the scene of the crime. But because no one had actually *witnessed* me setting the library on fire, I was able to avoid being sent to jail. Barely.

I caught giggles and whispers somewhere to my right, and then another folded piece of paper hit my arm. Annoyed, I was going to trash the note without reading it this time, but curiosity got the better of me, and I peeked quickly.

Did u really knife that guy in Juvie?

"Mr. Chase."

Miss Singer was stalking down the aisle toward me, her severe expression making her face look pinched behind her glasses. Or maybe that was just the dark, tight bun pulling at her skin, causing her eyes to narrow. Her bracelets clinked as she extended her hand and waggled her fingers at me. Her tone was no-nonsense. "Let's have it, Mr. Chase."

I held up the note in two fingers, not looking at her. She snatched it from my hand. After a moment, she murmured, "See me after class."

Damn. Thirty minutes into a new semester and I was already in trouble. This didn't bode well for the rest of the year. I slumped farther, hunching my shoulders against all prying eyes, as Miss Singer returned to the front and continued the lesson.

I remained in my seat after class was dismissed, listening to the sounds of scraping chairs and shuffling bodies, bags being tossed over shoulders. Voices surged around me, students talking and laughing with each other, gelling into their own little groups. As they began to file out, I finally looked up, letting my gaze wander over the few still lingering. A blond boy with glasses stood at Miss Singer's desk, rambling on while she listened with calm amusement. From the eager, puppy-dog look in his eyes, it was clear he was either suffering from major infatuation or was gunning for teacher's pet.

A group of girls stood by the door, clustered like pigeons, cooing and giggling. I saw several of the guys staring at them as they left, hoping to catch their eye, only to be disappointed. I snorted softly. *Good luck with that.* At least three of the girls were blonde, slender and beautiful, and a couple wore extremely short skirts that gave a fantastic view of their long, tanned legs. This was obviously the school's pom squad, and guys like me—or anyone who wasn't a jock or rich—had no chance.

And then, one of the girls turned and looked right at me.

I glanced away, hoping that no one noticed. Cheerleaders, I'd discovered, usually dated large, overly protective football stars whose policy was punch first, ask questions later. I did not want to find myself pressed up against my locker or a bathroom stall on my first day, about to get my face smashed in, because I'd had the gall to look at the quarterback's girlfriend. I heard more whispers, imagined fingers pointed my way, and then a chorus of shocked squeaks and gasps reached my corner.

"She's really going to do it," someone hissed, and then footsteps padded across the room. One of the girls had broken away from the pack and was approaching me. Wonderful.

Go away, I thought, shifting farther toward the wall. *I have nothing you want or need. I'm not here so you can prove that you're not scared of the tough new kid, and I do not want to get in a fight with your meathead boyfriend. Leave me alone.*

"Hi."

Resigned, I turned and stared into the face of a girl.

She was shorter than the others, more perky and cute than graceful and beautiful. Her long, straight hair was inky-black, though she had dyed a few strands around her face a brilliant sapphire. She wore sneakers and dark jeans, tight enough to hug her slender legs, but not looking like she'd painted them on. Warm brown eyes peered down at me as she stood with her hands clasped behind her, shifting from foot to foot, as if it was impossible for her to stay still.

"Sorry about the note," she continued, as I shifted back to eye her warily. "I told Regan not to do it—Miss Singer has eyes like a hawk. We didn't mean to get you in trouble." She smiled, and it lit up the room. My heart sank; I didn't want it to light up the room. I didn't want to notice anything about this girl, especially the fact that she was extremely attractive. "I'm Kenzie. Well, *Mackenzie* is my full name, but everyone calls me Kenzie. *Don't* call me Mac or I'll slug you."

Behind her, the rest of the girls gaped and whispered to each other, shooting us furtive glances. I suddenly felt like some kind of exhibit at the zoo. Resentment simmered. I was just a curiosity to them; the dangerous new kid to be stared at and gossiped about.

"And...you are...?" Kenzie prompted.

I looked away. "Not interested."

"Okay. Wow." She sounded surprised, but not angry, not yet. "That's...not what I was expecting."

"Get used to it." Inwardly, I cringed at the sound of my own voice. I was being a dick; I was fully aware of that. I was also fully aware that I was murdering any hope for acceptance in this place. You didn't talk this way to a cute, popular cheerleader without becoming a social pariah. She would go back to her friends, and they would gossip, and more rumors would spread, and I'd be shunned for the rest of the year.

Good, I thought, trying to convince myself. *That's what I want. No one gets hurt this way. Everyone can just leave me alone.*

Except...the girl wasn't leaving. From the corner of my eye, I saw her lean back and cross her arms, still with that lopsided grin on her face. "No need to be nasty," she said, seeming unconcerned with my aggressiveness. "I'm not asking for a date, tough guy, just your name."

Why was she still talking to me? Wasn't I making myself clear? I didn't want to talk. I didn't want to answer her questions. The longer I spoke to anyone, the greater the chance that *They* would notice, and then the nightmare would begin again. "It's Ethan," I muttered, still staring at the wall. I forced the next words out. "Now piss off."

"Huh. Well, aren't we hostile." My words were not having the effect I wanted. Instead of driving her off, she seemed almost...excited. What the hell? I resisted the urge to glance at her, though I still felt that smile, directed at me. "I was just trying to be nice, seeing as it's your first day and all. Are you like this with everyone you meet?"

"Miss St. James." Our teacher's voice cut across the room. Kenzie turned, and I snuck a peek at her. "I need to speak with Mr. Chase," Miss Singer continued, smiling at Kenzie. "Go to your next class, please."

Kenzie nodded. "Sure, Miss Singer." Glancing back, she caught me looking at her and grinned before I could look away. "See ya around, tough guy."

I watched her bounce back to her friends, who surrounded her, giggling and whispering. Sneaking unsubtle glances back at me, they filed through the door into the hall, leaving me alone with the teacher.

"Come here, Mr. Chase, if you would. I don't want to shout at you over the classroom."

I pulled myself up and walked down the aisle to slouch into a front-row desk. Miss Singer's sharp black eyes watched me over her glasses before she launched into a lecture about her no-tolerance policy for horseplay, and how she understood my situation, and how I could make something of myself if I just focused. As if that was all there was to it.

Thanks, but you might as well save your breath. I've heard this all before. How difficult it must be, moving to a new school, starting over. How bad my life at home must be. Don't act like you know what I'm going through. You don't know me. You don't know anything about my life. No one does.

If I had any say in it, no one ever would.

I got through my next two classes the same way—by ignoring everyone around me. When lunchtime rolled around, I watched the students filing down the hall toward the cafeteria, then turned and went in the opposite direction.

My fellow classmates were starting to get to me. I wanted to be outside, away from the crowds and curious looks. I didn't want to be trapped at a table by myself, dreading that someone would come up and "talk." No one would do it to be friendly, I was fairly certain. By now, that girl and her friends had probably spread the story of our first meeting through the whole school, maybe embellishing a few things, like how I called her awful names but somehow came on to her at the same time. Regardless, I didn't want to deal with angry boyfriends and indignant questions. I wanted to be left alone.

I turned a corner into another hall, intent on finding an isolated part of the school where I could eat in peace, and stumbled across the very thing I was trying to avoid.

A boy stood with his back to the lockers, thin shoulders hunched, his expression sullen and trapped. Standing in front of him were two larger boys, broad-shouldered and thick-necked, leering down at the kid they had pinned against the wall. For a second, I thought the kid had whiskers. Then he looked at me, quietly pleading, and through a mop of straw-colored hair, I caught a flash of orange eyes and two furred ears poking up from his head.

I swore. Quietly, using a word Mom would tear my head off for. These two idiots had no idea what they were doing. They couldn't See what he really was, of course. The "human" they had cornered was one of Them, one of the fey, or at least part fey. The term *half-breed* shot through my mind, and I clenched my fist around my lunch bag. Why? Why couldn't I ever be free of them? Why did they dog me every step of my life?

"Don't lie to me, freak," one of the jocks was saying, shoving the boy's shoulder back into the lockers. He had short, ruddy hair and was a little smaller than his bull-necked companion but not by much. "Regan saw you hanging around my car yesterday. You think it's funny that I nearly ran off the road? Huh?" He shoved him again, making a hollow clang against the lockers. "That snake didn't crawl in there by itself."

"I didn't do it!" the half-breed protested, flinching from the blow. I caught the flash of pointed canines when he opened his mouth, but of course, the two jocks couldn't see that. "Brian, I swear, that wasn't me."

"Yeah? So, you calling Regan a liar, then?" the smaller one asked, then turned to his friend. "I think the freak just called Regan a liar, did you hear that, Tony?" Tony scowled and cracked his knuckles, and Brian turned back to the half-breed. "That wasn't very smart of you, loser. Why don't we pay a visit to the bathroom? You can get reacquainted with Mr. Toilet."

Oh, great. I did not need this. I should turn around and walk away. *He's part faery,* my rational mind thought. *Get mixed up in this, and you'll attract Their attention for sure.*

The half-breed cringed, looking miserable but resigned. Like he was used to this kind of treatment.

I sighed. And proceeded to do something stupid.

"Well, I'm so glad this place has the same gorilla-faced morons as my old school," I said, not moving from where I stood. They whirled on me, eyes widening, and I smirked. "What's the matter, Daddy cut off your allowance this month, so you have to beat it out of the losers and freaks? Does practice not give you enough manhandling time?"

"Who the hell are you?" The smaller jock, Brian, took a menacing step forward, getting in my face. I gazed back at him, still smirking. "This your boyfriend, then?" He raised his voice. "You got a death wish, fag?"

Now, of course, we were beginning to attract attention. Students who had been averting their eyes and pretending not to see the trio against the locker began to hover, as if sensing violence on the air. Murmurs of "Fight" rippled through the crowd, gaining speed, until it felt as if the entire school was watching this little drama play out in the middle of the hall. The boy they'd been picking on, the half-breed, gave me a fearful, apologetic look and scurried off, vanishing into the crowd. *You're welcome,* I thought, resisting the urge to roll my eyes. Well, I had stepped into this pile of crap—I might as well go all out.

"New kid," grunted Brian's companion, stepping away from the lockers, looming behind the other. "The one from Southside."

"Oh, yeah." Brian glanced at his friend, then back at me. His lip curled in disdain. "You're that kid who shanked his cellmate in juvie," he continued, raising his voice for the ben- efit of the crowd. "After setting fire to the school and pulling a knife on a teacher."

I raised an eyebrow. *Really? That's a new one.*

Scandalized gasps and murmurs went through the student body, gaining speed like wildfire. This would be all over school tomorrow. I wondered how many more crimes I could add to my already lengthy imaginary list.

"You think you're tough, fag?" Bolstered by the mob, Brian stepped closer, crowding me, an evil smile on his face. "So you're an arsonist and a criminal, big deal. You think I'm scared of you?"

At least one more.

I straightened, going toe-to-toe with my opponent. "Arsonist, huh?" I said, matching his sneer with my own. "And here I thought you were as stupid as you look. Did you learn that big word in English today?"

His face contorted, and he swung at me. We were extremely close, so it was a nasty right hook, coming straight at my jaw. I ducked beneath it and shoved his arm as the fist went by, pushing him into the wall. Howls and cheers rose around us as Brian spun furiously and swung at me a second time. I twisted away, keeping my fists close to my cheeks, boxer style, to defend myself.

"Enough!"

Teachers descended from nowhere, pulling us apart. Brian swore and fought to get to me, trying to shove past the teacher, but I let myself be pulled off to the side. The one who grabbed me kept a tight hold of my collar, as if I might break free and throw a punch at him.

"Principal's office, Kingston," ordered the teacher, steering Brian down the hall. "Get moving." He glared back at me. "You, too, new kid. And you better pray you don't have a knife hidden somewhere on you, or you'll be suspended before you can blink."

As they dragged me off to the principal's office, I saw the half-faery watching me from the crowd. His orange eyes, solemn and grim, never left mine, until I was pulled around a corner and lost from view.

HALF-BREED

❀

I slumped in the chair in the principal's office, arms crossed, waiting for the man across the desk to notice us. The gold sign on the mahogany surface read *Richard S. Hill, Principal*, though the sign's owner hadn't given us more than a glance when we were brought in. He sat with his eyes glued to the computer screen, a small, balding man with a beaky nose and razor-thin eyebrows, lowered into a frown. His mouth pursed as he scanned the screen, making us wait.

After a minute or two, the jock in the chair next to mine blew out an impatient sigh.

"So, uh, do you need me anymore?" he asked, leaning forward as if preparing to stand. "I can go now, right?"

"Kingston," the principal said, finally glancing up. He blinked at Brian, then frowned again. "You have a big game this weekend, don't you? Yes, you can go. Just don't get into any more trouble. I don't want to hear about fights in the hallways, understand?"

"Sure, Mr. Hill." Brian stood, gave me a triumphant sneer, and swaggered out of the office.

Oh, that's fair. Jock-boy was the one who threw the first punch, but we don't want to jeopardize the team's chance of winning the game, do we? I waited for the principal to notice me, but he had gone back to reading whatever was on the computer. Leaning back, I crossed my legs and gazed longingly out the door. The ticking of the clock filled the small room, and students stopped to stare at me through the window on the door before moving on.

"You've quite the file, Mr. Chase," Hill finally said without looking up.

I suppressed a wince.

"Fighting, truancy, hidden weapons, arson." He pushed back his chair, and those hard black eyes finally settled on me. "Is there anything you'd like to add? Like assaulting the school's star quarterback on your very first day? Mr. Kingston's father is part of the school board, in case you did not realize."

"I didn't start that fight," I muttered. "He was the one who swung at me."

"Oh? You were just minding your own business, then?" The principal's sallow lips curled in a faint smile. "He swung at you out of nowhere?"

I met his gaze. "He and his football buddy were about to stick some kid's head down a toilet. I stepped in before they could. Jock-boy didn't appreciate me ruining his fun, so he tried smashing my face in." I shrugged. "Sorry if I like my face as it is."

"Your attitude does you no credit, Mr. Chase," Hill said, frowning at me. "And you should have gotten a teacher to take care of it. You're on very thin ice as it is." He folded pale, spiderlike hands on his desk and leaned forward. "Since it is your first day here, I'll let you go with a warning this time. But I will be watching you, Mr. Chase. Step out of line again, and I won't be so lenient. Do you understand?"

I shrugged. "Whatever."

His eyes glinted. "Do you think you're special, Mr. Chase?" A note of contempt had entered his voice now. "Do you think you're the only 'troubled youth' to sit in this office? I've seen your kind before, and they all go the same way—straight to prison, or the streets, or dead in the gutter somewhere. If that's the path you want, then, by all means, keep going down this road. Drop out. Get a dead-end job somewhere. But don't waste this school's time trying to educate you. And don't drag those who are going somewhere down with you." He jerked his head at the door. "Now get out of my office. And don't let me see you here again."

Fuming, I pulled myself upright and slid out the door.

The hallways were empty; everyone was back in their classrooms, well into postlunch stupor, counting down the minutes to the final bell. For a moment, I considered going home, leaving this sorry excuse of a new school and a clean start, and just accepting the fact that I would never fit in and be normal. No one would ever give me the chance.

But I couldn't go home, because Mom would be there. She wouldn't say anything, but she would look at me with that sad, guilty, disappointed expression, because she wanted so badly for me to succeed, to be normal. She was hoping that *this* time, things would work out. If I went home early, no matter the reason, Mom would tell me I could try again tomorrow, and then she would probably lock herself in her room and cry a little.

I couldn't face that. It would be worse than the lecture Dad would give me if he found out I skipped class. Plus, he'd been very fond of groundings lately, and I didn't want to risk another one.

It's just a couple more hours, I told myself and reluctantly started back to class, which would be the middle of trig by now, joy of joys. Why did every curriculum decide to teach math right after lunch when everyone was half-asleep? *You can survive a couple more hours. What else can happen, anyway?*

I should've known better.

As I turned a corner, I got that cold, prickly sensation on the back of my neck, the one that always told me I was being watched. Normally, I would've ignored it, but right then, I was angry and less focused than usual. I turned, glancing behind me.

The half-breed stood at the end of the hall next to the bathroom entrance, watching me in the frame. His eyes glowed orange, and the tips of his furry ears twitched in my direction.

Something hovered beside him, something small and humanoid, with buzzing dragonfly wings and dark green skin. It blinked huge black eyes at me, bared its teeth in a razor grin, then zipped into the air, flying up toward the ceiling tiles.

Before I could stop myself, my gaze followed it. The piskie blinked, startled, and I realized my slip-up.

Furious, I wrenched my stare down, but it was too late. *Dammit. Stupid, stupid mistake, Ethan.* The half-breed's eyes widened as he stared from me to the piskie, mouth gaping open. He knew. He knew I could see Them.

And now, They were aware, as well.

I managed to avoid the half-breed by going to class. When the last bell rang, I snatched up my backpack and hurried out the door, keeping my head down and hoping for a quick escape.

Unfortunately, he trailed me to the parking lot.

"Hey," he said, falling into step beside me as we crossed the lot. I ignored him and continued on, keeping my gaze straight ahead. He trotted doggedly to keep up. "Listen, I wanted to thank you. For what you did back there. Thanks for stepping in, I owe you." He paused, as if expecting me to say something. When I didn't, he added, "I'm Todd, by the way."

"Whatever," I muttered, not looking directly at him. He

frowned as if taken aback by the reaction, and I kept my expression blank and unfriendly. *Just because I rescued you from the jock and his goon doesn't mean we're buds now. I saw your little friend. You're playing with fire, and I want nothing to do with it. Go away.* Todd hesitated, then followed me in silence for a few steps, but he didn't leave.

"Uh, so," he continued, lowering his voice as we approached the end of the lot. I had parked my truck as far as I could from the Mustangs and Camaros of my fellow students, wanting it to avoid notice, as well. "When did you become able to see Them?"

My gut twisted. At least he didn't say *faeries* or *the fey,* because voicing their name out loud was a surefire way to attract their attention. Whether that was deliberate or ignorant on his part, I wasn't sure. "I don't know what you're talking about," I said coolly.

"Yes, you do!" He stepped in front of me, brow furrowed, and I had to stop. "You know what I am," he insisted, all subtlety gone. There was a hint of desperation in his eyes as he leaned forward, pleading. "I saw you, and Thistle caught you looking, too. You can see Them, and you can see what I really look like. So don't play dumb, okay? I know. We both do."

All right, this kid was pissing me off. Worse, the more I talked to him, the more attention I would draw from Them. His little "friends" were probably watching us right now, and that scared me. Whatever this half-breed wanted from me, it needed to end.

I sneered at him, my voice ugly. "Wow, you *are* a freak. No wonder Kingston picks on you. Did you not take your happy pills this morning?" Anger and betrayal flashed in Todd's orange eyes, making me feel like an ass, but I kept my voice mocking. "Yeah, I'd love to stay and chat with you and your imaginary friends, but I have real-world things to do. Why don't you go see if you can find a unicorn or something?"

His face darkened even more. I shoved past him and continued on, hoping he wouldn't follow. This time, he did not. But I hadn't gone three steps when his next words stopped me in my tracks.

"Thistle knows about your sister."

I froze, every muscle in my body coiling tight as my stomach turned inside out.

"Yeah, I thought you might be interested in that." Todd's voice held a note of quiet triumph. "She's seen her, in the Nevernever. Meghan Chase, the Iron Queen—"

I spun and grabbed the front of his shirt, jerking him forward off his feet. "Who else knows?" I hissed as Todd cringed, flattening his ears. "Who else has heard of me? Who knows I'm here?"

"I don't know!" Todd held up his hands, and short claws flashed in the sunlight. "Thistle is hard to understand sometimes, ya know? All she said was that she knew who you were—the brother of the Iron Queen."

"If you tell anyone…" I balled my fist, resisting the urge to shake him. "If you tell any of Them, I swear—"

"I won't!" Todd cried, and I realized then how I must have looked, teeth bared, eyes wild and crazy. Taking a deep breath, I forced myself to calm down. Todd relaxed, shaking his head. "Jeez, take it easy, man. So They know who you are—it's not the end of the world."

I sneered and shoved him backward. "You must be very sheltered, then."

"I was adopted," Todd shot back, catching himself. "How easy do you think it's been, pretending to be human when my own parents don't know what I am? No one here gets me, no one has any idea what I can do. They keep stepping on me, and I keep pushing back."

"So you *did* put a snake in Kingston's car." I shook my head in disgust. "I should've let him stick your head down a toilet this afternoon."

Todd sniffed and straightened the front of his shirt. "Kingston's a dick," he said, as if that justified everything. "He thinks he owns the school and has the teachers and the principal in his pocket. He believes he's untouchable." He smirked, orange eyes glittering. "Sometimes I like to remind him that he's not."

I sighed. *Well, it serves you right, Ethan. This is what happens when you get involved with Them. Even the half-fey can't keep themselves from pranking humans every chance they get.*

"The Invisible Folk are the only ones who understand me," Todd went on, as if trying to convince me. "They know what I'm going through. They're only too happy to help." His smirk grew wider, more threatening. "In fact, Thistle and her friends are making that jock's life very unpleasant right now."

A chill slid up my back. "What did you promise them?"

He blinked. "What?"

"They never do anything for free." I took a step forward, and he shrank back. "What did you promise them? What did they take?"

"What does it matter?" The half-breed shrugged. "The jerk had it coming. Besides, how much harm can two piskies and a boggart do?"

I closed my eyes. *Oh, man, you have no idea what you've gotten yourself into.* "Listen," I said, opening my eyes, "whatever bargains you've made, whatever contracts you've agreed to, stop. You can't trust them. They'll use you, because it's their nature. It's what they do." Todd raised a disbelieving eyebrow, and I scrubbed my scalp at his ignorance. How had he survived this long and not learned anything? "*Never* make a contract with Them. That's the first and most important rule. It doesn't ever go how you imagine, and once you've agreed to something, you're stuck. You can't ever get out of it, no matter what they ask for in return."

Todd still looked unconvinced. "Who made you the expert on all things faery?" he challenged, and I winced as he finally said the word. "You're human—you don't understand what it's like. So I made a few deals, promised a few things. What's that to you?"

"Nothing." I stepped back. "Just don't drag me into whatever mess you're creating. I want nothing to do with Them, or you, got it? I'd be happy if I never saw them again." And without waiting for an answer, I turned, opened my car door, and slammed it shut behind me. Gunning the engine, I squealed out of the parking lot, ignoring the half-breed's desolate figure as he grew smaller and smaller in my rearview mirror.

"How was school?" Mom asked as I banged through the screen door and tossed my backpack on the table.

"Fine," I mumbled, making a beeline for the fridge. She stepped out of the way with a sigh, knowing it was useless to talk to me when I was starving. I found the leftover pizza from last night and shoved two slices in the microwave while chewing on a cold third. Thirty seconds later, I was about to take my plate up to my room when Mom stepped in front of me.

"I got a call from the principal's office this afternoon."

My shoulders sank. "Yeah?"

Mom gestured firmly to the table, and I slumped into one of the chairs, my appetite gone. She sat down across from me, her eyes hooded and troubled. "Anything you want to tell me?"

I rubbed my eyes. No use trying to hide it, she probably already knew—or at least she knew what Hill told her. "I got into a fight."

"Oh, Ethan." The disappointment in her voice stabbed me like tiny needles. "On your first day?"

It wasn't my fault, I wanted to say. But I'd used that excuse so many times before, it seemed empty. Any excuse seemed empty now. I just shrugged and slouched farther in my seat, not meeting her eyes.

"Was it...was it Them?"

That shocked me. Mom almost never spoke of the fey, for probably the same reasons as me; she thought it might attract their attention. She would rather close her eyes and pretend they didn't exist, that they weren't still out there, watching us. It was one of the reasons I never talked openly to her about my problems. It just made her too frightened.

I hesitated, wondering if I should tell her about the half-breed and his invisible friends, lurking in the halls. But if Mom found out about them, she might pull me out of school. And as much as I hated going to class, I did not want to go through the whole "starting over" thing one more time.

"No," I said, fiddling with the edge of my plate. "Just these two dicks that needed a lesson in manners."

Mom gave one of her frustrated, disapproving groans. "Ethan," she said in a sharper voice. "It's not your place. We've gone over this."

"I know."

"If you keep this up, you'll be kicked out again. And I don't know where we can send you after that. I don't know..." Mom took a shaky breath, and covered her eyes with her hand.

Now I felt like a complete ass. "I'm sorry," I offered in a quiet voice. "I'll...try harder."

She nodded without looking up. "I won't tell your father, not this time," she murmured in a weary voice. "Don't eat too much pizza or you'll spoil your appetite for dinner."

Standing, I hooked my backpack over one shoulder and

took it and the plate into my room, kicking the door shut behind me.

Slumping to my desk, I ate my pizza while halfheartedly jiggling my laptop to life. The episode with Kingston, not to mention the talk with the half-breed, had made me edgy. I went to YouTube and watched videos of students practicing kali, trying to pick out the weaknesses in their attacks, poking holes in their defenses. Then, to keep myself occupied, I grabbed my rattan sticks from the wall and practiced a few patterns in the middle of my room, smacking imaginary targets with Brian Kingston's face, being careful not to hit the walls or ceiling. I'd put a couple of holes in the drywall already, by accident of course, before Dad made the rule that all practice must be done outside or in the dojo. But I was much better now, and what he didn't know wouldn't hurt him.

As I was finishing a pattern, I caught a flash of movement from the corner of my eye and turned. Something black and spindly, like a giant spider with huge ears, crouched on the windowsill outside, watching me. Its eyes glowed electric green in the coming darkness.

I growled a curse and started forward, but when the creature realized I'd spotted it, it let out an alarmed buzz and blinked out of sight. Yanking up the window, I peered into the darkness, searching for the slippery little nuisance, but it was gone.

"Damn gremlins," I muttered. Stepping back, I glared around my room, making sure everything was in place. I checked my lights, my clock, my computer; they all still worked, much to my relief. The last time a gremlin had been in my room, it had shorted out my laptop, and I'd had to spend my own money to get it fixed.

Gremlins were a special type of faery. They were Iron fey, which meant all my precautions and protections from the faery world didn't work on them. Iron didn't faze them, salt barriers didn't keep them out, and horseshoes over doors and windows did nothing. They were so used to the human world, so integrated with metal and science and technology, that the old charms and protection rituals were too outdated to affect them at all. I rarely had problems with Iron fey, but they were everywhere. I guessed even the Iron Queen couldn't keep track of them all.

The Iron Queen. A knot formed in my stomach. Shutting the window, I put my sticks away and dropped into the computer chair. For several minutes, I stared at the very top drawer of my desk, knowing what was inside. Wondering if I should torment myself further by taking it out.

Meghan. Do you even think of us anymore? I'd seen my half sister only a few times since she'd disappeared from our world nearly twelve years ago. She never stayed long; just a few hours to make sure everyone was okay, and then she was gone again. Before we moved, I could at least count on her to show up for my birthday and holidays. As I got older, those visits grew fewer and fewer. Eventually, she'd disappeared altogether.

Leaning forward, I yanked open the drawer. My long-lost older sister was another taboo subject in this household. If I so much as spoke her name, Mom would become depressed for a week. Officially, my sister was dead. Meghan wasn't part of this world anymore; she was one of Them, and we had to pretend she didn't exist.

But that half-breed knew about her. That could be trouble. As if I needed any more, as if being the delinquent, broody, don't-let-your-daughter-date-this-hooligan wasn't enough, now someone knew about my connection to the world of Faery.

Setting my jaw, I slammed the drawer shut and left the room, my thoughts swirling in a chaotic, sullen mess. I was human, and Meghan was gone. No matter what some half-breed faery said, I didn't belong to that world. I was going to stay on this side of the Veil and not worry about what was happening in Faery.

No matter how much it tried to drag me in.

CHAPTER THREE
FAERIES IN THE GYM BAG

Day two.

Of purgatory.

My "fight" with the school quarterback and my discussion in the principal's office hadn't gone unnoticed, of course. Fellow students stared at me in the halls, whispering to their friends, muttering in low undertones. They shied away from me as if I had the plague. Teachers gave me the evil eye, as if worried that I might punch someone in the head or pull a knife, maybe. I didn't care. Maybe Principal Hill had told them what had gone on in his office; maybe he'd told them I was a lost cause, because as long as I kept my head down, they ignored me.

Except for Miss Singer, who actually called on me several times during class, making sure I was still paying attention. I answered her questions about *Don Quixote* in monotones, hoping that would be enough to keep her off my back. She seemed pleasantly surprised that I'd read the homework assignment the night before, despite being somewhat distracted by the thoughts of gremlins lurking around my computer. Apparently satisfied that I could listen and stare out the window at the same time, Miss Singer finally left me alone, and I went back to brooding in peace.

At least Kingston and his flunky were absent today, though I did notice Todd in one of my classes, looking smug. He kept glancing at the quarterback's empty desk, smirking to himself and nodding. It made me nervous, but I swore not to get involved. If the half-breed wanted to screw around with the notoriously fickle Fair Ones, I wasn't going to be there when he got burned.

When the last bell rang, I gathered my backpack and rushed out, hoping to evade a repeat of the day before. I saw Todd as I went out the door, watching me as if he wanted to talk, but I quickly lost myself in the crowded hallway.

At my locker, I stuffed my books and homework into my pack, slammed the door—and came face-to-face with Kenzie St. James.

"Hey, tough guy."

Oh, no. What did she want? Probably to tear me a new one about the fight; if she was on the pom squad, Kingston was likely her boyfriend. Depending on which rumor you'd heard, I had either sucker-punched the quarterback or I'd threatened him in the hallway and had gotten my ass kicked before the teachers pulled us apart. Neither story was flattering, and I'd been wondering when someone would give me crap about it. I just hadn't expected it to be her.

I turned to leave, but she smoothly moved around to block my path. "Just a second!" she insisted, planting herself in front of me. "I want to talk to you."

I glared at her, a cold, hostile stare that had given redcaps pause and made a pair of spriggans back down once. Kenzie didn't move, her determined stance never wavering. I slumped in defeat. "What?" I growled. "Come to warn me to leave your boyfriend alone if I know what's good for me?"

She frowned. "Boyfriend?"

"The quarterback."

"Oh." She snorted, wrinkling her nose. It was kind of cute. "Brian's not my boyfriend."

"No?" That was surprising. I'd been so sure she was going to rip into me about the fight, maybe threaten to make me sorry if I hurt her precious football star. Why else would this girl want to talk to me?

Kenzie took advantage of my surprise and stepped closer. I swallowed and resisted the urge to step back. Kenzie was shorter than me by several inches, but that fact seemed completely lost on her. "Don't worry, tough guy. I don't have a boyfriend waiting to slug you in the bathrooms." Her eyes sparkled. "If it comes to that, I'll slug you myself."

I didn't doubt she'd try. "What do you want?" I asked again, more and more perplexed by this strange, cheerful girl.

"I'm the editor for the school paper," she announced, as if it was the most natural thing in the world. "And I was hoping you would do me a favor. Every semester, I interview the new students who started late, you know, so people can get to know them better. I'd love to do an interview with you, if you're up for it."

For the second time in thirty seconds, I was thrown. "You're an editor?"

"Well, more of a reporter, really. But since everyone else hates the technical stuff, I do the editing, too."

"For the paper?"

"That is generally what reporters report for, yes."

"But...I thought..." I gave myself a mental shake, collecting my scattered thoughts. "I saw you with the pom squad," I said, and it was almost an accusation. Kenzie's slender eyebrows rose.

"And, what? You thought I was a cheerleader?" She shrugged. "Not my thing, but thank you for thinking so. Heights and I don't really get along very well, and I can barely walk across the gym floor without falling down and bruising myself. Plus, I'd have to dye my hair blond, and that would just fry the ends."

I didn't know if she was serious or joking, but I couldn't stay. "Look, I have to be somewhere soon," I told her, which wasn't a lie; I had class tonight with my kali instructor, Guro Javier, and if I was late I'd have to do fifty pushups and a hundred suicide dashes—if he was feeling generous. Guro was serious about punctuality. "Can we talk later?"

"Will you give me that interview?"

"Okay, yes, fine!" I raised a hand in frustration. "If it will get you off my back, fine."

She beamed. "When?"

"I don't care."

That didn't faze her. Nothing did, it seemed. I'd never met someone who could be so relentlessly cheerful in the face of such blatant jack-assery. "Well, do you have a phone number?" she continued, sounding suspiciously amused. "Or, I could give you mine, if you want. Of course, that means you'd actually have to call me...." She gave me a dubious look, then shook her head. "Hmm, never mind, just give me yours. Something tells me I could tattoo my number on your forehead and you wouldn't remember to call."

"Whatever."

As I scribbled the digits on a scrap of paper, I couldn't help but think how weird it was, giving my phone number to a cute girl. I'd never done this before and likely never would again. If Kingston knew, if he even saw me talking to her, girlfriend or not, he'd probably try to give me a concussion.

Kenzie stepped beside me and stood on tiptoe to peer over my shoulder. Soft, feathery strands of her hair brushed my arm, making my skin prickle and my heart pound. I caught a hint of apple or mint or some kind of sweet fragrance, and for a second forgot what I was writing.

"Um." She leaned even closer, one slender finger pointing to the messy black scrawl on the paper. "Is this a six or a zero?"

"It's a six," I rasped, and stepped away, putting some distance between us. Damn, my heart was still pounding. What the hell was that about?

I handed over the paper. "Can I go now?"

She tucked it into the pocket of her jeans with another grin, though for just a moment she looked disappointed. "Don't let me stop you, tough guy. I'll call you later tonight, okay?"

Without answering, I stepped around her, and this time, she let me.

Kali was brutal. With the tournament less than a week off, Guro Javier was fanatical about making sure we would give nothing less than our best.

"Keep those sticks moving, Ethan," Guro called, watching me and my sparring partner circle each other, a rattan in each hand. I nodded and twirled my sticks, keeping the pattern going while looking for holes in my opponent's guard. We wore light padded armor and a helmet so that the sticks wouldn't leave ugly, throbbing welts over bare skin and we could really smack our opponent without seriously injuring him. That's not to say I didn't come home with nice purple bruises every so often—"badges of courage," as Guro called them.

My sparring partner lunged. I angled to the side, blocking his strike with one stick while landing three quick blows on his helmet with the other.

"Good!" Guro called, bringing the round to a close. "Ethan, watch your sticks. Don't let them just sit there, keep them moving, keep them flowing, always. Chris, angle out next time—don't just back up and let him hit you."

"Yes, Guro," we both said, and bowed to each other, ending the match. Backing to the corner, I wrenched off my helmet and let the cool air hit my face. Call me violent and aggressive, but I loved this. The flashing sticks, the racing adrenaline, the solid crack of your weapon hitting a vital spot on someone's armor...there was no bigger rush in the world. While I was here, I was just another student, learning under Guro Javier. Kali was the only place where I could forget my life and school and the constant, judging stares, and just be myself.

Not to mention, beating on someone with sticks was an awesome way to relieve pent-up aggression.

"Good class, everyone," Guro called, motioning us to the front of the room. We bowed to our instructor, touching one stick to our heart and the other to our forehead, as he continued. "Remember, the tournament is this Saturday. Those of you participating in the demonstrations, I would like you there early so you can practice and go over the forms and patterns. Also, Ethan—" he looked at me "—I need to talk to you before you leave. Class dismissed, everyone." He clapped his hands, and the rest of the group began to disperse, talking excitedly about the tournament and other kali-related things. I stripped off my armor, set it carefully on the mats and waited.

Guro gestured, and I followed him to the corner, gathering up punch mitts and the extra rattan sticks scattered near the wall. After stacking them neatly on the corner shelves, I turned to find Guro watching me with a solemn expression.

Guro Javier wasn't a big guy; in fact, I had an inch or two on him in my bare feet, and I wasn't very tall. I was pretty fit, not huge like a linebacker, but I did work out; Guro was all sinew and lean muscle, and the most graceful person I'd ever seen in my life. Even practicing or warming up, he looked like a dancer, twirling his weapons with a speed I had yet to master and feared I never would. And he could strike like a cobra; one minute he'd be standing in front of you demonstrating a technique, the next, you'd be on the ground, blinking and wondering how you got there. Guro's age was hard to tell; he had strands of silver through his short black hair, and laugh lines around his eyes and mouth. He pushed me hard, harder than the others, drilling me with patterns, insisting I get a technique close to perfect before I moved on. It wasn't that he played favorites, but I think he realized that I wanted this more, needed this more, than the other students. This wasn't just a hobby for me. These were skills that might someday save my life.

"How is your new school?" Guro asked in a matter-of-fact way. I started to shrug but caught myself. I tried very hard not to fall back into old, sullen habits with my instructor. I owed him more than a shrug and a one-syllable answer.

"It's fine, Guro."

"Getting along with your teachers?"

"Trying to."

"Hmm." Guro idly picked up a rattan and spun it through the air, though his eyes remained distant. He often did that stick twirling when thinking, demonstrating a technique, or even talking to us. It was habit, I guessed; I didn't think he even realized he was doing it.

"I've spoken to your mother," Guro continued calmly, and my stomach twisted. "I've asked her to keep me updated on your progress at school. She's worried about you, and I can't say I like what I've heard." The whirling stick paused for a moment, and he looked directly at me. "I do not teach kali for violence, Ethan. If I hear you've been in any more fights, or that your grades are slipping, I'll know you need to concentrate more on school than kali practice. You'll be out of the demonstration, is that clear?"

I sucked in a breath. *Great. Thanks a lot, Mom.* "Yes, Guro."

He nodded. "You're a good student, Ethan. I want you to succeed in other places, too, yes? Kali isn't everything."

"I know, Guro."

The stick started its twirling pattern again, and Guro nodded in dismissal. "Then I'll see you on Saturday. Remember, thirty minutes early, at least!"

I bowed and retreated to the locker room.

My phone blinked when I pulled it out, indicating a new message, though I didn't recognize the number. Puzzled, I checked voice mail and was greeted by a familiar, overly cheerful voice.

"Hey, tough-guy, don't forget you owe me an interview. Call me tonight, you know, when you're done robbing banks and stealing cars. Talk to you later!"

I groaned. I'd forgotten about her. Stuffing the phone into my bag, I slung it over my shoulder and was about to leave when the lights flickered and went out.

Oh, nice. Probably Redding, trying to scare me again. Rolling my eyes, I waited, listening for footsteps and snickering laughter. Chris Redding, my sparring partner, fancied himself a practical joker and liked to target people who kicked his ass in practice. Usually, that meant me.

I held my breath, remaining motionless and alert. As the silence stretched on, annoyance turned to unease. The light switch was next to the door—I could see it through a gap in the aisles, and there was no one standing there. I was in the locker room alone.

Carefully, I eased my bag off my shoulder, unzipped it and drew out a rattan stick, just in case. Edging forward, stick held out in front of me, I peered around the locker row. I was not in the mood for this. If Redding was going jump out and yell *"rah,"* he was going to get a stick upside the head, and I'd apologize later.

There was a soft buzz, somewhere overhead. I looked up just as something tiny half fell, half fluttered from the ceiling, right at my face. I leaped back, and it flopped to the floor, twitching like a dazed bird.

I edged close, ready to smack it if it lunged up at me again. The thing stirred weakly where it lay on the cement, looking like a giant wasp or a winged spider. From what I could tell, it was green and long-limbed with two transparent wings crumpled over its back. I stepped forward and nudged it with the end of the stick. It batted feebly at the rattan with a long, thin arm.

A piskie? What's it doing here? As fey went, piskies were usually pretty harmless, though they could play nasty tricks if insulted or bored. And, tiny or no, they were still fey. I was tempted to flick this one under the bench like a dead spider and continue on to my truck, when it raised its face from the floor and stared up at me with huge, terrified eyes.

It was Thistle, Todd's friend. At least, I thought it was the same faery; all piskies looked pretty much the same to me. But I thought I recognized the sharp pointed face, the puff of yellow dandelion hair. Its mouth moved, gaping wide, and its wings buzzed faintly, but it seemed too weak to get up.

Frowning, I crouched down to see it better, still keeping my rattan out in case it was just faking. "How did you get in here?" I muttered, prodding it gently with the stick. It swatted at the end but didn't move from the floor. "Were you following me?"

It gave a garbled buzz and collapsed, apparently exhausted, and I hesitated, not knowing what to do. Clearly, it was in trouble, but helping the fey went against all the rules I'd taught myself over the years. Don't draw attention to yourself. Don't interact with the Fair Folk. Never make a contract, and never accept their help. The smart thing to do would be to walk away and not look back.

Still, if I helped this once, the piskie would be in my debt, and I could think of several things I could demand in exchange. I could demand that she leave me alone. Or leave Todd alone. Or abandon whatever scheme the half-breed was having her do.

Or, better yet, I could demand that she tell no one about my sister and my connection to her.

This is stupid, I told myself, still watching the piskie crawl weakly around my rattan, trying to pull herself up the length of the stick. *You know faeries will twist any bargain to their favor, even if they owe you something. This is going to end badly.*

Oh, well. When had I ever been known for doing the smart thing?

With a sigh, I bent down and grabbed the piskie by the wings, lifting her up in front of me. She dangled limply, half-delirious, though from what I had no idea. Was it me, or did the faery seem almost...transparent? Not just her wings; she flickered in and out of focus like a blurry camera shot.

And then, I saw something beyond the piskie's limp form, lurking in the darkness at the end of the locker room. Something pale and ghostlike, long hair drifting around its head like mist.

"Ethan?"

Guro's voice echoed through the locker room, and the thing vanished. Quickly, I unzipped my bag and stuffed the piskie inside as my instructor appeared in the doorway. His eyes narrowed when he saw me.

"Everything all right?" he asked as I shouldered the bag and stepped forward. And, was it my imagination, or did he glance at the corner where the creepy ghost-thing was? "I thought I heard something. Chris isn't hiding in a corner ready to jump out, is he?"

"No, Guro. It's fine."

I waited for him to move out of the doorway so I wouldn't have to shoulder past him with my bag. My heart pounded, and the hair on the back of my neck stood up. Something was still in the room with me; I could feel it watching us, its cold eyes on my back.

Guro's eyes flicked to the corner again, narrowing. "Ethan," he said in a low voice, "my grandfather was a *Mang-Huhula*— you know what that means, yes?"

I nodded, trying not to seem impatient. The *Mang-Huhula* was the spiritual leader of the tribe, a faith-healer or fortune teller of sorts. Guro himself was a *tuhon,* someone who passed down his culture and practices, who kept the traditions alive. He'd told us this before; I wasn't sure why he was reminding me now.

"My grandfather was a wise man," Guro went on, holding my gaze. "He told me not to put your trust in only your eyes. That to truly see, sometimes you had to put your faith in the invisible things. You had to believe what no one else was willing to. Do you understand what I'm saying?"

I heard a soft slither behind me, like wet cloth over cement, and my skin crawled. It took all my willpower not to draw my rattan and swing around. "I think so, Guro."

Guro paused a moment, then stepped back, looking faintly disappointed. Obviously, I'd just missed something, or he could tell I was really distracted. But all he said was, "If you need help, Ethan, all you have to do is ask. If you're in trouble, you can come to me. For anything, no matter how small or crazy it might seem. Remember that."

The thing, whatever it was, slithered closer. I nodded, trying not to fidget. "I will, Guro."

"Go on, then." Guro stepped aside, nodding. "Go home. I'll see you at the tournament."

I fled the room, forcing myself not to look back. And I didn't stop until I reached my truck.

My phone rang as soon as I was home.

After closing my bedroom door, I dropped my gym bag on the bed, listening to the buzz of wings from somewhere inside. It seemed the piskie was still alive, though it probably wasn't thrilled at being zipped into a bag with used gym shorts and sweaty T-shirts. Smirking at the thought, I checked the trilling phone. Same unfamiliar number. I sighed and held it to my ear.

"God, you're persistent," I told the girl and heard a chuckle on the other end.

"It's a reporter skill," she replied. "If every newscaster got scared off by the threat of violence or kidnapping or death, there wouldn't be any news at all. They have to brave a lot to get their stories. Consider yourself practice for the real world."

"I'm so honored," I deadpanned. She laughed.

"So, anyway, are you free tomorrow? Say, after school? We can meet in the library and you can give me that interview."

"Why?" I scowled at the phone, ignoring the angry buzzing coming from my gym bag. "Just ask me your questions now and be done with it."

"Oh, no, I never do interviews over the phone if I can help it." The buzzing grew louder, and my bag started to shake. I gave it a thump, and it squeaked in outrage.

"Phone interviews are too impersonal," Kenzie went on, oblivious to my ridiculous fight with the gym bag. "I want to look at the person I'm interviewing, really see their reactions, get a glimpse into their thoughts and feelings. I can't do that over the phone. So, tomorrow in the library, okay? After the last class. Will you be there?"

A session alone with Kenzie. My heart beat faster at the thought, and I coldly stomped it down. Yes, Kenzie was cute, smart, popular and extremely attractive. You'd have to be blind not to see it. She was also obscenely rich, or her family was, anyway. The few rumors I'd heard said her father owned three mansions and a private jet, and Kenzie only went to public school because she wanted to. Even if I was anywhere near normal, Mackenzie St. James was way out of my league.

And it was better that way. I couldn't allow myself to get comfortable with this girl, to let my guard down for an instant. The second I let people get close to me, the fey would make them targets. I would not let that happen ever again.

My bag actually jumped about two inches off the bed, landing with a thump on the mattress. I winced and dragged it back before it could leap to the floor. "Sure," I said distractedly, not really thinking about it. "Whatever. I'll be there."

"Awesome!" I could sense Kenzie's smile. "Thanks, tough guy. See you tomorrow."

I hung up.

Outside, lightning flickered through the window, showing a storm was on its way. Grabbing my rattan stick, I braced myself and unzipped the gym bag in one quick motion, releasing a wave of stink and a furious, buzzing piskie into my room.

Not surprisingly, the faery made a beeline for the window but veered away when it noticed the line of salt poured along the sill. It darted toward the door, but an iron horseshoe hung over the frame and a coil of metal wire had been wound over the doorknob. It hummed around the ceiling like a frantic wasp, then finally drifted down to the headboard, alighting

on a bedpost. Crossing its arms, it gave me an annoyed, ex-
pectant look.

I smiled nastily. "Feeling better, are we? You're not getting
out of here until I say so, so sit down and relax." The piskie's
wings vibrated, and I kept my rattan out, ready to swat if it
decided to dive-bomb me. "I saved your life back there," I reminded the faery. "So I think you owe me something. That's
generally how these things work. You owe me a life debt, and
I'm calling it in right now."

It bristled but crossed its legs and sat down on the post,
looking sulky. I relaxed my guard, but only a little. "Sucks
being on that end of a bargain, doesn't it?" I smirked, enjoying my position, and leaned back against the desk.

The piskie glared, then lifted one arm in an impatient gesture that clearly said, *Well? Get on with it, then.* Still keeping it
in my sights, I crossed my room and locked the door, more to
keep curious parents out than annoyed faeries in. Life debt or
no, I could only imagine the trouble the piskie would cause
if she managed to escape to the rest of the house.

"Thistle, right?" I asked, returning to the desk. The piskie's
head bobbed once in affirmation. I wondered if I should ask
about Meghan but decided against it. Piskies, I'd discovered,
were notoriously difficult to understand and had the attention span of a gnat. Long, drawn-out conversations with them
were virtually impossible, as they tended to forget the question as soon as it was answered.

"You know Todd, then?"

The piskie buzzed and nodded.

"What did you do for him recently?"

The result was a garbled, high-pitched mess of words and
sentences, spoken so quickly it made my head spin. It was like
listening to a chipmunk on speed. "All right, enough!" I said,
holding up my hands. "I wasn't thinking." *Yes or no answers,*

Ethan, remember? The piskie gave me a confused frown, but I ignored it and continued. "So, were you following me today?"

Another nod.

"Why—"

The piskie gave a terrified squeal and buzzed frantically about the room, nearly smacking into me as it careened around the walls. I ducked, covering my head, as it zipped across the room, babbling in its shrill, squeaking voice. "Okay, okay! Calm down! Sorry I asked." It finally hovered in a corner, shaking its head, eyes bulging out of its skull. I eyed it warily.

Huh. That was...interesting. "What was that about?" I demanded. The piskie buzzed and hugged itself, wings trembling. "Something was after you tonight, wasn't it? That thing in the locker room—it was chasing you. Piss off an Iron faery, then?" The fey of the Iron Queen's court were the only creatures I could think of that could provoke such a reaction. I didn't know what it was like in the Nevernever, but here, the old-world faeries and the Iron fey still didn't get along very well. Generally, the two groups avoided each other, pretending the other didn't exist. But faeries were fickle and destructive and violent, and fights still broke out between them, usually ending fatally.

But the piskie shook its head, squeaking and waving its thin arms. I frowned. "It wasn't an Iron fey," I guessed, and it shook its head again, vigorously. "What was it?"

"Ethan?" There was a knock, and Dad's voice came through the door. "Are you in there? Who are you talking to?"

I winced. Unlike Mom, Dad had no problem invading my personal space. If it were up to him, I wouldn't even have a door. "On the phone, Dad!" I called back.

"Oh. Well, dinner is ready. Tell your friend you'll call back, okay?"

I grunted and heard his footsteps retreat down the hall.

The piskie still hovered in the corner, watching me with big black eyes. It was terrified, and even though it was fey and had probably played a million nasty pranks on unsuspecting humans, I suddenly felt like a bully.

I sighed. "You know what?" I told it, moving to the window. "Forget it. This was stupid of me. I'm not getting involved with any of you, life debt or no." Sweeping away the salt, I unlocked the window and pushed it open, letting in a blast of cool, rain-scented air. "Get out of here," I told the piskie, who blinked in astonishment. "You want to repay me? Whatever you're doing for that half-breed, stop it. I don't want you hanging around him, or me, ever again. Now beat it."

I jerked my head toward the window, and the piskie didn't hesitate. It zipped past my head, seeming to go right through the screen, and vanished into the night.

AN UNEXPECTED VISITOR

Storms always made me moody. More so than usual, anyway.

Don't know why; maybe they reminded me of my child-hood, back in the swamps. We'd gotten a lot of rain on our small farm, and somehow the drumming of water on the tin roof always put me to sleep. Or maybe because, when I was very small, I would creep out of bed and into my sister's room, and she would hold me as the thunder boomed and tell me stories until I fell asleep.

I didn't want to remember those days. They just reminded me that she wasn't here now, and she never would be again.

I loaded the last plate into the dishwasher and kicked it shut, wincing as a crash of thunder outside made the lights flicker. Hopefully, the power would stay on this time. Call me para-noid, but stumbling around in the dark with nothing but a candle made me positive that the fey were lurking in shadowy corners and darkened bathrooms, waiting to pounce.

I finished clearing the table, walked into the living room and flopped down on the couch. Dad had already gone to work, and Mom was upstairs, so the house was fairly still as I flipped on the television, turning up the volume to drown out the storm.

The doorbell rang.

I ignored it. It wasn't for me, that was for certain. I didn't have friends; no one ever came to my house to hang out with the weird, unfriendly freak. Most likely it was our neighbor, Mrs. Tully, who was friends with Mom and liked to glare at me through the slits in her venetian blinds. As if she was afraid I would throw eggs at her house or kick her yappy little dog. She liked to give Mom advice about what to do with me, claiming she knew a couple of good military schools that would straighten me right out. Most likely, she was huddled on our doorstep with an umbrella and a bag of extra candles, using the storm as an excuse to come in and gossip, probably about me. I snorted under my breath. Mom was too nice to tell her to take a hike, but I had no such convictions. She could just stay out there as far as I was concerned.

The doorbell rang again, and it sounded louder this time, more insistent.

"Ethan!" Mom called from somewhere upstairs, her voice sharp. "Will you get that, please? Don't leave whoever it is standing there in the rain!"

Sighing, I dragged myself upright and went to the door, expecting to see a plump old woman glaring disapprovingly as I yanked it open. It wasn't Mrs. Tully, however.

It was Todd.

At first, I didn't recognize him. He had on a huge camouflage jacket that was two sizes too big, and the hood had fallen over his eyes. When he raised a hand and shoved it back, the porch light caught his pupils and made them glitter orange. His hair and furry ears were drenched, and he looked even smaller than normal, huddled in that enormous coat. A bike lay on its side in the grass behind him, wheels spinning in the rain.

"Oh, good, this is the right house." Todd grinned at me, canines flashing in the dim light. A violet-skinned piskie peeked out of his hood, blinking huge black eyes, and I recoiled.

"Hey, Ethan!" the half-breed said cheerfully, peering past me into the house. "Nasty weather, isn't it? Uh, can I come in?"

I instantly shut the door in his face, leaving no more than a few inches open to glare at him through the crack. "What are you doing here?" I hissed. He flattened his ears at my tone, looking scared now.

"I need to talk to you," he whispered, glancing back over his shoulder. "It's important, and you're the only one who might be able to help. Please, you gotta let me in."

"No way." I kept a firm foot on the edge of the door, refusing to budge an inch as he pushed forward. "If you're in trouble with Them, that's your problem for getting involved. I told you before—I want nothing to do with it." I glared at the piskie who crouched beneath Todd's hood, watching it carefully. "Get lost. Go home."

"I can't!" Todd leaned in frantically, eyes wide. "I can't go home because *They're* waiting for me."

"Who?"

"I don't know! These weird, creepy, ghostly *things*. They've been hanging around my house since yesterday, watching me, and they keep getting closer."

A chill spread through my stomach. I gazed past him into the rainy streets, searching for glimmers of movement, shadows of things not there. "What did you do?" I growled, glaring at the half-phouka, who cringed.

"I don't know!" Todd made a desperate, helpless gesture, and his piskie friend squeaked. "I've never seen these type of fey before. But they keep following me, watching me. I think they're after us," he continued, gesturing to the fey on his shoulder. "Violet and Beetle are both terrified, and I can't find Thistle anywhere."

"So, you came *here*, to pull my family into this? Are you crazy?"

"Ethan?" Mom appeared behind me, peering over my shoulder. "Who are you talking to?"

"No one!" But it was too late; she'd already seen him.

Glancing past me, Todd gave a sheepish smile and a wave. "Um, hey, Ethan's Mom," he greeted, suddenly charming and polite. "I'm Todd. Ethan and I were supposed to trade notes this evening, but I sorta got caught in the rain on the way here. It's nothing—I'm used to biking across town. In the rain. And the cold." He sniffled and glanced mournfully at his bike, lying in the mud behind him. "Sorry for disturbing you," he said, glancing up with the most pathetic puppy dog eyes I'd ever seen. "It's late. I guess I'll head on home now...."

"What? In this weather? No, Todd, you'll catch your death." Mom shooed me out of the doorway and gestured to the half-phouka on the steps. "Come inside and dry off, at least. Do your parents know where you are?"

"Thank you." Todd grinned as he scurried over the threshold. I clenched my fists to stop myself from shoving him back into the rain. "And yeah, it's okay. I told my Mom I was visiting a friend's house."

"Well, if the rain doesn't let up, you're more than welcome to stay the night," Mom said, sealing my fate. "Ethan has a spare sleeping bag you can borrow, and he can take you both to school tomorrow in his truck." She fixed me with a steely glare that promised horrible repercussions if I wasn't nice. "You don't mind, do you?"

I sighed. "Whatever." Glancing at Todd, who looked way too pleased, I turned away and gestured for him to follow. "Come on, then. I'll get that sleeping bag set up."

He trailed me to my room, gazing around eagerly as he stepped through the frame. That changed when I slammed the door, making him jump, and turned to glare at him.

"All right," I growled, stalking forward, backing him up

to the wall. "Start talking. What's so damned important that you had to come here and drag my family into whatever mess you created?"

"Ethan, wait." Todd held up clawed hands. "You were right, okay? I shouldn't have been screwing around with the fey, but it's too late to go back and undo...whatever I did."

"What *did* you do?"

"I told you, I don't know!" The half-breed bared his canines in frustration. "Little things, nothing I haven't done before. Teensy contracts with Thistle and Violet and Beetle to help with some of my tricks, but that's all. But I think something bigger took notice of us, and now I think I'm in real trouble."

"What do you want *me* to do about it?"

"I just..." Todd stopped, frowning. "Wait a minute," he muttered, and pushed his hood back. It flopped emptily. "Violet? Where'd she go?" he said, stripping out of the coat and shaking it. "She was here a few minutes ago."

I smirked at him. "Your piskie friend? Yeah, sorry, she couldn't get past the ward on the front door. No faery can get over the threshold without my permission, and I wasn't about to set that thing free in my house. It doesn't work on half-breeds, sadly."

He looked up, eyes wide. "She's still outside?"

A tap came on the window, where a new line of salt had been poured across the sill. The dripping wet piskie stared through the glass at us, her small features pinched into a scowl. I grinned at her smugly.

"I knew it," Todd whispered, and dropped his wet jacket onto a chair. "I knew you were the right person to come to."

I eyed him. "What are you talking about?"

"Just..." He glanced at the piskie again. She pressed her face to the glass, and he swallowed. "Dude, can I...uh....let her in? I'm scared those things are still out there."

"If I refuse, are you going to keep bothering me until I say yes?"

"More or less, yeah."

Annoyed, I brushed away the salt and cracked open the window, letting the piskie through with a buzz of wings and damp air. Two faeries in my room in the same night; this was turning into a nightmare. "Don't touch anything." I glowered at her as she settled on Todd's shoulder with a huff. "I have an antique iron birdcage you can sit in if anything goes missing."

The piskie made irritated buzzing sounds, pointing at me and waving her arms, and Todd shook his head. "I know, I know! But he's the Iron Queen's brother. He's the only one I could think of."

My heart gave a violent lurch at the mention of the Iron Queen, and I narrowed my eyes. "What was that?"

"You have to help us," Todd exclaimed, oblivious to my sudden anger. "These things are after me, and they don't look friendly. You're the brother of the Iron Queen, and you know how to keep the fey out. Give me something to keep them away from me. The common wards are helping, but I don't think they're strong enough. I need something more powerful." He leaned forward, ears pricked, eyes eager. "You know how to keep Them away, right? You must, you've been doing it all your life. Show me how."

"Forget it." I glared at him, and his ears wilted. "What happens if I give you all my secrets? You would just use it to further your stupid tricks. I'm not revealing everything just to have it bite me in the ass later." His ears drooped even more, and I crossed my arms. "Besides, what about your little friends? The wards I know are for *all* fey, not just a select few. What happens to them?"

"We can get around that," Todd said quickly. "We'll make it work, somehow. Ethan, please. I'm desperate, here. What do you want from me?" He leaned forward. "Give me a hint. A tip. A note scribbled on a fortune cookie, I'll try anything. Talk to me this one time, and I swear I'll leave you alone after this."

I raised an eyebrow. "And your friends?"

"I'll make sure they leave you alone, as well."

I sighed. This was probably monumentally stupid, but I knew what it was like to feel trapped, not having anyone I could turn to. "All right," I said reluctantly. "I'll help. But I want your word that you'll stop all bargains and contracts after today. If I do this, no more 'help' from the Good Neighbors, got it?"

The piskie buzzed sadly, but Todd nodded without hesitation. "Deal! I mean…yeah. I swear."

"No more contracts or bargains?"

"No more contracts or bargains." He sighed and made an impatient gesture with a claw. "Now, can we please get on with it?"

I had major doubts that he could keep that promise—half fey weren't bound by their promises the way full fey were—but what else could I do? He needed my help, and if something *was* after him, I couldn't stand back and do nothing. Rubbing my eyes, I went to my desk, opened the bottom drawer and pulled out an old leather journal from under a stack of papers. After hesitating a moment, I walked forward and tossed it onto my bed.

Todd blinked. "What is that?"

"All my research on the Good Neighbors," I said, pulling a half-empty notepad off my bookshelf. "And if you mention it to anyone, I *will* kick your ass. Here." I tossed him the pad, and he caught it awkwardly. "Take notes. I'll tell you what you need to know—it'll be up to you to go through with it."

We stayed there for the rest of the evening, him sitting on

my bed scribbling furiously, me leaning against my desk reading wards, charms and recipes from the journal. I went over the common wards, like salt, iron and wearing your clothes inside out. We went over things that could attract the fey into a house: babies, shiny things, large amounts of sugar or honey. We briefly discussed the most powerful ward in the book, a circle of toadstools that would grow around the house and render everything inside invisible to the fey. But that spell was extremely complicated, required rare and impossible ingredients, and could be safely performed only by a druid or a witch on the night of the waning moon. Since I didn't know any local witches, nor did I have any powdered unicorn horn lying around, we weren't going to be performing that spell anytime in the near future. Besides, I told a disappointed Todd, you could put a wrought-iron fence around your house with less effort than the toadstool ring, and it would do nearly the same job in keeping out the fey.

"So," Todd ventured after a couple of hours of this. I sensed he was getting bored, and marveled that the half-phouka had lasted this long. "Enough talk about the fey already. Word around school is that you were a total douche to Mackenzie St. James."

I looked up from the journal, where I was making small corrections to a charm using ragwort and mistletoe. "Yeah? So what?"

"Dude, you'd better be careful with that girl." Todd put down his pen and gazed at me with serious orange eyes. The piskie buzzed from the top of my bookshelf to land on his shoulder. "Last year, some guy kept following her around, trying to ask her out. Wouldn't leave her alone even when she turned him down." He shook his shaggy head. "The whole football team took him out behind the bleachers to have 'a talk' about Kenzie. Poor bastard wouldn't even look at her after that."

"I have no interest in Kenzie St. James," I said flatly.

"Good to hear," Todd replied. "'Cause Kenzie is off-limits. And not just to people like you and me. Everyone at school knows it. You don't bother her, you don't start rumors about her, you don't hang around, you don't make yourself *unwanted*, or the Goon Squad will come and leave an impression of your face in the wall."

"Seems a little drastic," I muttered, intrigued despite myself. "What, did she have a nasty breakup with one of the jocks, and now he doesn't want anyone to have her?"

"No." Todd shook his head. "Kenzie doesn't have a boyfriend. She's *never* had a boyfriend. Not once. Why is that, you wonder? She's gorgeous, smart, and everyone says her dad is loaded. But she's never gone out with anyone. Why?"

"Because people don't want their heads bashed in by testosterone-ridden gorillas?" I guessed, rolling my eyes.

But Todd shook his head. "No, I don't think that's it," he said, frowning at my snort of disbelief. "I mean, think about it, dude—if Kenzie wanted a boyfriend, do you think anyone, even Chief Tool Kingston himself, would be able to stop her?"

No, I thought, *he wouldn't.* No one would. I had the distinct feeling that if Kenzie wanted something, she would get it, no matter how difficult or impossible it was. She had wheedled an interview out of *me*—that was saying something. The girl just didn't take no for an answer.

"Kinda makes you wonder," Todd mused. "Pretty girl like that, with no boyfriend and no interest in any guy? Do you think she could be—"

"I don't care," I interrupted, pushing thoughts of Mackenzie St. James to the back of my mind. I couldn't think about her. Because even if Kenzie was pretty and kind and had treated me like a decent human being, even though I was a total ass to her, I could not afford to bring someone else into my dangerous, screwed-up world. I was spending the evening teaching anti-faery charms to a piskie and a half-phouka; that was a pretty good indication of how messed up my life was.

A crash of thunder outside rattled the ceiling and made the lights flicker just as there was a knock on the door and Mom poked her head in. I quickly flipped the journal shut, and Todd snatched the notebook from where it lay on the bed, hiding the contents as she gazed down at us.

"How are you boys doing?" Mom asked, smiling at Todd, who beamed back at her. I kept a close eye on his piskie, making sure it didn't dart through the crack into the rest of the house. "Everything all right?"

"We're fine, Mom," I said quickly, wishing she would close the door. She frowned at me, then turned to my unwanted guest.

"Todd, it looks like it's going to storm all night. My husband is at work, so he can't drive you home, and I am not sending you out in this weather. It looks like you'll have to stay here tonight." He looked relieved, and I suppressed a groan. "Make sure you call your parents to let them know where you are, okay?"

"I will, Mrs. Chase."

"Did Ethan set you up with a sleeping bag yet?"

"Not yet." Todd grinned at me. "But he was just about to, right, Ethan?"

I glared daggers at him. "Sure."

"Good. I'll see you boys tomorrow morning, then. And Ethan?"

"Yeah?"

She gave me a brief look that said *be nice or your father will hear about this.* "It's still a school night. Lights out before too long, okay?"

"Fine."

The door clicked shut, and Todd turned to me, wide-eyed. "Wow, and I thought my parents were strict. I haven't heard 'lights out' since I was ten. Do you have a curfew, as well?" I gave him a hooded stare, daring him to go on, and he squirmed. "Um, so where's the bathroom, again?"

I rose, dug a sleeping bag from my closet, and tossed it and an extra pillow on the floor. "Bathroom's down the hall to the right," I muttered, returning to my desk. "Just be quiet—my dad gets home late and might freak out if he doesn't know about you. And the piskie stays here. It doesn't leave this room, got it?"

"Sure, man." Todd closed the notebook, rolled it up, and stuffed it in a back pocket. "I'll try some of these when I get home, see if any of them work. Hey, Ethan, thanks for doing this. I owe you."

"Whatever." I turned my back on him and opened my laptop. "You don't owe me anything," I muttered as he started to leave the room. "In fact, you can thank me by never mentioning this to anyone, ever."

Todd paused in the hallway. He seemed about to say something, but when I didn't look up, turned and left silently, the door clicking shut behind him.

I sighed and plugged my headphones into my computer, pulling them over my head. Despite Mom's insistence that I go to bed soon, sleep wasn't likely. Not with a piskie and a half-phouka sharing my room tonight; I'd wake up with my head glued to the baseboard, or find my computer taped to the ceiling, or something like that. I shot a glare at the piskie sitting on my bookshelf, legs dangling over the side, and she glared back, baring sharp little teeth in my direction.

Definitely no sleep for Ethan tonight. At least I had coffee and live-streaming to keep me company.

"Oh, cool, you like *Firefly?*" Todd came back into the room, peering over my shoulder at the computer screen. Grabbing a stool, he plunked himself down next to me, oblivious to my wary look. "Man, doesn't it suck that it was canceled? I seriously thought about sending Thistle with a few of her friends to jinx FOX until they put it on again." He tapped the side of his head, indicating my headphones. "Dude, turn it up. This is my favorite episode. They should've just stuck with the television series and not bothered with that awful movie."

I pulled the headphones down. "What are you talking about? *Serenity* was awesome. They needed it to tie up all the loose ends, like what happened with River and Simon."

"Yeah, after killing everyone that was important," Todd sneered, rolling his eyes. "Bad enough that they offed the preacher dude. Once Wash died I was done."

"That was brilliant," I argued. "Made you sit up and think, hey, if *Wash* died, no one was safe."

"Whatever, man. You probably cheered when Anya died on *Buffy,* too."

I smirked but caught myself. What was happening here? I didn't need this. I didn't need someone to laugh and joke and argue the finer points of Whedon films with me. *Friends* did that sort of thing. Todd was not my friend. More important, I wasn't anyone's friend. I was someone who should be avoided at all costs. Even someone like Todd was at risk if I didn't keep my distance. Not to mention the pain he could bring down on me.

"Fine." Pulling off the headphones, I set them on the desk in front of the half-breed, not taking my hand away. "Knock yourself out. Just remember..." Todd reached for the headphones, and I pulled them back. "After tonight, we're done.

You don't talk to me, you don't look for me, and you *definitely* don't show up at my front door. When we get to school, you'll go your way and I'll go mine. Don't ever come here again, got it?"

"Yeah." Todd's voice, though sullen, was resigned. "I got it."

I pushed myself to my feet, and he frowned, pulling the headphones over his furry ears. "Where are you going?"

"To make some coffee." I shot a glance at the piskie, now on my windowsill, staring out at the rain, and resigned myself to the inevitable. "Want some?"

"Ugh, usually that would be a 'no,'" Todd muttered, pulling a face. Following my gaze to the window, his ears flattened. "But, yeah, go ahead and make me a cup. Extra strong… black…whatever." He shivered as he watched the storm raging beyond the glass. "I don't think either of us will be getting much sleep tonight."

CHAPTER FIVE
THE GHOST FEY

❧

"Uh-oh," Todd muttered from the passenger seat of my truck. "Looks like Kingston is back."

I gave the red Camaro a weary look as we cruised past it in the parking lot, not bothering to think about what Todd might be implying. Hell, I was tired. Staying up all night as Todd watched reruns of *Angel* and *Firefly,* listening to the half-breed's running commentary and drinking endless cups of coffee to keep myself awake, wasn't high on my list of favorite things to do. At least one of us had gotten a few hours' sleep. Todd had finally curled up on the sleeping bag and started to snore, but the piskie and I had given each other evil glares until dawn.

Today was going to suck, big-time.

Todd opened the door and hopped out of the truck almost before I turned off the engine. "So, uh, I guess I'll see you around," he said, edging away from me. "Thanks again for last night. I'll start setting these up as soon as I get home."

Whatever, I wanted to say, but just yawned at him instead. Todd hesitated, as if he was debating whether or not to tell me something. He grimaced.

"Also, you might want to avoid Kingston today, man. I mean, like the plague. Just a friendly warning."

I gave him a wary look. Not that I had any intention of talking to Kingston, ever, but… "Why?"

He shuffled his feet. "Oh, just…because. See ya, Ethan." And he took off, bounding over the parking lot, his huge coat flapping behind him. I stared after him, then shook my head. *Why do I get the feeling I've just been had?*

Yep, the half-breed had definitely been hiding something, because Kingston was out for blood. I wouldn't have noticed, except he made a point of glaring at me all through class, following me down the hallway, cracking his knuckles and mouthing "you're dead, freak," at me over the aisles. I didn't know what his problem was. He couldn't still be pissed about that fight in the hallway, if you could even call it a fight. Maybe he was mad because he hadn't gotten to knock my teeth out. I ignored his unsubtle threats and made a point of not looking at him, vowing that the next time I ran into Todd, we were going to have a talk.

Other than glaring at me, Kingston left me alone in the halls to and from class. But I expected him to try something during lunch, so I found a hidden corner in the library where I could eat in peace. Not that I was afraid of the football star and his gorillas, but I wanted to go to that damn demonstration, and they weren't going to ruin it by getting me expelled.

The library was dim and smelled of dust and old pages. A No Food or Drink sign was plastered to the front desk, but I stuffed my sandwich under my jacket, slipped my soda can into my pocket, and retreated to the back. The head librarian stared as I walked past her desk, her hawk eyes glinting behind her glasses, but she didn't stop me.

Opening my soda, making sure it didn't hiss, I sank down on the floor between aisles M–N and O–P with a relieved sigh. Leaning against the wall, I gazed through the cracks in the books, watching students moving down the mazelike corridors. A girl came down my aisle once, book in hand, and came to an abrupt halt, blinking. I glared stonily, and she retreated without a word.

Well, my life had certainly reached a new low. Hiding out in the library so the star quarterback wouldn't try to stick my head through a wall or put his fist between my teeth. Return the favor, and I'd be expelled. Morosely, I finished the last of my sandwich and checked my watch. Still thirty-five minutes to class. Restless, I plucked a book off the shelf next to me and skimmed through it: *The History of Cheeses and Cheesemaking*. How fascinating.

As I put it back, my thoughts drifted to Kenzie. I was supposed to meet her here after school for that stupid interview. I wondered what she would ask, what she wanted to know. Why had she even singled me out, after I'd made it perfectly clear that I wanted nothing to do with her?

I snorted. Maybe that was the reason. She liked a challenge. Or maybe she was intrigued by someone who wasn't tripping over himself to talk to her. If you believed what Todd said, Mackenzie St. James probably had everything handed to her on a silver platter.

Stop thinking about her, Ethan. It doesn't matter why; after today you'll go back to ignoring her, same as everyone else.

There was a buzz somewhere overhead, the soft flutter of wings, and all my senses went rigidly alert.

Casually, I picked up the book again and pretended to flip through it while listening for the faery atop the shelves. If the piskie tried anything, it would be squashed like a big spider under *The History of Cheeses and Cheesemaking*.

The piskie squeaked in its excited, high-pitched voice, wings buzzing. I was tempted to glance up to see whether it was the piskie I'd saved in the locker room or Todd's little purple friend. If either were back to torture me after I just saved their miserable lives and stuck my neck out for the half-breed, I was going to be really annoyed.

"There you are!"

A body appeared at the end of the aisle, orange eyes glowing in the dim light. I suppressed a groan as the half-breed ducked into the corridor, panting. His ears were pressed flat to his skull, and his canines were bared as he flung himself down next to me.

"I've been looking everywhere for you," he whispered, peering through the books, eyes wild. "Look, you've got to help me. They're still after us!"

"Help you?" I glared at him, and he shrank back. "I've already helped you far more than I should have. You swore you would leave me alone after this. What happened to that?" Todd started to reply, and I held up my hand. "No, forget that question. Let me ask another one. Why does Kingston want to bash my head in today?"

He fiddled with the end of his sleeve. "Dude...you have to understand...this was before I knew you. Before I realized something was after me. If I'd known I'd be asking for your help...you can't get mad at me, okay?"

I waited, letting the silence stretch. Todd grimaced.

"Okay, so I...uh... might've asked Thistle to pay him back for what he did, but to make sure he didn't connect it to me. She put something in his shorts that...er...made him swell up and itch like crazy. That's why he wasn't here yesterday. But, the catch is, he knows someone did it to him."

"And he thinks it was me." Groaning, I leaned my head back and thumped it against the wall. So that's why the quarterback was on the warpath. I raised my head and glared at him. "Give me one good reason I shouldn't kick your ass right now."

"Dude, They are *here!*" Todd leaned forward again, apparently too panicked to take my threat seriously. "I've seen them, peering in through the windows, staring right at me! I can't go home while they're out there! They're just waiting for me to step outside."

"What do you want me to do about it?" I asked.

"Make them go away! Tell them to leave me alone." He grabbed my sleeve. "You're the brother of the Iron Queen! You have to do *something.*"

"No, I don't. And keep your voice down!" I stood and glared down at them both. "This is your mess. I told you before, I want nothing to do with Them, and your friends have caused me nothing but trouble since the day I got here. I stepped in front of Kingston for you, I let a piskie and a half-phouka into my room last night, and look where it got me. That's what I get for sticking my neck out."

Todd wilted, looking stunned and betrayed, but I was too angry to care. "I told you before," I growled, backing out of the aisle, "we're done. Stay away from me, you hear? I don't want you or your friends around me, my house, my family, my car, anything. I've helped you as much as I can. Now leave. Me. *Alone.*"

Without waiting for an answer, I whirled and stalked away, scanning the room for invisible things that might be lurking in the corners, ready to pounce. If the fey were hanging around the school like Todd said, I would have to up the ante on some of my protection wards, both for my truck and my person. Also, if Kingston was ready to put my head through a bathroom stall, I should probably head back to class and lay low until he and the gorilla squad cooled off a bit.

As I neared the librarian's desk, however, a faint, muffled sob came from one of the aisles behind me, and I stopped.

Dammit. Closing my eyes, I hesitated, torn between anger

and guilt. I knew what it was like, being hunted by the fey. I knew the fear, the desperation, when dealing with the Fair Folk who meant you harm. When you realized that it was just you against Them and no one could help you. When you realized *They* knew it, too.

Spinning on a heel, I walked back to the far aisle, cursing myself for getting involved one more time. I found Todd sitting where I had left him, huddled in the aisle looking miserable, the piskie crouched on his shoulder. They both glanced up when I approached, and Todd blinked, furry ears pricking hopefully.

"I'll drive you home," I said, watching his face light up with relief. "Last favor, all right? You have what you need to keep Them away from you—just follow the instructions I gave you and you'll be fine. Don't thank me," I said as he opened his mouth. "Just meet me here after class. I have this interview with the school reporter I have to do first, but it shouldn't take long. We'll leave when I'm done."

"School reporter?" Todd's smile shifted to an obnoxious leer in the space of a blink. "You mean St. James. So, she's got you wrapped around her little finger, too, huh? That didn't take long."

"You wanna walk home?"

"Sorry." The smirk vanished as quickly as it had come. "I'll be here. In fact, I think Violet and I are just going to stay right here until classes are over. You go do your interview thing. We'll be close, probably hiding under a table or something."

I made a mental note to check under the table before I did any interviews that afternoon, and left without another word. This time I did not look back.

Damn the fey. Why couldn't they leave me alone? Or Todd, for that matter? Why did they make life miserable for anyone caught up in their twisted sights? Human, half-breed, young, old, it didn't matter. I was no safer today than I had been thirteen years ago, just more paranoid and hostile. Was it always going to be like this, constantly looking over my shoulder, being alone so no one else got hurt? Was I ever going to be free of Them?

As I stepped through the library doors, my thoughts still on the conversation with the half-breed, something grabbed my shoulder and slammed me into the wall. My head struck the cement with a painful crack, expelling the air from my lungs. Stars danced across my vision for a second, and I blinked them away.

Kingston glared down at me, one fist in the collar of my shirt, pinning me to the wall. Two of his goons stood at his shoulders, flanking him like growling attack dogs.

"Hey there, asshole," Kingston's hot breath whipped at my face as he leaned close, reeking of smoke and spearmint. "I think we need to have a little talk."

The demonstration, Ethan. Keep it together. "What do you want?" I snarled, forcing myself not to move, not to shoot my arm up his neck, wrench his head down and drive my knee into his ugly mouth. Or grab the hand on my collar, spin around, and slam his thick face into the wall. So many options, but I kept myself still, not meeting his eyes. "I haven't done anything to you."

"Shut up!" His grip tightened, pressing me harder against the cement. "I know it was you. Don't ask me how, but I know. But we'll get to that in a minute." He brought his face close to mine, lips curling into a grim smile. "I hear you've been talking to Mackenzie."

You've got to be kidding me. All this time I've been saying "go away," *and this still happens?* "So what?" I challenged stupidly, making Kingston narrow his eyes. "What are you going to do, pee on her locker to let everyone know she's off-limits?"

Kingston didn't smile. His free fist clenched, and I kept a close eye on it in case it came streaking at my face. "She's off-limits to *you*," he said, dead serious now. "And unless you want me to make it so that all your food comes through a straw, you'll remember that. You don't talk to her, you don't hang around her, you don't even look at her. Just forget you ever heard her name, you got that?"

I would love to, I thought sourly. *If the girl would leave me alone.* But at the same time, something in me bristled at the thought of never talking to Kenzie again. Maybe I didn't respond well to threats, maybe Todd's unknown faeries had me itching for a fight, but I straightened, looked Brian Kingston right in the eye and said, "Piss. Off."

He tensed, and his two friends swelled up behind him like angry bulls. "Okay, freak," Kingston said, and that evil smirk came creeping back. "If that's how you want it. Fine. I still owe you for making me miss practice yesterday. And now, I'm gonna make you beg." The pressure on my shoulder tightened, pushing me toward the floor. "On your knees, freak. That's how you like it, right?"

"Hey!"

A clear, high voice rang through the hall, a second before I would've exploded, demonstration or no. Mackenzie St. James came stalking toward us, a stack of books under one arm, her small form tight with fury.

"Let him go, Brian," she demanded, marching up to the startled quarterback, a bristling kitten facing down a Rottweiler. "What the hell is your problem? Leave him alone!"

"Oh, hey, Mackenzie." Brian grinned at her, looking almost sheepish. *Taking your eyes off your opponent,* I thought. *Stupid move.* "What a coincidence. We were just talking about you to our mutual friend, here." He shoved me against the wall again, and I fought down a knee-jerk reaction to snap his elbow. "He's promised to be a lot nicer to you in the future, isn't that right, freak?"

"Brian!"

"Okay, okay." Kingston raised his hands and stepped away, and his cronies did the same. "Take it easy, Mac, we were just fooling around." He turned a sneer on me, and I glared back, daring him to step forward, to grab me again. "You got lucky, freak," he said, backing away. "Remember what I told you. You won't always have a little girl around to protect you." His friends snickered, and he winked at Kenzie, who rolled her eyes. "We'll see you around, real soon."

"Jerk," Kenzie muttered as they sauntered off down the hall, laughing and high-fiving each other. "I don't know what Regan sees in him." She shook her head and turned to me. "You okay?"

Embarrassed, fuming, I scowled at her. "I could've handled it," I snapped, wishing I could put my fist through a wall or someone's face. "You didn't have to interfere."

"I know, tough guy." She gave me a half smile, and I wasn't sure if she was being serious. "But Regan is fond of the big meathead, and I didn't want you to beat him up *too* badly."

I glared in the direction the jocks had gone, clenching my fists as I struggled to control my raging emotions, the urge to stalk down the hall and plant Kingston's face into the floor. *Why me?* I wanted to snap at her. *Why won't you leave me alone? And why do you have the entire football team ready to tear someone in half for looking at you funny?*

"Anyway," Kenzie continued, "we're still on for that interview, right? You're planning on showing up, I hope. I'm dying to know what goes on in that broody head of yours."

"I don't brood."

She snorted. "Tough guy, if brooding was a sport, you'd

have gold medals with scowling faces lining the walls of your room."

"Whatever."

Kenzie laughed. Sweeping past me, she pushed open the library door, pausing in the frame. "See you in a couple hours, Ethan."

I shrugged.

"I'm holding you to it, tough guy. Promise me you won't run off or conveniently forget."

"Yes." I blew out a breath as she grinned, and the door swung shut. "I'll be there."

I didn't go.

Not that I didn't try. Despite the incident in the hall—or maybe because of it—I wasn't about to let anyone tell me who I could or could not hang out with. Like I said, I don't respond well to threats, and if I was being honest with myself, I was more than a little curious about Mackenzie St. James. So after the last bell, I gathered my stuff, made sure the hall was clear of Kingston and his thugs, and headed toward the library.

About halfway there, I realized I was being followed.

The halls were nearly empty as I went by the cafeteria. The few bodies I passed were going the other way, to the parking lot and the vehicles that would take them home. But as I made my way through the quiet hallways, I got that strange prickle on the back of my neck that told me I wasn't alone.

Casually, I stopped at a water fountain, bending down to get a quick drink. But I slid my gaze off to the side, scanning the hall.

There was a shimmer of white at the edge of my vision, as something glided around a corner and stopped in the shadows, watching.

My gut tightened, but I forced myself to straighten and walk down the hall as if nothing was wrong. I could feel the presence at my back following me, and my heart began to thud in my chest. It was the same creature, the one that I'd seen in the locker room that night, when the piskie found me. What was it? One of the fey, I was certain, but I'd never seen this kind before, all pale and transparent, almost ghostlike. A bean sidhe, perhaps? But bean sidhes usually announced their presence with hair-raising shrieks and wails; they didn't silently trail someone down a dark corridor, being careful to stay just out of sight. And I certainly wasn't about to die.

I hoped.

What does it want with me? I paused at the library door, grasping the handle but not pulling it open. Through the small rectangular window, I saw the front desk, the librarian's gray head bent over the computer. Kenzie would be in there, somewhere, waiting for me. And Todd. I'd promised I would meet them both, and I hated breaking my word.

A memory flashed: one of myself, fleeing the redcaps, taking refuge in the library. Pulling a knife as I hunkered between the aisles, waiting for them. The sadistic faeries setting fire to the wall of books to flush me into the open. I escaped, but my rush to get out was taken as me fleeing the scene of the crime, leading to my expulsion from school.

I drew in a quiet breath, pausing in the door frame, anger and fear spreading through my stomach. No, I couldn't do this. If I went in, if They saw me talking to Kenzie, they could use her to get to me. I didn't know what They wanted, but I wasn't going to draw another person into my dangerous, messed-up life. Not again.

Releasing the handle, I stepped away and continued down the hall. I felt the thing follow me, and as I turned the corner, I thought I heard the library door creak open. I didn't look back.

I walked out to the parking lot, but I didn't stop there. Getting in my truck and driving home might lose my tail, but it wouldn't give me any answers as to why it was following me. Instead, I passed the rows of cars, stepped over the curb, and continued on to the football field. Thankfully, it was empty today. No practice, no screaming coaches, no armored jocks slamming into each other. If Kingston and his friends saw me sauntering casually across their turf in a very blatant show of *Screw you, Kingston, what are you gonna do about it?* they would try to bury me here. I wondered if anyone else could see me, and if they did, would they tell the quarterback I was figuratively pissing on his territory? I smirked at the thought, vaguely tempted to stop and make it literal, as well. But I had more important things to deal with, and a pissing contest with Kingston wasn't one of them.

Behind the bleachers, I stopped. A fence separated the field from a line of trees on the other side, so it was cool and shady here. I wished I had my knife. Something sharp, metal and lethal between me and whatever was coming my way. But I'd been caught with a knife before, and it had gotten me in a *lot* of trouble, so I'd left it at home.

Putting my back to the fence, I waited.

Something stepped around the bleachers, or rather, *shimmered* around the bleachers, barely visible in the sun. And even though it was a bright fall afternoon, with enough sunlight to melt away the chill, I suddenly felt cold. Sluggish. Like my thoughts and emotions were slowly being drained, leaving behind an empty shell.

Shivering, I gazed stonily at the thing hovering a few feet away. It was unlike any faery I'd seen before. Not a nymph, a sidhe, a boggart, a dryad, *anything* I recognized. Not to say I was an expert on the different types of faeries, but I'd seen more than most people, and this one was just…weird.

It was shorter than me by nearly a foot and so thin it didn't seem possible that its legs could hold it up. In fact, its legs ended in needle-sharp tips, so it looked as if it was walking on toothpicks instead of feet. Its face was hatchet thin, and its fingers were those same thin points, as if it could poke its nail right through your skull. The skeletons of what used to be wings protruded from its bony shoulders, broken and shattered, and it hovered a few inches off the ground, as if the earth itself didn't want to touch it.

For a few seconds, we just stared at each other.

"All right," I said in an even voice, as the creepy fey floated there, still watching me. "You followed me out here—you obviously wanted to see me. What the hell do you want?"

Its eyes, huge and multifaceted like an insect's, blinked slowly. I saw myself reflected a hundred times in its gaze. Its razor slit of a mouth opened, and it breathed:

"I bring a warning, Ethan Chase."

I resisted the urge to cringe. There was something very... wrong...about this creature. It didn't belong here, in the real world. The faeries I had seen, even the Iron fey, were still a part of reality, sliding back and forth between this realm and the Nevernever. *This* thing...it was as if its body was out of sync with the rest of world, the way it flickered and blurred, as if it wasn't quite there. Wasn't quite solid.

The faery raised one long, bony finger and pointed at me.

"Do not interfere," it whispered. "Do not become involved in what will soon happen around you. This is not your fight. We seek no trouble with the Iron Court. But if you meddle in our affairs, human, you put those you care about at risk."

"Your affairs? What *are* you?" My voice came out raspier than I wanted it to. "I'm guessing you're not from the Seelie or Unseelie Courts."

The faery's slitted mouth might've twitched into a smile.

"We are nothing. We are forgotten. No one remembers our names, that we ever existed. You should do the same, human."

"Uh-huh. So, you make a point of making certain I know you're there, of tracking me down and threatening my family, to tell me I should forget about you."

The faery drew back a step, gliding over the ground. "A warning," it said again and tossed something at my feet, something small and gray. "This is what will happen to those who interfere," it whispered. "Our return has just begun."

I crouched, still keeping a wary eye on the faery, and spared a glance at what lay on the ground.

A piskie. The same one I'd seen earlier that day with Todd, I was sure of it. But its skin was a dull, faded gray, as if all the color had been sucked out of it. Gently, I reached down and picked it up, cradling it in my palm. It rolled over and blinked, huge eyes empty and staring. It was still alive, but even as I watched, the faery's tiny body rippled and then…blew away. Like mist in the breeze. Leaving behind nothing at all.

My insides felt cold. I'd seen faeries die—they turned into leaves, branches, flowers, insects, dirt, and sometimes they did just vanish. But never like this. "What did you do to it?" I demanded, surging back to my feet.

The thing didn't answer. It shimmered again, going transparent, as if it, too, were in danger of blowing away on the wind. Raising its hands, it gazed at its fingers, watching as they flickered like a bad television channel.

"Not enough," it whispered, shaking its head. "Never enough. Still, it is something. That you can see me, talk to me. It is a start. Perhaps the half-blood will be stronger."

It drifted back. "We will be watching you, Ethan Chase," it warned, and suddenly turned, as if glimpsing something off to the side. "You do not want even more people hurt because of you."

More people? *Oh, no,* I thought, as it dawned on me what the faery was implying. The dead Thistle, the "half-blood" it mentioned. *Todd.* "Hey!" I snapped, striding forward. "Hold it right there. What are you?"

The faery smiled, rippled in the sunlight and drifted away, over the fence and out of sight. I would've given chase, but the sound of movement behind the bleachers caught my attention, and I turned.

Kenzie stood beside the benches, a notepad in one hand, staring at me. From the look on her face, she'd heard every word.

CHAPTER SIX
VANISHED

I ignored Kenzie and strode quickly across the football field, not looking back.

"Hey!" Kenzie cried, scrambling after me.

My mind was spinning. *Todd was right,* it whispered. *Something was after him. Damn, what* was *that thing? I've never seen anything like it before.*

My chest felt tight. It was happening again. It didn't matter what that thing was, the damned faeries were out to ruin my life and hurt everyone around me. I had to find Todd, warn him. I just hoped that he was okay; the half-breed might be annoying and ignorant, but he shouldn't have to suffer because of me.

"Ethan! Just a second! Will you please hold up?" Kenzie put on a burst of speed as we reached the edge of the field, blocking my path. "Will you tell me what's going on? I heard voices, but I didn't see anyone else. Was someone threatening you?" Her eyes narrowed. "You're not into anything illegal, are you?"

"Kenzie, get out of here," I snapped. The creepy faery could still be watching us. Or creeping closer to Todd. I had to get away from her, now. "Just leave me alone, okay? I'm not doing the damn interview. I don't give a crap about what you or this school or anyone else thinks of me. Put *that* in your article."

Her eyes flashed. "The parking lot is the other way, tough guy. Where are you going?"

"Nowhere."

"Then you won't mind if I come along."

"You're not coming."

"Why not?"

I swore. She didn't move, and my sense of urgency flared. "I don't have time for this," I growled, and brushed past her, sprinting down the hall toward the library. The girl followed, of course, but I wasn't thinking about her anymore. If that faery freak got close to Todd, if it did something to him like it had the piskie, it would be my fault. Again.

The librarian gave me the evil eye as I burst through the library doors, followed closely by the girl. "Slow down, you two," she barked as we passed the desk. Kenzie murmured an apology, but I ignored her, striding toward the back, searching for the half-breed in the aisles. Empty, empty, a couple making out in the history section, empty. My unease grew. Where *was* he?

"What are we looking for?" Kenzie whispered at my back.

I turned, ready to tell her to get lost, futile as it might be, when something under the window caught my eye.

Todd's jacket. Lying in a crumpled heap beneath the sill. I stared at it, trying to find an explanation as to why he would leave it behind. Maybe he just forgot it. Maybe someone stole it as a prank and ditched it here. A cold breeze whispered through the window, ruffling my clothes and hair. It was the only open window in the room.

Kenzie followed my gaze, frowned, then walked forward and picked up the jacket. As she did, something white fell out of the pocket and fluttered to the floor. A note, written on a torn half sheet of paper. I lunged forward to grab it, but Kenzie had already snatched it up.

"Hey," I said sharply, holding out a hand. "Give me that."

She dodged, holding the paper out of reach. Defiance danced in her eyes. "I don't see your name on it."

"It was for me," I insisted, stalking forward. She leaped away, putting a long table between us, and my temper flared. "Dammit, I'm not playing this game," I growled, keeping my voice down so the librarian wouldn't come stalking toward us. "Hand it over, now."

Kenzie narrowed her eyes. "Why so secretive, tough guy?" she asked, deftly maneuvering around the table, keeping the same distance between us. "Are these the coordinates for a drug deal or something?"

"What?" I grabbed for her, but she slid out of reach. "Of course not. I'm not into that crap."

"A letter from a secret admirer, then?"

"No," I snapped, and stopped edging around the table. This was ridiculous. Were we back in the third grade? I eyed her across the table, judging the distance between us. "It's not a love letter," I said, silently fuming. "It's not even from a girl."

"Are you sure?"

"Yes."

"Then you won't mind if I read it," she said and flipped open the note.

As soon as her attention left me, I leaped over the table and slid across the surface, grabbing her arm as I landed on the other side. She yelped in surprise and tried to jerk back, unsuccessfully. Her wrist was slender and delicate, and fit easily into my grasp.

For a second, we glared at each other. I could see my scowling, angry reflection in her eyes. Kenzie stared back, a slight smirk on her lips, as if this newest predicament amused her.

"What now, tough guy?" She raised a slender eyebrow. And, for some reason, my heart beat faster under that look.

Deliberately, I reached up and snatched the paper from her fingers. Releasing her, I turned my back on the girl, scanning the note. It was short, messy and confirmed my worst suspicions.

They're here! Gotta run. If you find this, tell my folks not to worry. Sorry, man. Didn't mean to drag you into this. —Todd.

I crumpled the note and shoved it into my jeans pocket. What did he expect me to do now? Go to his parents, tell them a bunch of creepy invisible faeries were out to get their son? I'd get thrown into the loony bin for sure.

I felt Kenzie's eyes on my back and wondered how much of the note she'd seen. Had she read anything in that split second it had taken me to get across the table?

"It sounds like your friend is in trouble," Kenzie murmured. Well, that answered *that* question. All of it, apparently.

"He's not my friend," I replied, not turning around. "And you shouldn't get involved. This is none of your business."

"The hell it's not," she shot back. "If someone is in trouble, we have to do something. Who's after him? Why doesn't he just go to the police?"

"The police can't help." I finally turned to face her. "Not with this. Besides, what would you tell them? We don't even know what's going on. All we have is a note."

"Well, shouldn't we at least see if he made it home okay?"

I sighed, rubbing my scalp. "I don't know where he lives," I said, feeling slightly guilty that I knew so little. "I don't have his phone number. I don't even know his last name."

But Kenzie sighed. "Boys," she muttered, and pulled out her phone. "His last name is Wyndham, I think. Todd Wyndham. He has a couple of classes with me." She fiddled with her phone without looking up. "Just a second. I'll Google it."

I tried to stay calm while she looked it up, though I couldn't stop scanning the room for hidden enemies. What were these transparent, ghostlike fey, and why had I not seen them before? What did they want with Todd? I remembered the piskie's limp body, an empty, lifeless husk before it disappeared, and shivered. Whatever they were, they were dangerous, and I needed to find the half-breed before they did the same to him. I owed him that, for not being there like I promised.

"Got it," Kenzie announced. "Or, at least, I have his house number." Glancing up from her phone, she looked at me and raised an eyebrow. "So, do you want to call them or should I?"

I dug out my phone. "I'll do it," I said, dreading the task but knowing I had to finish what I started.

She recited a string of numbers, and I punched them into my phone. Putting it to my ear, I listened to it ring once, twice, and on the third, someone picked up.

"Wyndham residence," said a woman's voice. I swallowed.

"Um, yeah. I'm a…friend of Todd's," I said haltingly. "Is he home?"

"No, he isn't back from school yet," continued the voice on the other end. "Do you want me to give him a message?"

"Uh, no. I was…um…hoping to catch him later today so we could…hang." I winced at how lame I sounded, and Kenzie giggled. I frowned at her. "Do you know his cell phone number?" I added as an afterthought.

"Yes, I have his number." Now the woman sounded suspicious. "Why do you want to know? Who is this?" she continued sharply, and I winced. "Are you one of those boys he keeps talking about? You think I don't notice when he comes home with bruises and black eyes? Do you think it's funny, picking on someone smaller then you? What's your name?"

I was tempted to hang up, but that would make me look even more suspicious, and it would get me no closer to Todd.

I wondered if he'd even told her that he spent the night at my house. "My name is Ethan Chase," I said in what I hoped was a calm, reasonable voice. "I'm just…a friend. Todd stayed at my place last night, during the storm."

"Oh." I couldn't tell if Todd's mother was appeased or not, but after a moment, she sighed. "Then, I'm sorry. Todd doesn't have many friends, none that have called the house, anyway. I didn't mean to snap at you, Ethan."

"It's fine," I mumbled, embarrassed. *I'm used to it.*

"One moment," she continued, and her voice grew fainter as she put the phone down. "I have his number on the fridge. Just a second."

A minute later, I thanked Todd's mom and hung up, relieved to have that over with. "Well?" asked Kenzie, watching expectantly. "Did you get it?"

"Yeah."

She waited a moment longer, then bounced impatiently. "Are you going to call him, then?"

"I'm getting to it." Truthfully, I didn't want to. What if he was perfectly fine, and that note was just a prank, revenge for some imagined slight? What if he was halfway home, laughing at how he pulled a fast one on the stupid human? Todd was half-phouka, a faery notorious for their mischievous nature and love of chaos. This could be a great, elaborate joke, and if I called him, he would have the last laugh.

Deep down, though, I knew those were just excuses. I hadn't imagined that creepy faery, or the dead piskie. Todd wasn't pretending to be terrified. Something was happening, something bad, and he was right in the middle of it.

And I didn't want to be drawn in.

Too late now, I suppose. Pressing in Todd's number, I put the phone to my ear and held my breath.

One ring.

Two rings.

Thr—

The phone abruptly cut off, going dead without sending me to voice mail. A second later, the dial tone droned in my ear.

"What happened?" Kenzie asked as I lowered my hand. "Is Todd all right?"

"No," I muttered, looking down at the phone, and the end call button at the bottom of the screen. "He's not."

I went home after that, having convinced Kenzie that there was nothing we could do for Todd right then. She was stubborn, refusing to believe me, wanting to call the police. I told her not to jump to conclusions as we didn't exactly know what was going on. Todd could've turned off his phone. He could be on his way home and was just running late. We didn't have enough evidence to start calling the authorities. Eventually, she caved, but I had the feeling she wouldn't let it go for long. I just hoped she wouldn't do anything that would attract Their attention. Hanging around me was bad enough.

Back home, I went straight to my room, locking the door behind me. Sitting at my desk, I opened the first drawer, reached all the way to the back, and pulled out the long, thin envelope inside.

Leaning back in the chair, I stared at it for a long while. The paper was wrinkled and brittle now, yellow with age, and smelled of old newspapers. It had one word written across the front: Ethan. My name, in my sister's handwriting.

Flipping it over, I opened the top and pulled out the letter within. I'd read it a dozen times before and knew it word for word, but I scanned the note one more time, a bitter lump settling in my throat.

Ethan,

I've started this letter a hundred times, wishing I knew the right words to say, but I guess I'll just come out and say it. You probably won't see me again. I wish I could be there for you and Mom, even Luke, but I have other responsibilities now, a whole kingdom that needs me. You're growing up so fast—each time I see you, you're taller, stronger. I forget, sometimes, that time moves differently in Faery. And it breaks my heart every time I come home and see that I've missed so much of your life. Please know that you're always in my thoughts, but it's best that we live our own lives now. I have enemies here, and the last thing I want is for you and Mom to get hurt because of me.

So, this is goodbye. I'll be watching you from time to time, and I'll do everything in my power to make sure you and Mom and Luke can live comfortably. But please, Ethan, for the love of all that's holy, do not try to find me. My world is far too dangerous; you of all people should know that. Stay away from Them, and try to have a normal life.

If there is an emergency, and you absolutely must see me, I've included a token that will take you into the Nevernever, to someone who can help. To use it, squeeze one drop of your blood onto the surface and toss it into a pool of still water. But it can only be used once, and after that, the favor is done. So use it wisely.

I love you, little brother. Take care of Mom for me.

—Meghan

I closed the letter, put it on the desk, and turned the envelope upside down. A small silver coin rolled into my open palm, and I closed my fingers around it, thinking.

Did I want to bring my sister into this? Meghan Chase, the freaking Queen of the Iron Fey? How many years had it been since I'd seen her last? Did she even remember us anymore? Did she care?

My throat felt tight. Pushing myself up, I tossed the coin on the desk and swept the letter back in the drawer, slamming it shut. No, I wasn't going to go crying to Meghan, not for this or anything. Meghan had left us; she was no longer part of this family. As far as I was concerned, she was Faery through and through. And I'd been through enough faery torment to last several lifetimes. I could handle this myself.

Even if it meant I had to do something stupid, something I'd sworn I would never do.

I was going to have to contact the fey.

THE EMPTY PARK

At 11:35 p.m., my alarm went off. I slapped it silent and rolled out of bed, already dressed, snatching my backpack from the floor. Creeping silently down the hall, I checked to see if Mom's light was off; sometimes she stayed up late, waiting for Dad to get home. But tonight, the crack under her door was dark, and I continued my quiet trek out the front door to the driveway.

I couldn't take my truck. Dad would be home later, and he'd know I was gone if he saw my truck was missing. Sneaking out in the middle of the night was highly frowned upon and tended to result in groundings, lectures and technology banishment. So I dug my old bike out of the garage, checked to see that the tires were still inflated and walked it down to the sidewalk.

Overhead, a thin crescent moon grinned down at me behind ragged wisps of cloud, and a cold autumn breeze sliced right through my jacket, making me shiver. That nagging, cynical part of me hesitated, reluctant to take part in this insanity. *Why are you getting involved?* it whispered. *What's the half-breed to you, anyway? Are you willing to deal directly with the fey because of him?*

But it wasn't just Todd now. Something strange was happening in Faery, and I had a feeling it was going to get worse. I needed to know what was going on and how I could defend myself from transparent ghost-fey that sucked the life right out of their victims. I didn't want to be left in the dark, not with those things out there.

Besides, Mr. Creepy Faery had threatened not only me but my family. And *that* pissed me off. I was sick of running and hiding. Closing my eyes, hoping They would leave me alone wasn't working. I doubted it ever had.

Hopping on my bike, I started pedaling toward the one place I'd always avoided until now. A place where, I hoped, I would get some answers.

If the damn fey wanted me as an enemy, bring it on. I'd be their worst nightmare.

Even in gigantic, crowded cities, where steel buildings, cars and concrete dominate everything, you can always find the fey in a park.

It doesn't have to be a big park. Just a patch of natural earth, with a few trees and bushes scattered about, maybe a little pond, and that's all they need. I'm told Central Park in New York City has hundreds, maybe thousands of faeries living there, and several trods to the Nevernever, all within its well-groomed perimeter. The tiny park three and a half miles from my house had about a dozen fey of the common variety—piskies, goblins, tree sprites—and no trods that I knew of.

I parked my bike against an old tree near the entrance and gazed around. It wasn't much of a park, really. There was a picnic bench with a set of peeling monkey bars and an old slide, and a dusty fire pit that hadn't been used in years. At least, not by humans. But the trees here were old, ancient things—huge oaks and weeping willows—and if you stared very hard be-

tween the branches, you sometimes caught flickers of movement not belonging to birds or squirrels.

Leaving the bike, I walked to the edge of the fire pit and
looked down. The ashes were cold and gray, days or weeks
old, but I had seen two goblins at this pit several weeks ago,
roasting some sort of meat over the fire. And there were several piskies and wood sprites living in the oaks, as well. The
local fey might not know anything about their creepy, transparent cousins, but it couldn't hurt to ask.

Crouching, I picked up a flat rock, dusted it off, and set
it in the center of the fire pit. Digging through my pack, I
pulled out a bottle of honey, stood and drizzled the golden
syrup onto the stones. Honey was like ambrosia to the fey;
they couldn't resist the stuff.

Capping the bottle, I tossed it into my pack and waited.

Several minutes passed, which was a surprise to me. I knew
the fey frequented this area. I was expecting at least a couple
of goblins or piskies to appear. But the night was still, the
shadows empty—until there was a soft rustle behind me, the
hiss of something moving over the grass.

"You will not find them that way, Ethan Chase."

I turned, calmly. *Rule number two: show no fear when dealing
with the Fair Folk.* I could have drawn my rattan sticks, and in
all honesty I really wanted to, but that might have been taken
as a sign of nervousness or unease.

A tall, slight figure stood beneath the weeping willow,
watching me through the lacy curtain. As I waited, a slender hand parted the drooping branches and the faery stepped
into the open.

It was a dryad, and the weeping willow was probably her
tree, for she had the same long green hair and rough, bark-
like skin. She was impossibly tall and slender, and swayed
slightly on her feet, like a branch in the wind. She observed

me with large black eyes, her long hair draped over her body, and slowly shook her head.

"They will not come," she whispered sadly, glancing at the swirl of honey at my feet. "They have not been here for many nights. At first, it was only one or two that went missing. But now—" she gestured to the empty park "—now there is no one left. Everyone is gone. I am the last."

I frowned. "What do you mean, you're the last? Where are all the others?" I gazed around the park, scanning the darkness and shadows, seeing nothing. "What the hell is going on?"

She drifted closer, swaying gently. I was tempted to step back but held my ground.

The dryad tilted her head to one side, lacy hair catching the moonlight as it fell. A large white moth flew out of the curtain and fluttered away into the shadows. "You have questions," the dryad said, blinking slowly. "I can tell you what you wish to know, but you must do something for me in return."

"Oh, no." I did step away then, crossing my arms and glaring at her. "No way. No bargains, no contracts. Find someone else to do your dirty work."

"Please, Ethan Chase." The dryad held out an impossibly slender hand, mottled and rough like the trunk of the tree. "As a favor, then. You must go to the Iron Queen for us. Inform her of our fate. Be our voice. She will listen to you."

"Go find Meghan?" I thought of the coin lying abandoned on my desk and shook my head. "You expect me to go into the Nevernever," I said, and my stomach turned just thinking about it. Memories crowded forward, dark and terrifying, and I shoved them back. "Go into Faery. With Mab and Titania and the rest of the crazies." I curled my mouth into a sneer. "Forget it. That's the *last* place I'll ever set foot in."

"You must." The dryad wrung her hands, pleading. "The courts do not know what is happening, nor would they care.

The welfare of a few half-breeds and exiles does not concern them. But you…you are the half brother of the Iron Queen—she will listen to you. If you do not…" The dryad trembled, like a leaf in a storm. "Then I'm afraid we will all be lost."

"Look." I stabbed a hand through my hair. "I'm just trying to find out what happened to a friend. Todd Wyndham. He's a half-breed, and I think he's in trouble." The dryad's pleading expression didn't change, and I sighed. "I can't promise to help you," I muttered. "I have problems of my own to worry about. But…" I hesitated, hardly believing I was saying this. "But if you can give me any information about my friend, then I'll…try to get a message to my sister. I'm still not promising anything!" I added quickly as the dryad jerked up. "But if I see the Iron Queen anytime in the near future, I'll tell her. That's the best I can offer."

The dryad nodded. "It will have to do," she whispered, shrinking in on herself. She closed her eyes as a breeze hissed through the park, rippling her hair and making the leaves around us sigh. "More of us have disappeared," she sighed. "More vanish with every breath. And they are coming closer."

"Who *are* they?"

"I do not know." The faery opened her eyes, looking terrified. "I do not know, nor do any of my fellows. Not even the *wind* knows their names. Or if it does, it refuses to tell me."

"Where can I find Todd?"

"Your friend? The half-breed?" The dryad took a step away, looking distracted. "I do not know," she admitted, and I narrowed my gaze. "I cannot tell you now, but I will put his name into the wind and see what it can turn up." She looked at me, her hair falling into her eyes, hiding half her face. "Return tomorrow night, Ethan Chase. I will have answers for you, then."

Tomorrow night. Tomorrow was the demonstration, the

event I'd been training for all month. I couldn't miss that, even for Todd. Guro would kill me.

I sighed. Tomorrow was going to be a long day. "All right," I said, stepping toward my bike. "I'll be here, probably some time after midnight. And then you can tell me what the hell is going on."

The dryad didn't say anything, watching me leave with unblinking black eyes. As I yanked my bike off the ground and started down the road, hoping I would beat Dad home, I couldn't shake the creeping suspicion that I wouldn't see her again.

THE DEMONSTRATION

The next day was Saturday, but instead of sleeping in like a normal person, I was up early and in the backyard, swinging my rattan through the air, smacking them against the tire dummy I'd set up in the corner. I didn't need the practice, but beating on something was a good way to focus, to forget the strangeness of the night before, though I still couldn't shake the eerie feeling whenever I remembered the dryad's last warning.

More of us have disappeared. More vanish with every breath. And they are coming closer.

"Ethan!"

Dad's voice cut through the rhythmic smacking of wood against rubber, and I turned to find him staring blearily at me from the patio. He wore a rumpled gray bathrobe, his face was grizzled and unshaven, and he did not look pleased.

"Sorry, Dad." I lowered the sticks, panting. "Did I wake you up?"

He shook his head, then stepped aside as two police officers came into the yard. My heart and stomach gave a violent lurch, and I tried to think of any crimes I might've committed without realizing it, or anything the fey might've pinned on me.

"Ethan?" one of them asked, as Dad watched grimly and

Mom appeared in the door frame, her hands over her mouth. "Are you Ethan Chase?"

"Yeah." I kept my arms at my sides, my sticks perfectly still, though my heart was going a mile a minute. The sudden thought of being arrested, being handcuffed in my own backyard in front of my horrified parents, nearly made me sick. I swallowed hard to keep my voice steady. "What do you want?"

"Do you know a boy named Todd Wyndham?"

I relaxed, suddenly aware of where this was going. My heart still pounded, but I kept my tone light, flippant, and I shrugged. "Yeah, he's in a few of my classes at school."

"You called his home yesterday afternoon, correct?" the policeman continued, and when I nodded, he added, "And he spent the night at your house the day before?"

"Yeah." I feigned confusion, looking back and forth between them. "Why? What's going on?"

The policemen exchanged a glance. "He's missing," one of them said, and I raised my eyebrows in fake surprise. "His mother reported that he didn't come home last night, and that she had received a call from Ethan Chase, a boy from his school, on the afternoon before his disappearance." His gaze flickered to the sticks in my hand, then back up to me, eyes narrowing slightly. "You wouldn't know anything about his whereabouts, would you, Ethan?"

I forced myself to be calm, shaking my head. "No, I haven't seen him since yesterday. Sorry."

It was pretty clear he didn't believe me, for his mouth thinned, and he spoke slowly, deliberately. "You have no clue as to what he was doing yesterday, no idea of where he could have gone?" When I hesitated, his voice became friendlier, encouraging. "Any information would be useful to us, Ethan."

"I told you," I said, firmer this time. "I don't know anything."

He gave an annoyed little huff, as if I was being deliberately evasive—which I was, but not for the reasons he thought. "Ethan, you realize we're only trying to help, don't you? You aren't protecting anyone if you hide information from us."

"I think that's enough." Dad suddenly came into the yard, bathrobe and all, glaring at the policemen. "Officers, your concern is appreciated, but I believe my son has told you all he knows." I blinked at Dad in shock as he came to stand beside me, smiling but firm. "If we find anything out, we'll be sure to call you."

"Sir, you don't seem to realize—"

"I realize just fine, officers," Dad said, his polite smile never wavering. "But Ethan has already given you his answer. Thank you for stopping by."

They looked irritated, but Dad wasn't a small man and had this stance that could be compared to a friendly but stubborn bull; you weren't going to get him to move once he'd made up his mind. After a lengthy pause—as if hoping I would fess up at the last second, perhaps—the officers gave curt nods and turned away. Muttering polite "ma'ams" to Mom, they swept by her, and she followed them, I assumed to the front door.

Dad waited a few seconds after the back door clicked shut before turning to me. "Todd Wyndham is the boy who came over the other night. Anything you'd like to tell me, son?"

I shook my head, not looking at him. "No," I muttered, feeling bad for lying, especially after he'd just gotten rid of the policemen for me. "I swear I don't know anything."

"Hmm." Dad gave me an unreadable look, then shuffled back into the house. But Mom appeared in the doorway again, watching me. I saw the fear on her face, the disappointment. She knew I was lying.

She hesitated a moment longer, as if waiting for me to confess, to tell her something different. But what could I say?

That the kid who'd spent the night with us was part faery, and this creepy new breed of fey were after him for some reason? I couldn't drag her into this; she would flip out for sure, thinking I was next. There was nothing either of them could do to help. So, I averted my gaze, and after a long, achingly uncomfortable pause, she slipped inside, slamming the door behind her.

I winced. Great, now they were both pissed at me. Sighing, I switched my rattan sticks to one hand and went in myself. I wished I could smack the tire dummy a while longer, but keeping a low profile seemed like a good idea now. The last thing I wanted was a grilling session where they would both ask questions I couldn't answer.

Mom and Dad were talking in the kitchen—probably about me—so I slipped into my room and gently closed the door.

My phone sat on the corner of my desk. For a second, I thought about calling Kenzie. I wondered what she was doing now, if the police had shown up on her doorstep, asking about a missing classmate. I wondered if she was worried about him…or me.

What? Why would she worry about you, you psychopath? You've been nothing but a jackass to her, and besides, you don't care, remember?

Angry now, I stalked to my bed and flopped down on it, flinging an arm over my face. I had to stop thinking of her, but my brain wasn't being cooperative this morning. Instead of focusing on the demonstration and the missing half-breed and the creepy Fey out to get us both, my thoughts kept going back to Kenzie St. James. The idea of calling her, just to see if she was all right, grew more and more tempting, until I jumped up and stalked to the living room, flipping on the television to drown out my traitorous thoughts.

★ ★ ★

The day passed in a blur of old action movies and commercials. I didn't move from the couch, afraid that if I went into my room, I'd see my unblinking phone and know Kenzie hadn't called me. Or worse, that she *had,* and I'd be tempted to call her back. I lounged on the sofa, the remains of empty chip bags, dirty plates and empty soda cans surrounding me, until late afternoon when Mom made an exasperated comment about rotting brains and bumps on logs or something, and ordered me to do something else.

Flipping off the television, I sat up, thinking. I still had a couple of hours till the demonstration. Wandering back to my room, I again noticed the phone on the corner of the desk. Nothing. No missed calls, texts, anything. I didn't know whether to be relieved or disappointed.

As I reached for it, though, it rang. Without checking the number, I snatched it up and put it to my ear.

"Hello?"

"Ethan?" The voice on the other end wasn't Kenzie, as I'd hoped, though it was vaguely familiar. "Is this Ethan Chase?"

"Yeah?"

"This…this is Mrs. Wyndham, Todd's mother."

My heart skipped a beat. I swallowed hard and gripped the phone tightly, as the voice on the other end continued.

"I know the police have already spoken to you," she said in a halting, broken voice, "but I…I wanted to ask you myself. You say you're Todd's friend…do you know what could have happened to him? Please, I'm desperate. I just want my son home."

Her voice broke at the end, and I closed my eyes. "Mrs. Wyndham, I'm sorry about Todd," I said, feeling like an ass. Worse than an ass, like a complete and utter failure, because I'd let another person down, because I couldn't protect them from the fey. "But I really don't know where he is. The last time we spoke was yesterday at school, before I talked to you, I swear." She gave a little sob, making my gut clench. "I'm really sorry," I said again, knowing how useless that sounded. "I wish I could give you better news."

She took a shaky breath. "All right, thank you, Ethan. I'm sorry to have bothered you." She sniffed and seemed about to say goodbye, but hesitated. "If...if you see him," she went on, "or if you find any information at all...will you let me know? Please?"

"Yeah," I whispered. "If I see him, I'll make sure he gets home, I promise."

After she hung up, I paced my room, not knowing what to do. I tried surfing online, watching YouTube, checking out various weapon stores, just to keep myself distracted, but it didn't help. I couldn't stop thinking of Todd, and Kenzie, caught in the twisted games of the fey. And it was partly my fault. Todd had been playing a dangerous game, and Kenzie was too stubborn to know when to back off, but the common denominator was me.

Now, one of them was gone and another family was torn apart. Just like last time.

Picking up my phone, I stuck it in my jeans pocket and snatched my keys from the desk. Grabbing my gym bag from the floor, I started to leave. Might as well head to the demonstration now; it was better than standing around here, driving myself crazy.

The silver coin on the desk glinted, and I paused. Sliding it into my palm, I stared at it, wondering where Meghan was, what she was doing. Did she ever think of me? Would she be disgusted, if she knew how I'd turned out?

"Ethan!" Mom's voice echoed from the kitchen. "Your

karate thing is tonight, isn't it? Do you want anything to eat before you go?"

I stuffed the coin in my pocket with the keys and left the room. "Kali, Mom, not karate," I told her, walking into the kitchen. "And no, I'll grab something on the way. Don't wait up for me."

"Curfew is still at eleven, Ethan."

Irritation flared. "Yeah, I know," I muttered. "It's been that way for five years. Why would it change now? It's not like I'm old enough to make my own decisions." Before she could say anything, I stalked past her and headed outside. "And, yes, I'll call if I'm going to be late," I threw back over my shoulder.

I could feel Mom's half angry, half worried gaze on my back as I slammed out the front door, making sure to bang it as I left. Stupid of me. If I had known what was going to happen at the demonstration that night, I would've said something much different.

The building was already full of people when I arrived. Tournaments had been going on for most of the afternoon, and shouts, *ki-yas,* and the shuffle of bare feet on mats echoed through the room as I ducked inside. Kids in their white gis tied with different colored belts threw punches and kicks within taped-off arenas; from the looks of it, it was the kempo students' turn on the mats.

I spotted Guro Javier and made my way over, weaving through students and onlookers, gritting my teeth as someone—a large kid with a purple belt—elbowed me in the ribs. I glared at him, and he smirked, as if daring me to try something. As if I'd start a fight with the brat in front of two hundred parents and about a dozen masters of various arts. Ignoring the kid's self-satisfied grin, I continued along the wall and stood next to my guro in the corner. He was watching the tournament with detached interest and gave a faint smile as I came up.

"You're very early, Ethan."

I shrugged helplessly. "Couldn't stay away."

"Are you ready?" Guro turned to me. "Our demonstration is after the kempo students are finished. Oh, and Sean sprained his ankle last night, so you're going to be doing the live weapon demo."

I felt a small, nervous thrill. "Really?"

"Do you need to practice?"

"No, I'll be fine." I thought back to the few times I'd handled Guro's real swords, which were short, single-edged blades similar to a machete. They were a little shorter then my rattan, razor sharp and about as deadly as they looked. They'd been in Guro's family for generations, and I was a bit in awe that I'd be wielding them tonight.

Guro nodded. "Go, get ready," he said, eyeing my holey jeans and T-shirt. "Warm up a bit if you want. We should start in about an hour."

I retreated to the locker room, changed into loose black pants and a white shirt, and carefully removed my wallet, keys and phone, ditching them in the side pocket of my gym bag. As I pulled my phone out, something bright tumbled to the floor, striking the ground with a ping.

The silver token. I'd forgotten about it. I stared at the thing, wondering if I should stuff it in my bag or just leave it on the floor. Still, it was my last connection to my sister, and even though Meghan didn't care about me, I didn't want to lose it just yet. I picked it up and slipped it into my pocket.

I stretched a bit, practiced several patterns empty-handed, making sure I knew what I was doing, then headed out to watch the tournament. The other kali students were starting to arrive, walking by me with brief nods and waves before flocking around Guro, but I didn't feel like socializing. Instead, I found an isolated corner behind the rows of chairs and leaned against it with my arms crossed, studying the matches.

"Ethan?"

The familiar voice caught me off guard. I jerked my head up as Kenzie slipped through the crowd and walked my way, a notebook in one hand and a camera around her neck. A tiny thrill shot through me, but I quickly squashed it.

"Hey," she greeted, giving me a friendly but puzzled smile. "I didn't expect to see you around. What are you doing here?"

"What are *you* doing here?" I countered, as though it wasn't obvious.

"Oh, you know." She held up her camera. "School paper stuff. A couple of the boys in our class take lessons here, and I'm covering the tournament. What about you?" Her eyes lit up. "Are you in the tournament? Will I actually get to see you fight?"

"I'm not fighting."

"But you do take something here, right? Kempo? Jujitsu?"

"Kali."

"What's that?"

I sighed. "A Filipino fighting style using sticks and knives. You'll see in a few minutes."

"Oh." Kenzie pondered this, then took a step forward, gazing up at me with thoughtful brown eyes. I swallowed the sudden dryness in my throat and leaned away, feeling the wall press against my back, preventing escape. "Well, you're just full of surprises, aren't you, Ethan Chase?" she mused with a small grin, cocking her head at me. "I wonder what other secrets are hiding in that broody head of yours."

I forced myself not to move, to keep my voice light and uncaring. "Is that why you keep hanging around me? You're curious?" I smirked and shook my head. "You're going to be disappointed. My life isn't that exciting."

I received a dubious look, and she took another step forward, peering into my eyes as if she could see the truth in them. My stomach squirmed as she leaned in. "Uh-huh. So, you keep your distance from everyone, take secret martial arts classes, and were expelled from your last school because the library mysteriously caught fire with you in it, and you're telling me your life isn't that exciting?"

I shifted uneasily. The girl was perceptive, I'd give her that. Unfortunately, she was now treading a little too close to the "exciting" part of my life, which meant I was either going to have to lie, pretend ignorance or pull the asshole card to drive her off. And right now, I didn't have it in me to be a jerk.

Meeting her gaze, I shrugged and offered a faint smile. "Well, I can't tell you all my secrets, can I? That would ruin my image."

She huffed, tossing her bangs. "Oh, fine. Be mysterious and broody. You still owe me an interview, you know." A wicked look crossed her face then, and she held up her notebook. "In fact, since you're not doing anything right now, care to answer a few questions?"

"Ethan!"

Strangely relieved and disappointed at the same time, I glanced up to see Guro waving me over. The rest of my classmates had gathered and were milling around nervously. It seemed the kempo matches were wrapping up.

Nice timing, Guro, I thought, and I didn't know if I was being serious or sarcastic. Pushing away from the wall, I turned to Kenzie with a helpless shrug. "I gotta go," I told her. "Sorry."

"Fine," she called after me. "But I'm going to get that interview, tough guy! I'll see you after your thing."

Guro raised an eyebrow as I came up but didn't ask who

the girl was or what I'd been doing. He never poked into our personal lives, for which I was thankful. "We're almost up," he said, and handed me a pair of short blades, their metal edges gleaming under the fluorescent lights. They weren't Guro's swords; these were different—a little longer, perhaps, the blades not quite as curved. I held them lightly, checking their weight and balance, and gave them a practice spin. Strangely enough, I felt they had been made especially for me.

I looked questioningly at Guro, and he nodded approvingly.

"I sharpened them this morning, so be careful," was all he said, and I backed away, taking my place along the wall.

The mats finally cleared, and a voice crackled over the intercom, introducing Guro Javier and his class of kali students. There was a smattering of applause, and we all went onto the mats to bow while Guro spoke about the origin of kali, what it meant, and how it was used. I could sense the bored impatience of the other students along the wall; they didn't want to see a demonstration, they wanted to get on with the tournament. I held my head high and kept my gaze straight ahead. I wasn't doing this for them.

There was a brief gleam of light along one side of the room: a camera flash. I suppressed a groan, knowing exactly who was taking pictures of me. Wonderful. If my photo ended up in the school paper, if people suddenly knew I studied a martial art, I could see myself being hounded relentlessly; people lining up to take a shot at the "karate kid." I cursed the nosy reporter under my breath, wondering if I could separate her from the camera long enough to delete the images.

The demonstration started with a couple of the beginner students doing a pattern known as Heaven Six, and the clacks of their rattan sticks echoed noisily throughout the room. I saw Kenzie take a few pictures as they circled the mats. Then the more advanced students demonstrated a few disarms, take-downs, and free-style sparring. Guro circled with them, explaining what they were doing, how we practiced, and how it could be applied to real life.

Then it was my turn.

"Of course," Guro said as I stepped onto the mats, holding the swords at my sides, "the rattan—the kali sticks—are proxies for real blades. We practice with sticks, but everything we do can be transferred to blades, knives or empty hands. As Ethan will demonstrate. This is an advanced technique," he cautioned, as I stepped across him, standing a few yards away. "Do not try this at home."

I bowed to him and the audience. He raised a rattan stick, twirled it once, and suddenly tossed it at me. I responded instantly, whipping the blades through the air, cutting it into three parts. The audience gasped, sitting straighter in their chairs, and I smiled.

Yes, these are real swords.

Guro nodded and stepped away. I half closed my eyes and brought my swords into position, one held vertically over one shoulder, the other tucked against my ribs. Balanced on the balls of my feet, I let my mind drift, forgetting the audience and the onlookers and my fellow students watching along the wall. I breathed out slowly and let my mind go blank.

Music began, drumming a rhythm over the loudspeakers, and I started to move.

I started slowly at first, both weapons whirling around me, sliding from one motion to the next. *Don't think about what you're doing, just move, flow.* I danced around the floor, throwing a few flips and kicks into the pattern because I could, keeping time with the music. As the drums picked up, pounding out a frantic rhythm, I moved faster, faster, whipping the blades around my body, until I could feel the wind from their passing, hear the vicious hum as they sliced through the air around me.

Someone whooped out in the audience, but I barely heard them. The people watching didn't matter; nothing mattered except the blades in my hands and the flowing motion of the dance. The swords flashed silver in the dim light, fluid and flexible, almost liquid. There was no block or strike, dodge or parry—the dance was all of these things, and none, all at once. I pushed myself harder than I ever had before, until I couldn't tell where the swords ended and my arms began, until I was just a weapon in the center of the floor, and no one could touch me.

With a final flourish, I spun around, ending the demonstration on one knee, the blades back in their ready position. For a heartbeat after I finished, there was absolute silence. Then, like a dam breaking, a roar of applause swept over me, laced with whistles and scraping chairs as people surged to their feet. I rose and bowed to the audience, then to my master, who gave me a proud nod. He understood. This wasn't just a demonstration for me; it was something I'd worked for, trained for, and finally pulled off—without getting into trouble or hurting anyone in the process. I had actually done something right for a change.

I looked up and met Kenzie's eyes on the other side of the mats. She was grinning and clapping frantically, her notebook lying on the floor beside her, and I smiled back.

"That was awesome," she said, weaving around the edge of the mat when I stepped off the floor, breathing hard. "I had no idea you could do...that. Congratulations, you're a certified badass."

I felt a warm glow of...something, deep inside. "Thanks," I muttered, carefully sliding the blades back into their sheaths before laying them gently atop Guro's bag. It was hard to give them up; I wanted to keep holding them, feeling their perfect weight as they danced through the air. I'd seen Guro practice with his own blades, and he looked so natural with them, as if they were extensions of his arms. I wondered if I'd looked the same out there on the mat, the shining edges coming so close to my body but never touching it. I wondered if Guro would ever let me train with them again.

Our instructor had called the last student to demonstrate knife techniques with him, and he had the audience's full attention now. Meanwhile, I caught several appreciative gazes directed at Kenzie from my fellow kali students, and felt myself bristle.

"Come on," I told her, stepping away from the others before Chris could jump in and introduce himself. "I need a soda. Want one?"

She nodded eagerly. Together, we slipped through the crowds, out the doors, and into the hallway, leaving the noise and commotion behind.

I fed two dollars into the vending machine at the end of the hall, choosing a Pepsi for myself, then a Mountain Dew at Kenzie's request. She smiled her thanks as I tossed it to her, and we leaned against the corridor wall, basking in the silence.

"So," Kenzie ventured after several heartbeats. She gave me a sideways look. "Care to answer a few questions now?"

I knocked the back of my head against the wall. "Sure," I muttered, closing my eyes. The girl wouldn't let me be until we got this thing over with. "Let's have at it. Though I promise, you're going to be disappointed by how dull my life really is."

"I somehow doubt that." Kenzie's voice had changed. It was uncertain, now, almost nervous. I frowned, listening to the flipping of notebook paper, then a quiet breath, as if she was steeling herself for something. "First question, then. How long have you been taking kali?"

"Since I was twelve," I said without moving. "That's...

what…nearly five years now." Jeez, had it really been that long? I remembered my first class as a shy, quiet kid, holding the rattan stick like it was a poisonous snake, and Guro's piercing eyes, appraising me.

"Okay. Cool. Second question." Kenzie hesitated, then said in a calm, clear voice, "What, exactly, is your take on faeries?"

My eyes flew open, and I jerked my head up, banging it against the wall again. My half-empty soda can dropped from my fingers and clanked to the floor, fizzing everywhere. Kenzie blinked and stepped back as I gaped at her, hardly believing what I'd just heard. *"What?"* I choked out, before I thought better of it, before the defensive walls came slamming down.

"You heard me." Kenzie regarded me intently, watching my reaction. "Faeries. What do you know about them? What's your interest in the fey?"

My mind spun. Faeries. Fey. She knew. How she knew, I had no idea. But she couldn't continue this line of questioning. This had to end, now. Todd was already in trouble because of Them. He might really be gone. The last thing I wanted was for Mackenzie St. James to vanish off the face of the earth because of me. And if I had to be nasty and cruel, so be it. It was better than the alternative.

Drawing myself up, I sneered at her, my voice suddenly ugly, hateful. "Wow, whatever you smoked last night, it must've been good." I curled my lip in a smirk. "Are you even listening to yourself? What kind of screwed-up question is that?"

Kenzie's eyes hardened. Flipping several pages, she held the notebook out to me, where the words *glamour*, *Unseelie* and *Seelie Courts* were underlined in red. I remembered her standing behind the bleachers when I faced that creepy transparent faery. My stomach went cold.

"I'm a reporter," Kenzie said, as I tried wrapping my brain around this. "I heard you talking to someone the day Todd disappeared. It wasn't hard to find the information." She flipped the notebook shut and stared me down, defiant. "Changelings, Fair Folk, All-Hallow's Eve, Summer and Winter courts, the Good Neighbors. I learned a lot. And when I called Todd's house this afternoon, he still wasn't there." She pushed her hair back and gave me a worried look. "What's going on, Ethan? Are you and Todd in some sort of pagan cult? You don't actually *believe* in faeries, do you?"

I forced myself to stay calm. At least Kenzie was reacting like a normal person should, with disbelief and concern. Of course she didn't believe in faeries. Maybe I could scare her away from me for good. "Yes," I smirked, crossing my arms. "That's exactly right. I'm in a cult, and we sacrifice goats under the full moon and drink the blood of virgins and babies every month." She wrinkled her nose, and I took a threatening step forward. "It's a lot of fun, especially when we bring out the crack and Ouija boards. Wanna join?"

"Very funny, tough guy." I'd forgotten Kenzie didn't scare easily. She glared back, stubborn and unmovable as a wall. "What's really going on? Are you in some kind of trouble?"

"What if I am?" I challenged. "What are you going to do about it? You think you can save me? You think you can publish one of your little stories and everything will be fine? Wake up, Miss Nosy Reporter. The world's not like that."

"Quit being a jerkoff, Ethan," Kenzie snapped, narrowing her eyes. "You're not really like this, and you're not as bad as you think you are. I'm only trying to help."

"No one can help me." Suddenly, I was tired. I was tired of fighting, tired of forcing myself to be someone I wasn't. I didn't want to hurt her, but if she continued down this path, she would only rush headlong into a world that would do its best to tear her apart. And I couldn't let that happen. Not again.

"Look." I sighed, slumping against the wall. "I can't explain it. Just…leave me alone, okay? Please. You have no idea what you're getting into."

"Ethan—"

"Stop asking questions," I whispered, drawing away. Her eyes followed me, confused and sad, and I hardened my voice. "Stop asking questions, and stay the hell away from me. Or you're only going to get hurt."

"Advice you should have followed yourself, Ethan Chase," a voice hissed out of the darkness.

TOKEN TO THE NEVERNEVER

They were here.

The creepy, transparent fey, floating a few inches off the tile floors, drifting toward us down the hall. Only now there were a whole lot of them, filling the corridor, their bony fingers and shattered wings making soft clicking sounds as they eased closer.

"We told you," one whispered, regarding me with shiny black eyes, "we told you to forget, to not ask questions, to not interfere. You were warned, and you chose to ignore us. Now, you and your friend will disappear. No one will endanger our lady's return, not even the mortal kin of the Iron Queen."

"Ethan?" Kenzie gave me a worried look, but I couldn't tear my eyes away from the ghostly faeries, creeping toward us. She glanced back down the hall, then turned to stare at me again. "What are you looking at? You're starting to freak me out."

Backing away, I grabbed Kenzie's wrist, ignoring her startled yelp, and fled back into the main room.

"Hey!" She tried to yank free as I bashed through the doors, nearly knocking down three students in white gis. "Ow! What the hell are you doing? Let go!"

We were starting to attract attention, despite the noise of battle and sparring, and several parents turned to give me the evil eye. I pulled Kenzie into the corner where I'd left my bag and released her, watching the door we'd just come through. She glared at me, rubbing her wrist. "Next time, a little warning would be nice." When I didn't answer, she frowned and dropped her wrist. "Are you okay? You look like you're about to hurl. What's going on?"

The creepy fey drifted through the door frame, rising over the crowd like skeletal wraiths, black eyes scanning the floor. No one saw them, of course. They flickered, fading from sight for just a second before, as one, their faceted black eyes locked onto me.

I whispered a curse. "Kenzie," I muttered, as the fey started to float toward us. "We have to get out of here. Will you trust me, just this once, without asking any questions?" She opened her mouth to protest, and I whirled on her frantically. "Please!"

Her jaw snapped shut. Whether it was from the look on my face or something else, she nodded. "Lead the way."

Shouldering my bag, I fled along the wall with Kenzie right behind me, weaving through students and watching parents, until we reached the back of the dojo. The fire door stood slightly ajar, propped open to let in the cool autumn air, and I lunged toward it.

Just as I hit the metal bar, pushing it open, something struck my arm, sending a flaring pain up my shoulder. I stifled a yell and staggered down the steps, dragging Kenzie with me, seeing the hatchet-face of the faery glaring at me from behind the door.

"Ethan," Kenzie gasped as I pulled her across the back lot. It had rained again, and the pavement smelled like wet asphalt. Puddles glimmered under the streetlamps, pooling in cracks and potholes, and we splashed our way through the black, oily water.

"Ethan!" Kenzie called again. She sounded frantic, but all

my thoughts were on getting to my truck around front. "Oh, my God! Wait a second. Look at your arm!"

I looked back, and my skin crawled. Where the faery had hit me, the entire sleeve of my shirt was soaked with red. I pushed back the sleeve, revealing three long, vivid slashes across my triceps. Blood was starting to trickle down my arm.

"What the hell?" Kenzie gasped, as the pain suddenly hit like a hot knife peeling back my skin. I gritted my teeth and clamped a hand over the wound. "Something tore the crap out of your arm. You need to go to the hospital. Here." She reached for me, putting a gentle hand on my uninjured shoulder. "Give me your bag."

"No," I rasped, backing away. They were coming down the stairs now, pointed stick legs skipping over the puddles. One of them stared at me and raised a thin, bloody claw to his mouth slit, licking the blood with a pale, wormlike tongue.

The sound of movement rippled behind us, and I turned to see more of them floating around the corner of the building, spreading out and trapping us between them.

My stomach felt tight. Is this what had happened to Todd, surrounded on all sides by creepy transparent fey, torn apart with long needle fingers?

I shivered, trying to be calm. My rattan sticks were in my bag, feeble weapons against so many, but I had to do something.

For just a moment, I caught a reflection of myself in the puddle at my feet, grim-faced and hollow-eyed. There was a dark smear on my cheek, my own blood, from where I'd rubbed my face after touching the wound....

Wait. Blood. Standing water.

The fey drifted closer. I stuck my hand into my pocket, and my bloody fingers closed around the silver coin. Pulling it out, I faced Kenzie, who was giving me that worried, bewildered stare, still insisting we go to a doctor.

"Kenzie," I said, taking her hand as the clicking around us grew very loud in my ears, "do you believe in faeries?"

"What?" She blinked at me, looking confused and almost angry that I'd brought up something so ridiculous. "Do I… no! Of course not, that's crazy."

I closed my eyes. "Then, I'm sorry," I whispered. "I didn't want to do this. But try not to freak out when we get there."

"Get…where?"

The circle of fey hissed and flowed toward us, claws reaching out, mouths gaping. Praying this would work, I squeezed Kenzie's hand in a death grip and flung the token into the puddle at my feet.

A flash of blinding white, a ripple of energy with no sound. I felt my stomach pulled inside out, the ground spinning under my feet, and held my breath. The mad hisses and clicking of the transparent fey cut out, and suddenly I was falling.

I hit the ground on my stomach, biting my lip as the gym bag landed on my shoulder and sent a flare of pain up my arm. Beside me, I heard Kenzie's breathless yelp as she thumped to the dirt and lay there, gasping.

"What…what in the hell?" she panted, and I heard her struggle to get up. "What just happened? Where are we?"

"Well, well," answered a cool, amused voice from somewhere above us. "And here you are again. Ethan Chase, your family does have a knack for getting into trouble."

PART II

CHAPTER TEN
CAVE OF THE CAIT SITH

I jerked upright, pushing off the bag. The motion sent a blaze of agony across my back and shoulder. Clenching my jaw, I struggled to my feet and searched for the source of the elusive voice. We were in some sort of a cave with a sandy bottom and a small pool near the back. Along the walls, enormous spotted toadstools glowed with eerie luminance. Tiny glowing balls, like blue and green fireflies, drifted over the pool, throwing rippling splashes of light over the cavern, but I couldn't see anyone besides Kenzie and myself.

"Who's there?" Kenzie demanded, in a far more steady voice than I'd expect. "Where are you? Show yourself."

"As usual, you mortals have not the slightest ability to see what is right in front of your faces," continued the voice in a bored tone, and I thought I heard a yawn. "Very well, humans. Up here, if you would."

There was a shimmer of movement along the far wall. I followed it up to a rocky shelf about fifteen feet off the ground. For a moment, the shelf appeared empty. Then, two glowing yellow eyes blinked into existence, and a second later a large gray cat sat there with its tail curled around itself, peering down on us haughtily.

"There." It sighed, sounding exceptionally weary, as if it had held this entire conversation before. "See me now?"

A memory flickered to life—the image of a metal tower, crumbling all around us, and a furry gray cat leading us to safety. A name hovered at the edge of my mind, eluding me for the moment, but the image of the golden-eyed cat was clear. Of course, it hadn't changed a bit.

Kenzie took two staggering steps backward, staring at the feline as if in a daze. "O-kay," she breathed, shaking her head slightly. "A cat. A cat that talks. I'm going crazy." She glanced at me. "Or you slipped something into my drink at the tournament. One or the other."

"How predictable." The cat sighed again and stuck its hind leg into the air to lick its toes. "I believe there is nothing wrong with your eyes or ears, human. My previous statement still stands."

I glared at it. "Lay off, cat," I said. "She's never seen one of you before, let alone been *here*." My arm throbbed, and I sank onto a nearby rock. "Dammit, I don't why *I'm* here. Why am I here? I was hoping I'd never see this place again."

"Please," the cat said in that annoyingly superior voice, eyeing me over its leg. "Why are you even surprised, human? Your last name is Chase, after all. I was expecting your arrival any day now." It sniffed and glanced at Kenzie, who was still staring at it openmouthed. "Minus the girl, of course. But I am sure we can work around that. First things first, however." The golden eyes shifted to me. "You are dripping blood everywhere, human. Perhaps you should try to put a stop to that. We would not want to attract anything nasty, would we?"

I exhaled, hard. Well, here I was, in the Nevernever. Nothing to be done now but try to get out as quickly as I could. Pulling my bag toward me, I tugged it open and rifled through it one-handed, biting my lip as pain continued to claw at my shoulder. Blood still oozed sluggishly down my arm, and the left side of my shirt was spattered with red.

"Here." Kenzie suddenly knelt across from me, stopping

my hand. "Don't hurt yourself. Let me do it." Taking off her camera, she started going through the bag. "You have gauze in here somewhere, right?"

"I can get it," I said quickly, not wanting her to see my old clothes and smelly belongings. I reached forward, but she gave me such a fierce glare that I sat back with a grimace, leaving her to it. Setting her jaw, she rummaged around, pushing aside rattan sticks and old T-shirts, pulling out a rag and the roll of gauze I kept for sports-related injuries. Her lips were pressed in a thin line, her eyes hard and determined, as if she was going to take care of this little problem before she faced anything else. For a second, I felt a weird flicker of pride. She was taking things remarkably well.

"Take off your shirt."

I blinked, feeling my face heat. "Uh. What?"

"Shirt, tough guy." She gestured to my blood-spattered T-shirt. "I don't think you're going to want it after this, anyway. Off."

Her words were almost too flippant, like someone forcing a smile after a horrible tragedy. I hesitated, more out of concern than embarrassment—though there was that, too. "You sure you're okay with this?"

"Oh, do as she says, human." The cat thumped its tail. "Otherwise we will be here all night."

Gingerly, I eased off my shirt and tossed the bloodied rag aside. Kenzie soaked the cloth in the pool, wrung it out, and crouched behind me in the sand. For a moment, she hesitated, and I tensed, suddenly feeling highly exposed—half-naked and bleeding in front of a strange girl and a talking cat. Then her fingers brushed my skin, cool and soft, and my stomach turned into a pretzel.

"God, Ethan." She laid one palm gently against my shoulder, leaning in to examine the tears down my arm. I closed my eyes, forcing myself to relax. "These are nasty. What the hell was after you, demon cougars?"

I sucked in a ragged breath. "You wouldn't believe me if I told you."

"Oh, I'm willing to believe just about anything right now." She pressed the cloth to the jagged claw marks, and I set my jaw. We were both silent as she dabbed blood off my shoulder and wrapped the gauze around my arm. I could sense Kenzie was still a little dazed from the whole situation. But her fingers were gentle and sure, and I shivered each time they touched my skin, leaving goose bumps behind.

"There," she said, dusting off her knees as she stood. "That should do it. Those first aid sessions in Ms. Peters's class didn't go to waste, at least."

"Thanks," I muttered. She gave me a shaky smile.

"No problem." She watched as I reached into my bag and pulled out another T-shirt, shrugging into it with a grimace. "Now, before I start screaming, will someone—you or the talking cat or a freaking flying goat, I don't care—please tell me what the hell is going on?"

"Why are mortals so boring?" the cat asked, landing on the sandy floor without a sound. Padding toward us, it leaped atop a flat rock and observed us both critically, waving its tail, before its gaze settled on the girl. "Very well, I will be the voice of reason and sanity once again. Listen closely, human, for I will explain this only once." It sat down with a sniff, curling its tail around its feet. "You are in the Nevernever, the home of the fey. Or, as you mortals insist upon calling them, faeries. Yes, faeries are real," it added in its bored tone, as Kenzie took a breath to speak. "No, mortals cannot normally see them in the real world. Please save all unnecessary questions until I am finished.

"You are here," it continued, giving me a sideways look, "because Ethan Chase apparently cannot stay out of trouble with the fey and has used a token to bring you both into the Nevernever. More important, into my home—one of them, anyway. Which begs the question…" The cat blinked and looked at me now, narrowing its eyes. "Why *are* you here, human? The token was to be used only in the most dire circumstances. By your wounds, I would guess something was chasing you, but why drag the girl into this, as well?"

"I didn't have a choice," I said, avoiding Kenzie's eyes. "They were after her, too."

"They?" asked Kenzie.

I scrubbed my good hand over my face. "There's something out there," I told the cat. "Something different, some type of fey I've never seen before. They're killing off exiles and half-breeds, and they've taken a friend of mine, a half-phouka named Todd Wyndham. When I tried to find out more…"

"They came to silence you," the cat finished solemnly.

"Yeah. Right in the open. In front of a couple hundred people." I felt Kenzie's gaze on me and ignored her. "So," I asked the cat, "do you know what's going on?"

The cat twitched an ear. "Perhaps," it mused, managing to look bored and thoughtful all at once. "There have been strange rumors circling the wyldwood. They have me curious." It yawned and casually licked a foot. "I believe it is time to pay a visit to the Iron Queen."

I stood up. "No," I said a little too forcefully, though the cat didn't even look up from its paw. "I can't go to Meghan. I have to get home! I have to find Todd and see if my family is all right. They're gonna freak out if I don't come back soon." I remembered what Meghan said about time in the Nevernever, and groaned. "God, they're probably freaking out right now."

"The Iron Queen needs to be informed that you are here," the cat said, calmly rubbing the paw over his whiskers. "That was the favor—should you ever use that token, I would bring you to her. Besides, I believe she will be most interested in what is happening in the mortal world, and this new type of fey. I think one of the courts needs to know about this, do you not agree?"

"Can't you at least take Kenzie home?"

"That was not the bargain, human." The cat finally looked at me, unblinking. "And, were I you, I would think long and hard about sending her back alone. If these creatures are still out there, they could be waiting for you both to return."

A chill ran down my back. I glanced at Kenzie and found her looking completely lost as she stared from me to the cat and back again. "I have no idea what's going on here," she said matter-of-factly, though her eyes were a bit glazed. "I just hope that when I wake up, I'm not in a padded room with a nice man in a white suit feeding me pills."

I sighed, feeling my life unravel even more. *I'm sorry, Kenzie,* I thought, as she hugged herself and stared straight ahead. *I didn't want to drag you into this, and this is the very last place I want to be. But the cat's right; I can't send you back alone, not with those things out there. They already got Todd; I won't let them have you, too.*

"All right," I snapped, glaring at the feline. "Let's go see Meghan and get this over with. But I'm not staying. I have to get home. I have a friend who's in trouble, and I have to find him. Not even Meghan can help me with that."

The cat sneezed several times, curling his whiskers in mirth. I didn't see what was so funny. "This should be most amusing," it said, hopping down from the rock. "I suggest you remain here for the night," it continued as he padded away over the sand. "Nothing will harm you in this place, and I am in no mood to lead wounded humans around the wyldwood in the dark. We will start out for the Iron Realm in the morning."

"How long will it take to get there?" I asked, but there was no answer. Frowning, I glanced around the cave. The cat was gone.

Oh, yeah, I thought, remembering something then, from long ago. *Grimalkin. He does that.*

Kenzie still seemed unnaturally quiet as I sat down and started fishing in my bag, taking stock of what I had. Rattan sticks, extra clothes, bottled water, a smashed box of energy bars, a container of aspirin and a couple of small, secret items I kept handy for pests of the invisible variety. I wondered if my little charms would work in the Nevernever, the fey's home territory. I would find out soon enough.

I shook four painkillers into my palm and tossed them back, swallowing them with a grimace, then sliding the bottle into my pocket. My shoulder still ached, but against all odds, it seemed to be nothing more than a flesh wound. I just hoped the strange, creepy fey didn't have venomous claws.

"Here," I muttered, pulling out a slightly crushed energy bar, offering it to the girl sitting across from me. She blinked and stared at it blankly. "We should probably eat something. You don't want to take anything anyone offers you here. No food, drinks, gifts, anything, got it? Oh, and never agree to do someone a favor, or make any kind of deal or say 'thank you.'" She continued to watch me without expression, and I frowned. "Hey, are you listening to me? This is important."

Great, she's gone into shock. What am I supposed to do now? I stared at her, wishing I had never pulled her into this, wishing we could both just go home. I was worried for my parents; what would they say when they found out yet another child of theirs had disappeared from the face of the earth? *I'm not Meghan,* I promised, not knowing if it was to Mom, to Kenzie or myself. *I'll get us home, I swear I will.*

The girl still wasn't responding, and waggling the energy bar at her was getting me nowhere. I sighed. "Kenzie," I said, firmer this time, leaning forward over the bag. "Mackenzie. Hey!"

She jumped when I got right up in her face and grabbed her arm, jerking back with a startled look. I let her go, and she blinked rapidly, as if coming out of a trance.

"You all right?" I asked, sitting back, watching her cautiously. She stared at me for an uncomfortable moment, then took a deep breath.

"Yeah," she finally whispered, making me sag in relief. "Yeah, I'm good. I'm fine. I think." She gazed around the cave, as if making sure it was still there. "The Nevernever," she murmured, almost to herself. "I'm in the Nevernever. I'm in freaking Faeryland."

I watched her carefully, wondering what I would do if she started to scream. But then, sitting there on the log in the middle of the Nevernever, Kenzie did something completely unexpected.

She smiled.

It wasn't big or obvious. Just a faint, secret grin, a flicker of excitement crossing her face, as if this was something she'd been waiting for her whole life, only she hadn't known it. It raised the hairs on the back of my neck. Normal human beings did not react well to being dropped into an imaginary place with creatures that existed only in fairy tales. I was expecting fear, anger, rationalization. Kenzie's eyes nearly glowed with anticipation.

It made me very nervous.

"So," she said brightly, turning back to me, "tell me about this place."

I gave her a wary look. "You do realize we're in the *Nevernever,* home of *the fey*. Faeries? Wee folk? Leprechauns and pixies and Tinkerbell?" I held out the food bar again, watching her reaction. "Isn't this your cue to start explaining how faeries don't exist?"

"Well, I'm a reporter," Kenzie said, accepting the food package and fiddling with a corner. "I have to face facts. And it occurs to me that one of two things is happening right now. One, you slipped something into my drink at the dojo, and I'm having a really whacked-out dream. And if that's the case, I'll wake up soon and you'll go to jail and we'll never see each other again."

I winced.

"Or two…" She took a deep breath and gazed around the cavern. "This…is really happening. It's kind of silly to tell the talking cat he doesn't exist when he's sitting right there arguing with you."

I kept quiet, chewing on granola. You couldn't fault her reasoning, though she was still far more pragmatic and logical than I'd expected. Still, something about her reaction didn't feel right. Maybe it was her complete lack of fear and skepticism, as if she desperately wanted to believe that this was really happening. As if she didn't care at all about leaving what was real and sane and normal behind.

"Anyway," Kenzie went on, looking back at me, "you've been here before, right? From the way that cat was talking to you, it was like you knew each other."

I shrugged. "Yeah," I said, staring at the ground between my knees. Memories—the bad memories I tried so hard to forget—crowded in. Fangs and claws, poking at me. Glowing eyes and shrieking, high-pitched laughter. Lying in utter darkness, the stench of rust and iron clogging my nose, waiting for my sister to come. "But it was a long time ago," I muttered, shoving those thoughts away, locking them in the farthest corner of my mind. "I barely remember it."

"How long have you been able to see…um…faeries?"

I flicked a glance at her. She sat with her knees drawn to her chest, leaning against a rock, watching me gravely. The fluorescent toadstools on the walls gave off a black light effect, making the blue in her hair glow neon bright. I caught myself staring and looked down at the floor again.

"All my life." I hunched a little more. "I can't remember a time when I couldn't see them, when I didn't know they were there."

"Can your parents—?"

"No." It came out a bit sharper than I'd intended. "No one in my family can see them. Just me."

Except my sister, of course. But I didn't want to talk about her.

"Hmm." Kenzie rested her chin on her knees. "Well, this explains a lot about you. The secrecy, the paranoia, the weirdness at the tournament." My face heated, but Kenzie didn't seem to notice. "So how many…faeries…are out there in the real world?"

"Sure you want to know?" I challenged, smiling bitterly. "You might end up like me, mean and paranoid, staring at corners and out windows for things that aren't there. There's a reason no one ever talks about the fey, and not just because it draws their attention. Because normal people, the ones who can't see Them, will label you *weird* or *crazy* or *freak,* and will either treat you like you have the plague or will want to throw you in a cell."

"I never thought of you like that," Kenzie said softly.

Anger burned suddenly. At myself, for dragging her into this. At Kenzie, for being too damn stubborn to leave me alone, for refusing to stay away and not hate me like any normal, sane person would. And at myself, again, for allowing her to get this close, for wanting to be near someone. I had let down my guard the tiniest bit, and now look where we were.

"Well, maybe you should have," I said, standing and glaring down at her. "Because now you're stuck here with me. And I really don't know if we're going to make it out of here alive."

"Where are you going?" Kenzie asked as I stalked away toward the mouth of the cave. Ignoring her, hoping she wouldn't come after me, I walked to the entrance, just a foot or so from the edge of the cave, so I could see Faery for myself.

Peering into the darkness, I shivered. The wyldwood stretched away before me, tangled and ominous in the shadows. I couldn't see the sky through the canopy of leaves and branches, but I could see glimmers of movement far, far above, lights or creatures floating through the trees.

"Going somewhere?" came a voice above my head. Grimalkin sat in a tangle of roots that curled lazily from the ceiling. His huge eyes seemed to hover in the darkness.

"No," I muttered, giving him a cautious look. Grimalkin had helped my sister in the past, but I didn't know him well, and he was still fey. Faeries never did anything for free; his agreeing to guide us through the wyldwood into the Iron Realm was just part of a deal.

"Good. I would hate to have you eaten before we even started," he purred, raking his claws across the wood. "You appear to have the same recklessness as your sister, always rushing into things without thinking them through."

"Don't compare me to Meghan," I said, narrowing my eyes. "I'm not like her."

"Indeed. She, at least, had a pleasant personality."

"I'm not here to make friends." The cat was bugging the hell out of me, but I refused to let it show. "This isn't a reunion. I just want to get to the Iron Realm, talk to Meghan and go home." *Todd is still out there, counting on me.*

The cat stretched lazily on the branch. "Desire what you will, human," he said with a knowing, half-lidded stare. "With your family, I have found that it is never as easy as that."

INTO THE WYLDWOOD

I didn't think I'd sleep, but I must've dozed off, because the next thing I knew, I was waking up on the sandy floor of the cave, and my shoulder was killing me. Pulling out the aspirin, I popped another three pills, crunched them down with a grimace and looked around for Kenzie and Grimalkin.

Unsurprisingly, the cat was nowhere to be seen, but a faint gray light was seeping in from the cave mouth, and the glowing fungi along the walls had dimmed, looking like ordinary toadstools now. I wondered how much time had passed, if a year had already flown by in the mortal world and my parents had given up all hope of ever seeing me again.

Grimacing, I struggled upright, cursing myself for falling asleep. Anything could've happened while I'd been out: something could've snuck up on me, stolen my bag, convinced Kenzie to follow it down a dark tunnel. Where was she, anyway? She didn't know about Faery, how dangerous it could be. She was far too trusting, and anything in this world could grab her, chew her up and spit her out again.

I spun, searching frantically, until I saw her sitting cross-legged near the entrance.

Talking to Grimalkin.

Oh, great. I hurried over, hoping she hadn't promised the cat anything she would regret, or we would regret, later. "Kenzie," I said as I swept up. "What are you doing? What are you two talking about?"

She glanced up at me, smiling, and Grimalkin yawned widely as he bent to lick his paws. "Oh, you're up," she said. "Grimalkin was just telling me a little about the Nevernever. It's fascinating. Did you know there's a whole huge city on the ocean floor that stretches for miles? Or that the River of Dreams supposedly runs to the End of the World before falling off the edge?"

"I don't want to know," I said. "I don't want to be here any longer than we have to, so don't think we're staying for the tour. I just want to go to the Iron Realm, talk to Meghan, and go home. How's that part coming along, cat?"

Grimalkin sniffed. "Your friend is far better company than you," he stated, and scrubbed the paw over his head. "And if you are so eager to get to the Iron Realm, we will leave whenever you are ready. However—" he peeked up at me, twitching his tail "—be absolutely sure you have everything you need, human. We will not be coming back to this place should you leave something behind."

I walked back to my gym bag, wondering what to leave. I couldn't take the whole bag, that was obvious. It was bulky and heavy, and I wasn't going to tote it across the Nevernever if I didn't have to. Besides, my arm still hurt like hell, so I wouldn't be carrying anything much larger than a stick.

I pulled out my rattan, the gauze, two bottles of water, and the last three power bars, then rifled around the side pocket for one more thing. Kenzie wandered over and knelt on the other side, watching curiously.

"What are you looking for?"

"This," I muttered, and pulled out a large, slightly rusted key, something I'd found half buried in the swamp when I was a kid. It was ancient, bulky and made of pure iron. I'd kept it as a lucky charm and a faery deterrent ever since.

"Here," I said, holding it out to her. It dangled from an old string, spinning lazily between us. I'd meant to get a chain for it but kept putting it off. "Keep this close," I told her as she stared at it curiously. "Iron is the best protection you can have against the creatures that live here. It's poison to them—they can't even touch it without being burned. It won't keep them away completely, but they might think twice about biting your head off if they smell that around your neck."

She wrinkled her nose, whether from the thought of having to wear a rusty old key or having her head bitten off, I didn't know. "What about you?" she asked.

I reached into my shirt and pulled out the iron cross on the chain. "Already have one. Here." I jiggled the key at her. "Take it."

She reached out, and my fingers brushed hers as they closed around the amulet, sending a rush of warmth up my arm. I jerked and nearly dropped the key, but she didn't pull back, her touch lingering on mine, watching me over our clasped hands.

"I'm sorry, Ethan."

I blinked and quickly pulled my hand back, frowning in confusion. My heart was pounding again, but I ignored it. "Why?"

"For not believing you at the tournament." She looped the heavy key around her neck, where it clinked softly against the camera. "I thought you might be into something dangerous and illegal, and had gotten Todd into trouble because of it. And that the faery thing was a cover for something else. I never thought they could be real." Her solemn gaze met mine over the gym bag. "They were at the tournament, weren't they?" she asked. "The faeries that grabbed Todd. That's what was chasing us, and you were trying to get us out." Her gaze flicked to my bandaged arm, and her brow furrowed. "I'm sorry for that, too."

I started to reply, but Kenzie rose and briskly dusted herself off, as if not wanting an answer. "Come on," she said in an overly cheerful voice. "We should get going. Grim is giving us the evil eye."

She started to walk away but paused very briefly, her fingers touching my shoulder as she passed. "Also...thanks for saving my life."

I sat there a moment, listening to Kenzie's footsteps pad quietly over the sand. What just happened here? Kenzie had nothing to apologize for. It wasn't her fault we were here, stuck in the Nevernever for who knew how long, that a bunch of ghostly, homicidal faeries were after us. Her life had been fairly normal before I came along. If anything, she should hate me for dragging her into this mess. I certainly hated myself.

My shoulder still prickled where she'd touched it.

An extremely loud yawn came from the mouth of the cave. "Are we going to start this expedition sometime in the next century?" Grimalkin called, golden eyes blinking in annoyance. "For someone who is in such a hurry to leave, you certainly are taking your time."

I rose, snatched my rattan sticks and water from the floor, and walked toward the cave entrance, leaving the bag behind. It, along with my dirty clothes and equipment, would have to stay in Faery. Hopefully it wouldn't stink up Grimalkin's home *too* badly.

"Finally." The cat sighed as I came up. He stood, tail waving, and sauntered to the mouth of the cave, looking out at the wyldwood beyond. "Ready, humans?"

"Hey, Grimalkin." Kenzie suddenly brought up her camera. "Smile."

The cat snorted. "That silly toy will not work here, mortal," he said as Kenzie pressed the button and discovered just that. Nothing happened. Frowning, she pulled back to look at it, and Grimalkin sniffed.

"Human technology has no place in the Nevernever," he stated. "Why do you think there are no pictures of dragons and goblins floating about the mortal world? The fey do not photograph well. We do not photograph at all. Magic and technology cannot exist together, except perhaps in the Iron Realm. And even there, your purely human technology will not work as you expect. The Iron Realm, for all its advancement, is still a part of the Nevernever."

"Well, shoot." Kenzie sighed and let the camera drop. "I was hoping to write a book called *My Trip to Faeryland*." Now how am I going to convince myself that I'm not completely loony?"

Grimalkin sneezed with laughter and turned away. "I would not worry about that, mortal. No one ever leaves the Nevernever completely sane."

The cave entrance vanished as soon as we stepped through, changing to a solid wall of stone when we looked back. Kenzie jumped, then reached out to prod the rock, a look of amazement and disbelief crossing her face.

"Better get used to things like that," I told her as she turned forward again, looking a bit stunned. "Nothing ever makes sense around here."

"I'm starting to see that," she murmured as we made our way down the rocky slope after Grimalkin. The cat trotted briskly ahead, neither slowing down nor glancing back to see if we were still there, and we had to scramble to keep up. I wondered if Meghan had had this same problem when she first came to the Nevernever.

Meghan. Flutters of both nerves and excitement hit my stomach, and I firmly shoved them down. I was going to see my sister, the queen of the Iron Fey. Would she remember me? Would she be angry that I'd come here, after she'd told me not to look for her? Maybe she didn't want to see me at all. Maybe she was glad to be rid of her human ties.

That thought sent a chill through me. Would she even be the same Meghan I remembered? I had so many memories of her, and she was always the same: the steady older sister who looked out for me. When we got to the Iron Realm, would I find the Iron Queen was insane and cruel like Mab, or fickle and jealous like Titania? I hadn't met the fey queens, of course, but the stories I'd heard about them told me everything I needed to know. Which was to stay far, far away from them both.

"How old were you when you first came here?"

Kenzie voiced the question just as Grimalkin vanished into the dark gray undergrowth. Alarmed, I stared hard between the trees until I spotted him again and hurried to catch up. Except he did the same damn thing a minute later, and I growled a curse, scanning the bushes. Catching sight of a bushy tail, I hurried forward, Kenzie trailing doggedly beside me. I kept silent, hoping Kenzie would forget the question. No such luck.

"Ethan? Did you hear me? How old were you the last time you came to this place?"

"I don't want to talk about it," I said curtly, dodging a bush with vivid blue thorns. Kenzie stepped deftly around it, keeping pace with me.

"Why?"

"Because." I searched for the cat, ignoring her gaze, and tried to hold on to my temper. "It's none of your business."

"News flash, Ethan—I'm stuck in Faeryland, same as you. I think that makes it my business—"

"I was four!" I snapped, turning to glare at her. Kenzie blinked. "The fey took me from my home when I was four and used me as *bait* so my sister would come rescue me. They stuck me in a cage and poked at me until I screamed, and when she finally did come, they took her away and turned her into one of Them. I have to pretend I don't have a sister, that I don't see anything weird or strange or unnatural, that my parents aren't terrified to let me do anything because they're scared the fey will steal me again! So, excuse me for not wanting to talk about myself or my screwed-up life. It's kind of a sore subject, okay?"

"Oh, Ethan." Kenzie's gaze was horrified and sympathetic, which was not what I was expecting. "I'm so sorry."

"Forget it." Embarrassed, I turned away, waving it off. "It's just…I've never told anyone before, not even my parents. And being back here—" I gestured to the trees around us "—it's making me remember everything I hated about this place, about Them. I swore I'd never come back. But, here I am and…" Exhaling, I kicked a rock into the undergrowth, making it rattle noisily. "And I managed to pull you in, as well."

Just like Samantha.

"Humans." Grimalkin appeared overhead, in the branches of a tree. "You are making too much noise, and this is not a safe place to do so. Unless you wish to attract the attention of every hungry creature in the area, I suggest attempting to continue on in silence." He sniffed and regarded us without hope. "Give it your best shot at least, hmm?"

We walked for the rest of the afternoon. At least, I thought we did. It was hard to tell time in the endless gray twilight of the wyldwood. My watch had, of course, stopped, and our phones were dead, so we trailed Grimalkin as best we could for several hours as the eerie, dangerous land of the fey loomed all around us. Shadows moved among the trees, keeping just out of sight. Branches creaked, and footsteps shuffled through

the leaves, though I never saw anything. Sometimes I thought
I heard voices on the wind, singing or whispering my name.

The colors of the wyldwood were weird and unnatural;
everything was gray and murky, but then we'd pass a single
tree that was a vivid, poisonous green, or a bush with huge
purple berries hanging from the branches. Except for a few
curious piskies and one hopeful will-o'-the-wisp, I didn't see
any faeries, which made me relieved and nervous at the same
time. It was like knowing a grizzly was stalking you through
the woods, only you couldn't see it. I knew They were out
there. I didn't know if I was happy that they were staying out
of sight, or if I'd rather they try something now and get it
over with.

"Careful through here," Grimalkin cautioned. We picked
our way through a patch of thick black briars with thorns as
long as my hand, shiny and evil-looking. "Do not take your
eyes from the path. Pay attention to what is happening at
your feet."

Bones hung in the branches and littered the ground at the
base of the bushes, some tiny, some not. Kenzie shuddered
whenever we passed one, clutching the key around her neck,
but she followed the cat through the branches without a word.

Until a vine snaked around her ankle.

She pitched forward with a yelp, right toward a patch of
nasty looking thorns. I caught her before she could impale
herself on the spikes. She gasped and clung to my shirt while
the offending vine slithered back into the undergrowth.

"You okay?" I asked. I could feel her shaking against me,
her heart thudding against my ribs. It felt…good…to hold her
like this. Her small body fit perfectly against mine.

With a start, I realized what I was doing and released her
quickly, drawing back. Kenzie blinked, still trying to process what had happened, then glared down at the briar patch.

"It…the branch…it *tried* to trip me, didn't it?" she said, sounding incredulous and indignant all at once. "Jeez, not even the plant life is friendly. What did I ever do to it?"

We stepped out of the briar patch, and I looked around for Grimalkin. He had vanished once more, and I stared hard into the trees, searching for him. "Here's a hint," I told Kenzie, narrowing my eyes as I peered into the undergrowth and shadows. "And it might save your life. Just assume that everything here—plant, animal, insect, toadstool, whatever—is out to get you."

"Well, that's not very friendly of them. They don't even know me."

"If you're not going to take this seriously—"

"Ethan, I was just nearly impaled by a bloodthirsty killer bush! I think I'm taking this fairly well, considering."

I glanced back at her. "Whatever. Just remember, nothing in the Nevernever is friendly to humans. Even if the fey appear friendly, they all have ulterior motives. Not even the cat is doing this for free. And if they can't get what they want, they'll take something anyway or try to kill you. You can't trust the fey, ever. They'll pretend to be your friend and stab you in the back when it's most convenient, not because they're mean, or spiteful or hateful, but because it's their nature. It's just how they are."

"You must hate them a great deal," Kenzie said softly.

I shrugged, abruptly self-conscious. "You haven't seen what I have. It's not without cause, trust me." Speaking of which, Grimalkin still hadn't appeared. "Where's that stupid cat?" I muttered, starting to get nervous and a little mad. "If he's gone off and left us—"

A branch rustled somewhere in the woods behind us. We both froze, and Kenzie looked over warily.

"That sounded a little too big for a cat…"

Another branch snapped, closer this time. Something was coming. Something big and fast.

"Humans!" Grimalkin's voice echoed from nowhere, though the urgency in it was plain. "Run! Now!"

Kenzie jumped. I tensed, gripping my weapons. Before we could even think about moving, the bushes parted and a huge reptilian creature spilled out of the brambles into the open.

At first, I thought it was a giant snake, as the scaly green body was close to twenty feet long. But its head was more dragon than serpent, and two short, clawed forearms stuck out of its sides, just behind its shoulder blades. It raised its head, a pale, forked tongue flicking the air, before it reared up with a hiss, baring a mouthful of needlelike teeth.

Kenzie gasped, and I yanked her into the trees as the monster lunged, barely missing us. The snap of its jaws echoed horribly in my ears. We ran, weaving around trees, tearing through bramble and undergrowth, hearing the crashing of twigs and branches at our heels as it followed.

I dodged behind a thick trunk, pulling Kenzie behind me, and raised my sticks as the monster's head slithered around, forked tongue tasting the air. When it turned, I brought the rattan down across its snout as hard as I could, striking the rubbery nose three times before the thing hissed and pulled back with blinding speed. As it drew away, I spotted a place where we could make our stand and yanked Kenzie toward it.

"What is that thing?" Kenzie cried as I pulled her into a cluster of trees, their trunks grown close together to form a protective cage around us. No sooner had I squeezed through than the monster's head appeared between a crack, snapping narrow jaws at me. I whacked it across the head with my sticks, and it pulled back with a screech. I saw its scaly body through the circle of trees, coiling around us like a snake with a mouse, and fought to remain calm.

"Kenzie," I panted, trying to track the thing's head through the branches. My arms shook, and I focused on staying loose, holding my sticks in front of me. "Stay in the center as much as you can. Don't go near the edge of the trees."

The thing lunged again, snaking through the trunks, snapping at me. Thankfully, its body was just a bit too wide to maneuver at top speed, and I was able to dodge, cracking it in the skull as I did. Hissing, it pulled back, trying from a different, higher angle. I ducked, stabbing it in the throat, wishing I had a knife or a blade instead of wooden sticks. It gave an angry gurgle and backed out, eyeing me evilly through the trunks.

"Ethan!" Kenzie yelled, as the monster darted close again, "behind you!"

Before I could turn, a heavy coil snaked around my waist, slamming me back into a tree trunk, pinning me there. I struggled, cursing myself for focusing solely on the monster's head instead of the whole creature. My right arm was pinned to my side; I raised my left as the head snaked through the trees and came at me again. Timing it carefully, I stabbed up with the tip, jamming it into a slitted yellow eye.

Screeching, the monster drew back. With a hiss, it tightened its coils around my chest, cutting off my air. I gasped for breath, punching the end of my rattan into the monster's body, trying to struggle free. It only squeezed harder, making my ribs creak painfully. My lungs burned, and my vision began to go dark, a tunnel of hazy light that started to shrink. The creature's head drifted closer; its tongue flicked out to brush my forehead, but I didn't have the strength to raise my weapon.

And then, Kenzie stepped up and brought her iron key slashing down across the monster's hurt eye.

Instantly, the coils loosened as the monster reared up, screaming this time. Gasping, I dropped to my knees as it writhed and thrashed, scraping the side of its face against the trunk, snapping branches and smashing into the trees. A flailing coil struck Kenzie, knocking her back several feet. I heard her gasp as she hit the ground, and tried to push myself upright, but the ground was still spinning and I sagged to my knees again.

Cursing, I struggled to get up, to put myself between Kenzie and the snake in case it turned on her. But the iron key to the face seemed to have killed its appetite for humans. With a final wail, the monster slithered off. I watched it vanish into the undergrowth, then sagged in relief.

"Are you all right?" Kenzie dropped beside me, placing a slender hand on my arm. I could feel it shaking. I nodded, still trying to suck air into my burning lungs, feeling as if they'd been crushed with a vise.

"I'm fine," I rasped, pulling myself to my feet. Kenzie rose, dusting herself off, and I stared at her in growing astonishment. That thing had had me on the ropes, seconds away from being swallowed like a big mouse. If she hadn't been there, I'd be dead right about now.

"Kenzie, I…" I hesitated, grateful, embarrassed and angry all at once. "Thanks."

"Oh, no problem," Kenzie replied with a shaky grin, though her voice trembled. "Always happy to help with any giant snake monster issues that pop up."

I felt a weird pull somewhere in my stomach, and the sudden crazy urge to draw her close, to make sure we were both still alive. Uncomfortable, I retreated a step. "Sorry about your camera," I muttered.

"Huh? Oh." She held up the device, now very broken from the fall, and gave a dramatic sigh. "Well, it wasn't working anyway. Besides…" She reached out and gently squeezed my arm. "I owed you one."

My mouth was dry again. "I'll replace it. Once we get back
to the real world—"

"Don't worry about it, tough guy." Kenzie waved it off.
"It's just a camera. And I think surviving an attack by a giant
snake monster was more important."

"Lindwurm," came a voice above our heads, and Grimalkin appeared in the branches, peering down at us. "That," he
stated imperiously, "was a lindwurm, and a rather young one at
that. An adult would have given you considerably more trouble." He flicked his tail and dropped to the ground, wrinkling
his nose as he gazed at us. "There might be others around, as
well, so I suggest we keep moving."

I glared at the cat as we maneuvered through the trees
again, wincing as my bruised ribs twinged. "You couldn't
have warned us any earlier?"

"I tried," Grimalkin replied with a sniff. "But you were too
busy discussing hostile vegetation and how faeries are completely untrustworthy. I practically had to yell to get your
attention." He glanced over his shoulder with a distinct I-
told-you-so expression. "Next time, when I suggest you move
silently through a dangerous part of the Nevernever, perhaps
you will listen to me."

"Huh," Kenzie muttered, walking along beside me. "You
know, if all cats are like him, I'm kinda glad they don't talk."

"That you know of, human," Grimalkin returned mysteriously, and continued deeper into the wyldwood.

CHAPTER TWELVE
THE BORDER

"The Iron Realm is not far, now."

I glanced up from where I sat on a fallen log, hot, sweaty and still sore from the recent battle. Kenzie slumped beside me, leaning against my shoulder, making it hard to concentrate on what the cat was saying. I didn't mind the contact—she was exhausted and probably just as sore—but I wasn't used to having anyone this close, touching me, and it was… distracting. I don't know how long we'd been walking, but it felt like the hours were stretching out just for spite. The wyldwood never changed; it was still as dark, murky and endless as it had been when we started. I didn't even know if we were walking in circles. Since fighting the lindwurm thing, I'd seen a wood sprite, several more piskies and a single goblin who might've given us trouble if he'd been with his pack. The short, warty fey had grinned evilly as it tried to block our path, but I'd drawn my weapons and Kenzie had stepped up beside me, glaring, and the goblin had suddenly decided it had other places to be. A will-o'-the-wisp had trailed us for several miles, trying to capture our attention so it could get us lost, but I'd told Kenzie to ignore the floating ball of light, and it eventually had given up.

I broke the last energy bar in half and handed the bigger part

to Kenzie, who sat up and took it with a murmur of thanks.
"How far?" I asked Grimalkin, biting into my half. The cat
began grooming his tail, ignoring me. I resisted the urge to
throw a rock at him.

I glanced at Kenzie. She sat hunched forward, her forearms
resting on her knees, chewing methodically. There were circles
under her eyes and a streak of mud across her cheek, but she
hadn't complained once through the entire march. In fact, she
had been very quiet ever since the fight with the lindwurm.

She saw me looking and managed a tired smile, bumping
her shoulder against mine. "So, we're almost there, huh?"
she said, brushing a strand of hair from her face. "I hope it's
less…woodsy than this place. Do you know much about it?"

"Unfortunately," I muttered. Machina's tower, the gremlins, the iron knights, the stark, blasted wasteland. I remembered it all as if it was yesterday. "It's not as woodsy, but the
Iron Realm isn't pleasant, either. It's where the Iron fey live."

"See, that's where I'm confused," Kenzie said, shifting to
face me. "Everything I researched said faeries are allergic to
iron." She held up the iron key. "That's why this thing worked
so well, right?"

"Yes," I said. "And they are. At least, the normal faeries
are. But the Iron fey are different. The fey—the entire Nevernever, actually—comes from us, from our dreams and imagination, as cheesy as that sounds. The traditional faeries are the
ones you read about in the old myths—Shakespeare and the
Grimm Brothers, for example. But, during the past hundred
years or so, we've been…er…dreaming of other things. So,
the Iron fey are a little more modern."

"Modern?"

"You'll see when we get there."

"Huh," Kenzie said, considering. "And you said the place
is ruled by a queen?"

"Yeah," I said, quickly standing up. "The Iron Queen."

"Any idea what *she's* like?" Kenzie stood, too, unaware of my burning face. "I've read about Queen Mab and Titania, of course, but I've never heard of the Iron Queen."

"I dunno," I lied and walked over to Grimalkin, who was watching with amused golden eyes, the hint of a smile on his whiskered face. I shot a warning glare at the feline, hoping he would remain silent. "Come on, cat. The sooner we get there, the sooner we can leave."

We started off again, pushing through the trees, following the seemingly tireless cait sith as he glided through the undergrowth. Kenzie walked next to me, her eyes weary and dull, barely looking up from the ground. A tiny faery with a mushroom cap peeked at us from a nearby branch, but she didn't even glance at it a second time. Either the overwhelming weirdness of the Nevernever had driven her to a kind of numb acceptance or she was too tired to give a crap.

The tangled woods started to thin as the gray twilight was finally fading, giving way to night. Fireflies or faery lights began appearing through the trees, blinking yellow, blue and green.

Grimalkin stopped at the base of a tall black tree and turned to face us. I frowned as he swatted at a blue light, which zipped off into the woods with a buzz.

"Why are we stopping? Shouldn't we get out of the wyldwood before night falls and the really nasty things start coming out?"

"You do not know where you are, do you?" Grimalkin purred. I gave him an irritated look, and he yawned. "Of course not. This," he stated, waving his tail languidly, "is the border of the Iron Realm. You are at the very edge of the Iron Queen's territory."

"What, right here?" I looked around but couldn't see anything unusual. Just black woods and a few blinking lights. "How can you tell? There's nothing here."

"One moment," the cat mused, a smug grin in his voice. "It should not be long."

I sighed. "We don't really have time for…"

I trailed off, as the tree behind Grimalkin flickered, then blazed with light. Kenzie gasped as neon lights erupted along the branches, like Christmas bulbs or those fiberglass trees in department stores. There were no wires or extension cords; the bulbs were growing right out of the branches. As the tree lit up, a swarm of multicolored fireflies spiraled up from the leaves and scattered to all parts of the forest, drifting around us like stray fireworks.

I blinked, dazzled by the display. Around us, the trees glimmered silver; trunks, leaves, branches and twigs shining as if they were made of polished metal. They reflected the drifting lights and turned the woods into a swirling galaxy of stars.

"Ethan," Kenzie breathed, staring transfixed at her arm. A tiny green bug perched on her wrist, blinking erratically. Its fragile body glittered in its own light, metallic and shiny, before it buzzed delicate transparent wings and zipped away into the woods. Kenzie held up her hand, and several more tiny lights hovered around her, landing on her fingers and making them glow.

For a second, I couldn't look away. My heartbeat picked up, and my mouth was suddenly dry, watching the girl in the center of the winking cloud, smiling as the tiny lights landed in her hair or perched on her arm.

She was beautiful.

"Okay," I muttered, tearing my gaze away before she noticed I was staring, "I can admit it—that's pretty cool."

Grimalkin sniffed. "So pleased you approve," he said. I frowned at him through the swirling lights, waving away several bugs drifting around my face. It occurred to me that we were on our own, now. Like the rest of the normal fey, Grimalkin couldn't set foot in the Iron Realm. Meghan's kingdom was still deadly to the rest of the Nevernever—only the Iron fey could live there without poisoning themselves. Grimalkin was showing us the border because he planned to leave us here.

"How far to the Iron Queen from here?" I asked.

The cat flicked a bug off his tail. "Still a few days by foot. Do not worry, though. Beyond this rise is a place that will take you to Mag Tuiredh, the site of the Iron Court, much faster than humans can walk."

"I suppose this is where you leave," I said.

"Do not be ridiculous, human." The cat yawned and stood up. "Of course I am coming with you. Besides your being highly amusing, the favor dictates that I see you all the way to Mag Tuiredh and dump you at the Iron Queen's feet. After that, you become her problem, but I will see you there, first."

"You can't go into the Iron Realm. It'll kill you."

Grimalkin gave me a bored look, turned and stalked off. Past the border and into the Iron Realm.

I hurried after him, Kenzie on my heels. "Wait," I said, catching up to him, frowning. "I *know* the Iron Realm is deadly to normal fey. How are you doing this?"

Grimalkin paused, looking over his shoulder with glowing, half-lidded eyes. His tail waved lazily. "There are things about this world that you do not realize, human," he purred. "Events that took place years ago, when the Iron Queen rose to power, still shape this world today. You do not know as much as you think you do. Besides…" He blinked, raising his head imperiously. "I am a cat."

And that was the end of it.

The fireflies continued to light up the forest as we walked on, blinking through leaves and branches, glinting off the trunks. Trees with flickering light bulbs illuminated the path to wherever Grimalkin was taking us. Kenzie kept staring at them, the amazement and disbelief back on her face.

"This…is impossible," she murmured once, brushing her fingers over a glittering trunk. Small glowing bulbs sprouted overhead like clusters of Christmas lights. Streetlamps grew right out of the dirt, lighting the path. "How…how can this be real?"

"This is the Iron Realm," I told her. "It's still Faery, just a different flavor of crazy."

Before she could answer, the trees fell away, and we found ourselves at the top of a rise, staring down at the lights of a small village on the edge of a massive lake. It looked sort of like a gypsy town or a carnival, all lit up with torches and strings of colored lights. Thatched huts stood on posts rising out of the water, and wooden bridges crisscrossed the spaces between. Creatures of all shapes and sizes roamed the walkways above the water.

At the edge of the town, a railroad arched away over the lake, vanishing to a point somewhere on the horizon.

"What is this place?" I muttered, as Kenzie pressed close to my back, peering over my shoulder. Grimalkin sat down and curled his tail over his feet.

"This is a border town, one of many along the edge of the Iron Realm. I forget its exact name, if it even has one. Many Iron fey gather here, for one reason." He raised a hind leg and scratched an ear. "Do you see the railroad, human?"

"What about it?"

"That will take you straight to Mag Tuiredh, the site of the Iron Court and the seat of the Iron Queen's power. It costs nothing to board, and anyone may use it. The railroad was one of the first improvements the queen made when she took the throne. She wished for everyone to have a safe way to travel to Mag Tuiredh from anywhere in the Iron Realm."

"We're going down there?" Kenzie asked, her eyes big as she stared at the creatures roaming about the bridges. Grimalkin sniffed.

"Do you see another way to get to the railroad, human?"

"But...what about the faeries?"

"I doubt they will bother you," the cat replied, unconcerned. "They see many travelers through this part of town. Do not speak to anyone, get on the train, and you will be fine." He raised a hind leg to scratch his ear. "That is where I will meet you, when you finally decide to show up."

"You're not coming?"

Grimalkin curled his whiskers in distaste. "Outside of Mag Tuiredh, I try to avoid contact with the denizens of the Iron Realm," he said in a lofty voice. "It circumvents tiresome, unnecessary questions. Besides, I cannot hold your hands the entire way to the Iron Queen." He sniffed and stood up, waving his tail. "The train will arrive soon. Do try not to miss it, humans."

Without another word, he disappeared.

Kenzie sighed, muttering something about impossible felines. And I realized, suddenly, that she looked very pale and tired in the moonlight. There were shadows under her eyes, and her cheeks looked hollow, wasted. Her normal boundless energy seemed to have deserted her as she rubbed her arm and gazed down the slope, shivering in the cold breeze.

"So," she said, turning to me. Even her smile looked weary as she stood at the edge of the rise, the wind ruffling her hair. "Head into the creepy faery town, talk to the creepy faery conductor and board the creepy faery train, because a talking cat told us to."

"Are you all right?" I asked. "You don't look so good."

"Just tired. Come on, let's go already." She backed up a step, avoiding my eyes, but as she turned, I saw something in the moonlight that made my stomach clench.

"Kenzie, wait!" Striding forward, I caught her arm as gently as I could. She tried squirming from my grip, but I pulled back her sleeve to reveal a massive purple stripe, stretching from her shoulder almost to her elbow. A dark, sullen blotch marring her otherwise flawless skin.

I sucked in a horrified breath. "When did you get this?" I demanded, angry that she hadn't told me, and that I hadn't noticed it until now. "What happened?"

"It's fine, Ethan." She yanked her arm back and tugged her sleeve down. "It's nothing. I got it when we were fighting the lindwurm thing."

"Why didn't you say anything?"

"Because it's not a big deal!" Kenzie shrugged. "Ethan, trust me, I'm all right. I bruise easily, that's all." But she didn't look at me when she said it. "I get them all the time, now can we please go? Like Grim said, we don't want to miss the train."

"Kenzie…" But she was already gone, dropping down the rise without looking back, striding merrily toward the lights and the railroad and the town of Iron fey. I blew out a frustrated breath and hurried to catch up.

After picking our way down the slope, we entered the town. Kenzie gazed around in wonder, her weariness forgotten, while I gripped my rattan and tensed every time something came near.

Iron fey surrounded us, weird, crazy and nightmarish. Creatures made entirely of twisted wire. A well-dressed figure in a top hat, holding the leash of a ticking clockwork hound. An old woman with the body of a giant spider scuttled past, her metallic, needlelike legs clicking over the wood. Kenzie let out a squeak and squeezed my hand, nearly crushing my fingers, until the spider-thing had disappeared.

We were getting stared at. Despite what Grimalkin said, the Iron fey *were* taking notice of us, and why not? It wasn't every day two humans strolled through their town, looking decidedly mortal and un-fey. Strangely enough, no one tried to stop us as we maneuvered the swaying bridges and walkways, passing shacks and odd-looking stores, feeling glowing fey eyes on my back.

Until we reached a large, circular deck where several walkways converged. I could see the railroad at the edge of town, stretching out over the lake. But as we headed toward it, a hunched figure dressed in rags suddenly reached out and grabbed Kenzie's wrist as she passed, making her yelp.

I spun, whipping my rattan down, striking the arm that held her, and the faery let go with a raspy cry. Shaking its fingers, it crept forward again, and I shoved Kenzie behind me, meeting the faery with my sticks raised.

"Humans," it hissed, and several rusty screws dropped out of its rags as it circled. "Humans have something for me, yes? A pocket watch? A lovely phone?" It raised its head, revealing a face put together with bits and pieces of machinery. One eye was a glowing bulb, the other the head of a copper screw. A mouth made of wires smiled at us as the thing eased forward. "Stay," it urged, as Kenzie recoiled in shock. "Stay and share."

"Back off," I warned, but a crowd was forming now, fey that had simply been watching before easing forward. They surrounded us on the platform, not lunging or attacking, but preventing us from going any farther. I kept an eye on both them and the machine-scrap faery; if they wanted a fight, I'd be happy to oblige.

"Stay," urged the faery in rags, still circling us, smiling. "Stay and talk. We help each other, yes?"

A piercing whistle rent the air, drawing the attention of several fey. Moments later, an enormous train appeared over the lake, trailing billowing clouds of smoke as it chugged closer. Bulky and massive, leaking smoke and steam everywhere, it pulled into the station with a roar and a screech of rusty gears before shuddering to a halt.

Several faeries began making their way toward the huge, smoking engine, as a copper-skinned faery in a conductor's uniform stepped out front, waving them forward. The crowd thinned a bit, but not enough.

"Dammit, I don't want to have to fight our way out," I growled, keeping an eye on the fey surrounding us. "But we need to get to that train now." The faery in rags eased closer, as if he feared we would turn and run. "This one isn't going to let us go," I said, feeling my muscles tense, and gripped my weapons. "Kenzie, stay back. This could get ugly."

"Wait." Kenzie grabbed my sleeve, a second before I would've lunged forward and cracked the fey in the skull. Pulling me to the side, she stepped forward and stripped off her camera. "Here," she told the ragged fey, holding it out. "You want a trade, right? Is this good enough?"

The Iron faery blinked, then reached out and snatched the camera, wire lips stretched into a grin. "Ooooh," it cooed, clutching it to its chest. "Pretty. So generous, little human." It shook the camera experimentally and frowned. "Broken?"

"Um…yeah," Kenzie admitted, and I tensed, ready to step in with force if the thing took offense. "Sorry."

The faery grinned again. "Good trade!" it rasped, tucking the camera into its robes. "Good trade. We approve. Luck on your travels, little humans."

With a hissing cackle, it hobbled down a walkway and vanished into the town.

The crowd began to disperse, and I slowly relaxed. Kenzie

pushed her hair back with a shaking hand and sighed in relief. "Well, there go the pictures for this week's sports article," she said wryly. "But, if you think about it, that camera has more than paid for itself today. I'm just sad no one will get to see your mad kali skills."

I lowered my sticks. That was twice now that Kenzie's quick thinking had gotten us out of trouble. Another few seconds, and I would've been in a fight. With a faery. In the middle of a faery town.

Not one of my smarter moments.

"How did you know what it wanted?" I asked as we headed toward the station again. Kenzie gave me an exasperated look.

"Really, Ethan, you're supposed to know this stuff. Faeries like gifts, all the Google articles say so. And since we don't have any jars of honey or small children, I figured the camera was the best bet." She chuckled and rolled her eyes at me. "This doesn't have to be a fight all the way to the Iron Queen, tough guy. Next time, let's try talking to the faeries before the sticks come out."

I would've said something, except...I was kind of speechless.

We boarded the train without trouble, receiving only a brief glare from the conductor, and made our way to a deserted car near the back. Hard wooden pews sat under the windows, but there were a few private boxes as well, and after a few minutes of searching, we managed to find an empty one. Sliding in behind Kenzie, I quickly shut the doors, locked them and lowered the blind over the window.

Kenzie sank down on one of the benches, leaning against the glass. I followed her gaze, seeing the glittering metal of the tracks stretch out over the dark waters until they were lost from view.

"How long do you think it'll be before we're there?" Kenzie asked, still gazing out the window. "What is this place called again?"

"Mag Tuiredh," I replied, sitting beside her. "And I don't know. Hopefully not long."

"Hopefully," Kenzie agreed, and murmured in a softer voice, "I wonder what my dad is doing right now?"

With a huff, the train began to move, chugging noisily at first, then smoothing out as it picked up speed. The lights of the village fell away until nothing could be seen outside the window but the flat, silvery expanse of the lake and the stars glittering overhead.

"I hope Grimalkin made it on," Kenzie said, her voice slurred and exhausted. She shifted against the window, crossing her arms. "You think he's here like he said he would be?"

"Who knows?" I watched her try to get comfortable for a few seconds, then scooted over, closing the distance between us. "Here," I offered, pulling her back against my shoulder. With everything she'd done for us, the least I could do was let her sleep. She leaned into me with a grateful sigh, soft strands of hair brushing my arm.

"I wouldn't worry about the cat," I went on, shifting to give her a more comfortable position. "If he made it, he made it. If not, there's nothing we can do about it."

She didn't say anything for a while, closing her eyes, and I pretended to watch the shadows outside the window, hyper-aware of her head on my shoulder, her slim hand on my knee.

"Mool onyurleg, m'surry," Kenzie mumbled, sounding half-asleep.

"What?"

"I said, if I drool on your leg, I'm sorry," she repeated. I chuckled at that, making her crack an eye open.

"Oh, wow, the broody one can laugh after all," she murmured, one corner of her mouth curling up. "Maybe we should alert the media."

Smirking, I looked down, ready to give a smart-ass reply.

And suddenly, my breath caught at how close our faces were, her lips just a few inches from mine. If I ducked my head just slightly, I would kiss her. Her hair was brushing my skin, the feathery strands tickling my neck, and the fingers on my leg were very warm. Kenzie didn't move, continuing to watch me with a faint smile. I wondered if she knew what she was doing, or if she was waiting to see what I would do.

I swallowed and carefully tilted my head back, removing the temptation. "Go to sleep." I told her. She sniffed.

"Bossy." But her eyes closed, and a few minutes later, a soft snore escaped her parted lips. I crossed my arms, leaned back, and prepared for a long, uncomfortable ride to Mag Tuiredh.

When I opened my eyes, it was light, and the sky through the window was mottled with sun and clouds. Groggily, I scanned the rest of the car, wondering if any faeries had crept up on us while I was asleep, but it seemed we were still alone.

My neck ached, and part of my leg was numb. I had drifted off with my chin on my chest, arms still crossed. I started to stretch but froze. Kenzie had somehow curled up on the tiny bench and was sleeping with her head on my leg.

For a few seconds, I watched her, the rise and fall of her slim body, the sun falling over her face. Seeing her like that filled me with a fierce protectiveness, an almost painful desire to keep her safe. She mumbled something and shifted closer, and I reached down, brushing the hair from her cheek.

Realizing what I was doing, I pulled my hand back, clenching my fists. Dammit, what was happening to me? I could not be falling for this girl. It was dangerous for the both of us. When we did go back to the mortal world, Kenzie would return to her old life and her old friends and her family, and I would do the same. She did not need someone like me hanging around, someone who attracted chaos and misery, who couldn't stay out of trouble no matter how hard he tried.

I'd already ruined one girl's life. I would not do that again. Even if I had to make her hate me, I would not do to Kenzie what I'd done to Sam.

"Hey," I said, jostling her shoulder. "Wake up."

She groaned, hunching her shoulders against my prodding. "Two more minutes, Mom."

It was mean, but I scooted away from her, letting her head thump to the bench. "Ow!" she yelped, sitting up and rubbing her skull. "What the hell, Ethan?"

I nodded out the window, ignoring the immediate stab of remorse. "We're almost there."

Kenzie still frowned at me, but when she looked out the glass, her eyes went wide.

Mag Tuiredh. The Iron Court. I'd never been there, never seen it. I'd only learned of the city from stories, rumors I'd heard over years of existing among the fey. Meghan herself had never told me where she lived and ruled from, though I'd asked her countless times before she disappeared. She didn't want me to know, to imagine it, to get ideas in my head that might lead me there, looking for her.

I had imagined it, of course. But as an ugly monstrosity, the images tainted by the memory of a stark black tower in the center of a blasted wasteland. The city at the end of the railroad tracks was anything but.

It was old, even from this distance, I could see that. Stone walls and mossy roofs, vines coiled around everything. Trees pushing up through rock, roots draped and curled around stone. Some of the buildings were huge—massively huge.

Not sprawling so much as they looked as if they were built by a race of giants.

But the city *gleamed,* too. Sunlight glinted off metal spires, lights glimmered in the haze and steam, glass windows caught the faint rays and reflected them back into the sky. It reminded me of a city under construction, with sleek metal towers rising up among the ancient moss- and vine-covered buildings. And above it all, gleaming spires stabbing into the clouds, the silhouette of a huge castle stood proud and imposing over Mag Tuiredh, like a glittering mountain.

The home of the Iron Queen.

The train came to a wheezing, clanking, chugging halt at the station. Gazing out the window, I narrowed my eyes. There were a lot more Iron fey here than at the tiny border town on the lake, a lot of guards and faeries in armor. Knights with the symbol of a great iron tree on their breastplates stood at attention or roamed the streets in pairs, keeping an eye on the populace.

"Well?" came a familiar voice from behind us, and we jerked around. Grimalkin sat on the bench across from us, watching us lazily. "Are you just going to sit there until the train starts moving again?"

"Where do we go from here?" Kenzie asked, peeking out the window again. "I guess we can't hail a taxi, right?"

Grimalkin sighed.

"This way," he said, walking along the edge of the bench before dropping to the ground. "I will take you to the Iron Queen's palace."

The palace, I thought, as we followed Grimalkin down the aisle toward the doors up front. I knew the huge castle must be hers. It was just hard to imagine Meghan living in a palace now. *Must be nice. Better than a rundown farmhouse or little home in the suburbs, anyway.*

Following Grimalkin, we stepped through the doors and walked down the steps into the hazy streets of Mag Tuiredh.

Aside from the crowds of fey, it was difficult to believe we were still in the Nevernever. Mag Tuiredh reminded me a little of Victorian England—the steampunk version. The streets were cobblestone and lined with flickering lanterns in hues of blue and green. Carriages stood at the edge of the sidewalks, pulled by strange, mechanical horses of bright metal and copper gears. Buildings crowded the narrow streets, some stony and vine-ridden and Gothic, others decidedly more modern. Pipes crisscrossed the sky overhead, leaking steam that trickled to the ground in lacy curtains. And, of course, there were the Iron fey, looking as if they'd stepped straight out of an alchemist's nightmare.

They stared at us as if *we* were the nightmares, the monsters, watching and whispering as we trailed Grimalkin through the cobblestone paths. The cat was nearly invisible in the haze and falling steam, as difficult to glimpse as a shadow in the wyldwood. I kept a tight grip on my weapons, glaring back at any fey who gave me a funny look. We were even more conspicuous here than we'd been at the border village. I hoped we could get to Meghan before anyone stepped up to challenge the two humans strolling through the middle of the faery capital.

Yeah, that wasn't going to happen.

As we passed beneath a stone archway, clanking footsteps rang out and a squad of faery knights stepped up to block our path. Weapons drawn, they surrounded us, a ring of bristling steel, their faces cold and hard beneath their helmets. I pulled Kenzie close, trying to keep her behind me, swinging my own weapons into a ready stance. Grimalkin, I noticed, had disappeared, and I cursed him under my breath. Fey gathered behind the knights, watching and murmuring, as the tension swelled and unspoken violence hung thick on the air.

"Humans." A knight stepped forward, pointing at me with his sword. He had a sharp face, pointed ears, and was covered head to toe in plate mail. His expression beneath the open helmet was decidedly unfriendly. "How did you get into Mag Tuiredh? Why are you here?"

"I'm here to see the Iron Queen," I returned, not lowering my weapons, though I had no idea what I could do against so many armored knights. I didn't think beating on them with a pair of wooden sticks would penetrate that thick steel. Not to mention, they had very sharp swords and lances, all pointed in our direction. "I don't want any trouble. I just want to talk to Meghan. If you tell her I'm here—"

An angry murmur went through the ranks of fey. "You cannot just walk into the palace and demand an audience with the queen, mortal," the knight said, swelling indignantly. "Who are you, to demand such things, to speak as if you know her?" He leveled his sword at my throat before I could reply. "Surrender now, intruders. We will take you to the First Lieutenant. He will decide your fate."

"Hold!" ordered a voice, and the knights straightened immediately. The ranks parted, and a faery came through, glaring at them. Instead of armor, he wore a uniform of black and gray, the silhouette of the same iron tree on his shoulder. His spiky black hair bristled like porcupine quills, and neon strands of lightning flickered and snapped between them.

As he came into the circle, he nodded to me in a genuine show of respect, before turning on the knight. Violet eyes glimmered as he stared him down. "What is the meaning of this?"

"First Lieutenant!" The knight jerked to attention as the

rest of the knights did the same. "Sir! We have apprehended these two mortal intruders. They were on their way to the palace, saying they wished an audience with the Iron Queen. We thought it best if we brought them to you. The boy claims to know her—"

"Of course he does!" the faery snapped, scowling, and the knight paled. "I know who he is, though it is apparent that you do not."

"Sir?"

"Stand down," said the First Lieutenant, and raised his voice, addressing all the faeries watching this little spectacle. "All of you, stand down! Bow to your prince!"

Uh. What?

THE IRON PRINCE

"Prince?"

I could feel Kenzie's disbelieving stare as all the fey surrounding us, knights, civilians and guards alike, lowered their heads and bent at the waist or sank to their knees. Including the First Lieutenant, who put a fist over his heart as he bowed. I wanted to tell them all to stop, to not bother, but it was too late.

Oh, great. I can already hear the questions this is going to bring on.

"Prince Ethan," the lieutenant said, straightening again. The knights sheathed their weapons, and a glare from a few of the armored fey quickly dispersed the crowd. "This is a surprise. Please excuse my guards. We were not expecting you. Are you here to see your sister?"

"Sister?" Kenzie echoed behind me, her voice climbing several octaves. I resisted the urge to groan.

"It's...Glitch, right?" I asked, dragging the name up from memory. Glitch was something of a legend even in the real world, the rebel Iron faery who'd joined with Meghan in defeating the false king. I'd seen him once or twice in the past, hanging around the house like a worried bodyguard when Meghan came to visit. I didn't mind his presence that much; it was another figure I hated, another faery who sometimes waited in the shadows for his queen to return, who never came into the house. He was a legend, too, even more so than Glitch, as one of the three who had taken down the false king and stopped the war. He was also the only normal fey (besides Grimalkin, apparently) who could survive in the Iron Realm. The rumors of how he'd accomplished such an impossible task were long and varied, but the reason behind it was always the same. Because he'd fallen in love with the Iron Queen and would do anything to be with her.

Including take her away from her family, I thought as the old, familiar anger spread through my chest. *Including making sure she never leaves Faery. It's because of you that she stayed, and it's because of you that she's gone. If you hadn't shown up that night to take her back, she would still be in the real world.*

But Glitch was still waiting for an answer and probably wouldn't appreciate my feelings concerning his boss. "Yeah, I came to see Meghan," I said, shrugging. "Sorry, we couldn't call ahead of time. She probably doesn't know I'm here."

Glitch nodded. "I will inform her majesty right away. If you and your...friend—" the faery lieutenant glanced at Kenzie "—would come with me, I will take you to the Iron Queen."

He gestured for us to follow, and we trailed him down the cobblestone paths as crowds of iron fey parted for us, bowing as we passed. The knights fell into rank behind us, their clanking echoing through the streets. I tried to ignore them and the way my stomach squirmed with every step that brought us closer to the palace and the Iron Queen.

"If you don't mind my asking, sire," Glitch continued, glancing back. His purple eyes regarded us with curious appraisal. "How did you cross over from the mortal world?"

"My doing," purred another familiar voice, and Grimalkin appeared, walking along the edge of a stone wall. Glitch looked up and sighed.

"Hello again, cat," he said, not sounding entirely pleased.

"Why am I not surprised to see you involved? What have you been scheming lately?"

The cat very deliberately ignored that question, pretending to be occupied with the tiny glittering moths that flitted around the streetlamps. Glitch shook his head, making the lightning in his hair flicker, then stopped at a corner and raised an arm.

A horse and carriage pulled up, both looking decidedly mechanical, the horse's body made of shifting copper gears and bright metal. The driver, green-skinned beneath his black-and-white coat, tipped his top hat at us. The clockwork dog sitting beside him thumped a wiry tail.

Grimalkin observed the carriage from atop the stone wall and wrinkled his nose.

"I believe I will find my own way to the palace," he stated, blinking in a bored manner as he looked down at me. "Human, please attempt to stay out of trouble for the last leg of the journey. Mag Tuiredh is not *that* big a place to become lost in. Do not make me have to come find you again."

Glitch's spines bristled. "I will make sure the prince gets to the palace, cait sith," he snapped, sounding indignant. "Any kin of the Iron Queen in Mag Tuiredh becomes my top priority. He will be perfectly safe here, I assure you."

"Oh, well, if you say so, Lieutenant, then it must be true." With a sniff, the cat disappeared, dropping off the wall and vanishing midleap.

Sighing, Glitch pulled open the door and nodded for us to get in. I climbed aboard, and Kenzie followed as the First Lieutenant helped her up the steps, then closed the door behind us.

"I will ride ahead and meet you at the palace," he told us through the window, and stepped back to the curb. "The queen will be informed of your arrival right away. Welcome to Mag Tuiredh, Prince Ethan."

He bowed once more, and the carriage started to move, taking his figure from sight. I stared out the window, watching the city of Mag Tuiredh scroll by, feeling Kenzie's gaze piercing my back. I knew it wouldn't be long before she started asking questions, and I was right.

"Prince?" she said softly, and I closed my eyes. "You're the prince of this place? You never told me that."

I sighed, turning to meet her bewildered, accusing gaze. "I didn't think it was important."

"Not *important?*" Kenzie's eyes bugged, and she threw up her hands. "Ethan, you're a freaking prince of Faeryland, and you didn't think that was important?"

"I'm not a real prince," I insisted. "It's not like you think. I'm not part faery, I'm just…related to the queen." Kenzie stared at me, waiting, and I stabbed my fingers through my hair. "The Iron Queen…" I sighed again and finally came out with it. "She's my half sister, Meghan."

Her mouth dropped open. "And you couldn't have mentioned that earlier?"

"No, I didn't want to talk about it!" I turned away to stare out the window again. Mag Tuiredh looked both bright and dark in the hazy light, a glittering realm of shadows and steam, stone and metal. "I haven't seen Meghan in years," I said in a quieter voice. "I don't know what she's like anymore. She told me to stay away from her, that she was cutting my whole family out of her life. Comes with being a faery queen, I guess." I heard the bitterness in my voice and struggled to control it. "I didn't want you to associate me with…Them," I told Kenzie. "Not like that."

Kenzie was quiet for a moment. Then, "So…when you were kidnapped, and your sister went into the Nevernever to rescue you…"

"Long story short, she became the Iron Queen, yeah."

"And...you blame them for taking her away. That's why you hate them."

My throat felt suspiciously tight. I swallowed hard to open it. "No," I growled, clenching my fist against the window-sill. "I blame her."

The Iron Queen's palace soared over the rest of the build-ings in the city, a huge pointed structure of glass, stone and steel. Banners emblazoned with the great iron tree flapped in the wind, and the path to the front gate was lined with enor-mous oaks, forming a tunnel of branches, leaves and lights. It was the strangest castle I'd ever seen, not really ancient or completely modern but caught somewhere between the two. It had mossy stone turrets, crawling with vines, but also tow-ers of shining glass and steel, catching the sunlight as they stabbed toward the sky. A pair of Iron knights bowed their heads as the carriage rolled through the gate into the court-yard, so apparently we were expected.

Past the gates, the road circled a massive green lawn strewn with metal trees, their leaves and branches glittering like tinsel as the light caught them. The stone walls of the castle rose up on either side, patrolled by more Iron knights. A small pond sat in the center of the courtyard, making me wonder what kind of fish swam beneath those waters. Iron goldfish, per-haps? Metallic turtles? I smirked at the thought.

Movement under one of the trees caught my attention. Two figures circled each other beneath the branches of a silver pine, a pair of swords held in front of them. One was easily rec-ognizable as an Iron knight, his armor and huge broadsword gleaming as he bore down on his opponent.

The other combatant was smaller, slighter and not wear-ing any armor as he danced around the much larger knight. He looked about my age, with bright silver hair tied back in a ponytail and an elegant curved blade in his hand.

And he knew how to move. Long years of watching Guro Javier made me appreciate a skilled fighter when I saw one. This kid reminded me of him: flowing, agile, deadly accurate. The knight lunged at him, stabbing at his head. He stepped aside, disarmed the knight faster than thought and pointed the blade at his throat.

Damn. He might even be faster than me.

As the carriage clopped past the fighters, the boy raised a hand to his opponent and turned to watch us.

The eyes under his silver brows were far too bright, a piercing ice-blue that made my skin crawl. He was fey, and *gentry,* that much was certain. I didn't need to see the tips of his pointed ears to know that. He watched me with a faint, puzzled smile, until the carriage took us around a bend in the road and he was lost from view.

We came to the steps of the palace and lurched to a halt. A tiny creature with a wrinkled face, carrying an enormous pile of junk on his hunched shoulders, stood waiting with a squad of knights as the carriage clanked and groaned and finally stilled.

"Prince Ethan," it squeaked as we climbed down from the carriage. It had an odd accent, as if English wasn't its first language. "Welcome to Mag Tuiredh. My name is Fix, and I will be your escort to the throne room. Please, come with me. The Iron Queen is expecting you."

My stomach churned, but I swallowed my nervousness and followed the creature across the road, up the steps and through the massive iron doors to the palace.

Things sort of went to hell from there.

Meghan's castle was pretty impressive, even I had to admit. I was expecting it to be old and slightly run-down on the inside, but the interior was bright and cheerful and very modern. Though it did have a few strange features that reminded you that this was still Faery, no matter what. The hallway of trees, for one, with glowing bulbs lighting the way through metal branches. And the computer mice that scurried over the floors on tiny red feet, chased by gremlins and clockwork hounds. One wall was covered in enormous brass and copper gears that, from what I could tell, served no purpose except to fill the air with deafening creaks, ticks and groans.

Kenzie stayed close to me as we followed the Iron faery through the hallways, but she couldn't stop staring at our surroundings, her eyes wide with amazement. I refused to be as captivated, glaring at the Iron fey passing us in the halls, trying to keep track of directions in this huge place. Fix finally led us down a long, brightly lit corridor, where Glitch bowed to me as we passed him in the hall. A pair of massive arching doors stood at the end of the corridor, flanked on all sides by armored knights.

"This is the queen's throne room," Fix explained as we stopped at the doors. "She and the Prince Consort are expecting you. Are you ready?"

My palms felt clammy, my stomach turning cartwheels. I nodded, and Fix pushed both doors open at once.

A huge, cathedral-like room greeted us as we stepped through the frame. Decorative pillars, twisted with vines and coils of tiny lights, soared up to a vaulted glass ceiling that showed off sun and sky. Our footsteps echoed in the empty chamber as we followed the guide down the strip of red carpet. The room was obviously used for large gatherings, but except for me, Kenzie and Fix, the floor appeared empty.

A large metal throne stood on a dais at the end of the room, and I noticed Grimalkin sitting on a corner step, calmly washing a paw. Rolling my eyes, I looked up at the throne itself.

And...there she was. Not sitting on the throne, but standing beside it, her fingers resting lightly on the arm.

My sister, Meghan Chase. The Iron Queen.

She looked exactly as I remembered. Even though it had been years since I'd seen her last, and back then she had been taller than me, she still had the same long, pale hair, the same blue eyes. She even wore jeans and a white shirt, much like she had when she'd lived at home. Nothing had changed. This Meghan could be the same girl who'd rescued me from Machina's tower, thirteen years ago.

My throat ached, and a flood of confusing emotions made my stomach feel tight. I didn't know what I would say to my sister now that I was finally here. *Why did you leave us? Why don't I ever see you anymore?* Useless questions. I already knew the answer, much as I hated it.

"Ethan." Her voice, so familiar, flowed across the room and drew me forward as if I was a little kid once more. Meghan smiled down at me, and any fears I had that she had changed, that she was some distant faery queen, were gone in an instant. Stepping from the dais, she walked up and, without hesitation, pulled me into a tight hug.

The dam broke. I hugged her back tightly, ignoring everyone else in the room, not caring what they thought. This was Meghan, the same Meghan who had looked out for me, who'd gone into the Nevernever to bring me home. And despite my anger, despite all those dark moments when I thought I hated her, she was still my sister.

Come home, I wanted to tell her, knowing it was useless. *Mom and Dad miss you. It's not the same since you left. And I'm tired of pretending you're dead, that I don't have a sister. Why did you always choose them instead of me?*

I couldn't say any of those things, of course. I'd tried, when I was younger, to get her to stay, or to at least visit more often. It had never worked; no matter how much I begged, pleaded or cried, she would always vanish back into the Nevernever,

leaving us behind. I knew she would never abandon her kingdom, not even for family. Not even for me.

Meghan drew back, smiling, holding me at arm's length.
I noticed with a strange thrill that I was taller than her now.
A weird sensation—the last time I'd seen my sister, she'd had
several inches on me. It really had been a long time.

"Ethan," she said again, with such undeniable affection I
instantly felt guilty for thinking the worst of her. "It's good to
see you." One hand rose, brushing hair from my eyes. "God,
you've gotten so tall."

I held her gaze. "And you haven't changed a bit."

Guilt flickered across her face, just for a moment. "Oh,"
she whispered, "you'd be surprised."

I didn't know what she meant by that, but my stomach
twisted. Meghan was immortal now, I reminded myself. She
looked the same, but who knew what she had done in the
time she had been the Iron Queen.

"Regardless," Meghan went on, her expression shifting to
puzzled concern. "Why are you here, Ethan? Grim told me
you were in the Iron Realm, that you had used his token. Is
something wrong at home?" Her fingers tightened on my
arms. "Are Mom and Luke okay?"

I nodded. "They're fine," I said, freeing myself and stepping back. "At least, they were fine when I left."

"How long ago was that?"

"About two days? Faery time?" I shrugged, nodding to the
gray lump of fur on the dais. "Ask him. The cat had us tromping all over the wyldwood. I don't know how long it's been
in the real world."

"They're probably worried sick." Meghan sighed, giving
me a stern look, then seemed to notice Kenzie hovering behind me. She blinked, and her brow furrowed. "And you

brought someone with you." She beckoned Kenzie forward.
"Who is this?"

"Kenzie," I replied as the girl stepped around me and dropped
into a clumsy curtsy. "Mackenzie St. James. She's one of my
classmates."

"I see." I caught the displeasure in her voice, not directed
at Kenzie, but that I would bring someone into the Nevernever, perhaps. "And did she know anything about us before
you dropped her into this world?"

"Oh, sure," I said flatly. "I talk about seeing invisible faeries every day, to whoever will listen. That always goes over
so well."

Meghan ignored the jab. "Are you all right?" she asked
Kenzie, her voice gentle. "I know it's a lot to take in. I was
about your age when I first came here, and it was...interest-
ing, to say the least." She gave her a sympathetic smile. "How
are you holding up?"

"I'm okay, your...uh...your majesty," Kenzie said, and
jerked her thumb in my direction. "Ethan sort of gave me
the crash course in everything Faery. I'm still waiting to see
if I wake up or not."

"We'll get you home soon," Meghan promised, and turned
back to me. "I assume this visit wasn't just to say 'hi,' Ethan,"
she said in a firmer voice. "That token was only supposed to
be used in emergencies. What's going on?"

"Wish I knew." I crossed my arms defensively. "I didn't
want to come here. I would've been perfectly happy never
seeing this place again." I paused to see if my words affected
her. Except for a slight tightening of her eyes, her expression
remained the same. "But there's a bunch of creepy fey hanging around the real world that I've never seen before, and they
really didn't give me a choice."

"What do you mean, they didn't give you a choice?"

"I mean they kidnapped a friend of mine, a half-phouka, right from school, in broad daylight. And when I tried to find him, they came after us. Me and Kenzie both."

Meghan's eyes narrowed, and the air around her went still, like the sky before a storm. I could suddenly *feel* the power flickering around the Iron Queen, like unseen strands of lightning, making the hairs on my neck stand up. I shivered and took a step back, resisting the urge to rub my arms.

In that instant, I knew exactly how she had changed.

But the flare of energy died down, and Meghan's voice remained calm as she continued. "So, you came here," she went on, glancing from me to Kenzie and back again. "To escape them."

I nodded shakily.

The Iron Queen regarded me intently, thinking. "And you said they were a type of faery you've never seen before," she questioned, and I nodded again. "A new species, like the Iron fey?"

"No. Not like the Iron fey. These things are…different. It's hard to explain." I thought back to that night at the dojo, the ghostly, transparent faeries, the way they'd flickered in and out, as if they couldn't quite hold on to reality. "I don't know *what* they are, but I think they might be kidnapping exiles and half-breeds." I remembered the dead piskie, and my stomach churned. Todd might already be gone. "A dryad told me all the local fey are disappearing. Something is happening, but I don't know what they want. I don't even know what they are."

"And you're sure of this?"

"These things tried to kill me a couple days ago. Yeah, I'm sure."

"All right," Meghan said, turning from me. "If you say you've seen them, I believe you. I'll call a meeting with Summer and Winter, tell them there could be a new group of fey on the rise. If these faeries are killing off exiles and half-breeds, it could just be a matter of time before they start eyeing the Nevernever." She paced back to her throne, deep in thought. "Mab and Oberon will be skeptical, of course," she said in a half weary, half exasperated voice. "They're going to want proof before they act on anything."

"What about Todd?" I asked.

She turned back with an apologetic look. "I'll put out feelers in the mortal realm," she offered, "see if the gremlins or hacker elves can turn anything up. But my first responsibility is to my own kingdom, Ethan. And you."

I didn't like where this was going. It didn't sound as if she would try terribly hard to find Todd, and why would she? She was a queen who'd just been informed her entire kingdom could be threatened soon. The life of a single half-breed wasn't a high priority.

Meghan glanced at Kenzie, who looked confused but still trying to follow along as best she could. "I'll have someone take you home," she said kindly. "I'm sorry you had to go through all this. You should also be aware that time in the Nevernever flows differently than time in the mortal realm, which means you've probably been missing for several days now."

"Right," said Kenzie, a little breathlessly. "So, I'll have to make up a really good story for when I get home. I don't think 'stuck in Faeryland' is going to go over well."

"Better than the alternative," I told her. "At least you can lie and they'll believe you. After this, my parents aren't going to let me out of the house until I'm thirty."

Meghan gave me a sad smile. "I'll send someone over to explain what's happened," she said, and my nervousness increased. "But Ethan, I can't let you go home just yet. Until we figure out what's going on, I have to ask you to stay here, in Mag Tuiredh."

CHAPTER FOURTEEN
KEIRRAN

"Screw that!"

I glared at Meghan, feeling the walls of the Iron Court close in. She watched me sadly, though her stance and the determined look on her face didn't change.

"No way," I said. "Forget it. You can't keep me here. I have to get home! I have to find Todd. And to see if Mom and Dad are all right. You said it yourself—they're probably going crazy by now."

"I'll send someone to explain what's going on," Meghan said again, her voice and expression unyielding. "I'll go myself, if I must. But I can't send you home yet, Ethan. Not when something out there is trying to kill you."

"I'm fine!" I protested, somehow feeling like a toddler again, arguing to stay up one more hour. "Dammit, I'm not four anymore, Meghan. I can take care of myself."

Meghan's gaze hardened. Striding up to me, she reached out and pulled up my sleeve, revealing the filthy, bloody bandages wrapped around my arm. I jerked back, scowling, but it was too late.

"You're not as invincible as you think, little brother," Meghan said firmly. "And I won't put Mom and Luke through that again. They've been through enough. I can at least tell them that you're safe and that you'll be home soon. Please understand, I don't want to do this to you, Ethan. But you can't leave just yet."

"Try to stop me," I snarled, and whirled around intending to stalk out of the throne room. A stupid move, but my anger—at myself, at the fey, the Nevernever, everything— had emerged full force, and I wasn't thinking rationally. "I'll find my own way home."

I didn't make it out of the room.

A figure melted out of the shadows in the corner, stepping in front of the door, a sharp silhouette against the light. He moved like darkness itself, silent and smooth, dressed all in black, his eyes glittering silver as he blocked my exit. I hadn't noticed him until now, but as soon as he appeared, my gut contracted with hatred and the blood roared in my ears. A memory flickered to life: a scene of moonlight and shadows, and sitting on the couch with Mom and Meghan as the door slowly creaked open, spilling his shadow across the floor. Of this faery, stepping into the room, his eyes only for my sister. He'd said that it was time; he'd spoken of bargains and promises, and Meghan hadn't resisted. She'd followed him out the door and into the night, and from then on, nothing was the same.

I took a deep breath, trying to calm my shaking hands. How many nights in kali had I imagined fighting this very demon, taking my rattan and smashing in his inhumanly pretty face, or stabbing him repeatedly with my knife? Wild fantasies— I stood no chance against someone like him, even I realized that. And I knew Meghan…cared for him. Loved him, even. But this was the fey responsible for the state of our sad, broken family. If he'd never come to our house that night, Meghan would still be home.

I raised my weapons and spoke through gritted teeth. "Get. The hell. Out of my way, Ash."

The dark faery didn't move. "You hate me, I can understand that," Ash said, his voice low and soothing. "But you're being irrational. Meghan is only trying to keep you safe."

Rage and frustration flared, thirteen years of hurt, fear and anger, all bursting to the surface at once. "You know, I don't remember asking her to!" I seethed, knowing I was way out of line and not caring. "Where was she when I was growing up, when I couldn't go to sleep because I could hear faeries outside my window? Where was she when they followed me to the school bus, when they chased me into the library and set it on fire, trying to flush me out? Or when I ruined a girl's life, because the damned fey can't seem to leave me alone? Where was she then, Ash?"

"Enough."

I shivered, looking back. Meghan's voice had changed. It was now steely with authority, and the girl who faced me when I turned around was no longer my sister. The Iron Queen stood there, blue eyes flashing in the aura of power that glowed around her.

"That's enough," she said again, quietly, as the magic flickered and died. "Ethan, I'm sorry, but I've made my decision. You'll remain in the Iron Court until we can find out what's going on. You'll be a guest in the palace, but please don't try to leave the grounds." She exhaled, her shoulders slumping wearily. "Let's hope we can figure this out quickly."

"You'll keep your own brother hostage?" I spat at her. "Against his will?"

"If I must." Meghan didn't flinch as she stared at me, solemn and grave. "You can be angry with me all you want, Ethan. I'm not going to lose you."

I sneered, lowering my weapons. "It's a little late, sister. You lost me a long time ago, when you walked out on us."

It was a low blow, meant to hurt her, and I was sorry as soon as I said it. Meghan's lips pressed together, but other than that, she didn't respond. I did feel a sharp chill at my back, and realized I was pushing Ash dangerously, as well, speaking to his queen like that. My relation to Meghan was likely the only thing keeping him from drawing his sword and demanding I apologize.

Good, I thought. *How does it feel, Ash? Not being able to do anything? Being forced to just watch events unfold around you? Pretty damn frustrating, huh?*

The Iron Queen turned back to the throne. "Grimalkin," she said softly, and the cat raised his head from where he'd been curled up in the corner, blinking sleepily. "Will you be able to take Mackenzie home? You know the way, right?"

Crap. I'd forgotten about Kenzie. Again. What did she think of all of this—this morbid family drama, with me at my very worst, lashing out at everyone around me?

God, she must think I'm an absolute freak.

Grimalkin yawned, but before he could reply, Kenzie stepped forward. "No," she said, and Meghan glanced back in surprise. I blinked at her, as well. "I'd like to stay, please. If Ethan isn't going home, then I'm not leaving, either."

"Kenzie, you don't have to stay," I muttered, though the thought of her leaving made me realize how alone I really was. "Go home. I'll be fine."

She shook her head. "No, it's partially my fault that we're here. I'm not going anywhere until we can leave together."

I wanted to argue, but at the same time, a part of me desperately wanted her to stay. It was selfish, that small piece that didn't want to be alone, even among those who were supposed to be family. Because, even though Meghan was my sister, she was still the Iron Queen, still fey, and I was a human intruder in her world.

Meghan nodded. "I won't force you," she said, annoying me that Kenzie had a choice and I didn't get one. "Stay if you wish—it might be safer for you here, anyway. Though I'm not sure when this issue will be resolved. You may be with us for some time."

"That's all right." Kenzie glanced at me and smiled bravely. "It's been several days in the real world, right? I might as well stay. I probably can't dig myself any deeper."

Ash moved, gliding into the room to stand by Meghan's side. I noticed he watched her carefully, as if she were the only person in the room, the only presence that mattered. I could be a gnat on the wall for all he cared. "I'll tell Glitch to send a message to the other courts," he said. "With Elysium approaching, we'll need to call this gathering soon."

Meghan nodded. "Grimalkin," she called, and the cat sauntered up, blinking lazily. "Will you please show Ethan and Kenzie to the guest quarters? The rooms in the north wing over the garden should be empty. Ethan…" Her clear blue eyes fixed on me, though they seemed tired and weary now. "For now, just stay. Please. We'll talk later, I promise."

I shrugged, not knowing what to say, and when the silence stretched between us, the queen nodded in dismissal. We followed Grimalkin out of the throne room and into the hall, where the motionless Iron knights lined the corridor. I glanced back at my sister as the doors started to close and saw her standing in the center of the room, one hand covering her face. Ash reached out, silently drawing her into him, and then the doors banged shut, hiding them from view.

You really are a jackass, aren't you? Guilt and anger stabbed at every part of me. *You haven't seen Meghan in years, and when you finally get to talk to her, what do you do? Call her names and try to make her feel guilty. Yeah, that's great, Ethan. Pushing people away is the only thing you know how to do, isn't it? Wonder what Kenzie thinks of you now?*

I stole a glance at her as we made our way down the halls of the Iron Court. Gremlins scuttled over the walls, laughing and making the lights flicker, and Iron knights stood like metal statues every dozen or so feet. I could feel their eyes on us as we passed, as well as the curious stares of the gremlins and every other Iron faery in the castle. If I wanted to get out of here unseen, it was going to be challenging to impossible.

Kenzie saw me looking at her and smiled. "Your sister seems nice," she offered as Grimalkin turned a corner without slowing down or looking back. "Not what I was expecting. I didn't think she would be our age."

I shrugged, grateful for the shift of focus, the chance to talk about something other than what had happened in the throne room. "She's not. Well, technically that's not right. I guess she is, but…" I struggled to explain. "When I saw her last, several years ago, she looked exactly the same. She doesn't age. None of them do. If I live to be a hundred years old, she still won't look a day over sixteen."

"Oh." Kenzie blinked. A strange look crossed her face, that same look I had seen back in Grimalkin's cave; thoughtful and excited, when she should have been disbelieving and terrified. "So, what about us? If we stay in the Nevernever, do we stop aging, too?"

I narrowed my eyes, not liking this sudden interest or the thought of staying here. But Grimalkin, sitting at a pair of doors facing each other across the wide hall, raised his head and yawned.

"Not to the extent that you are immortal," he explained, eying us lazily. "Humans in the Nevernever do age, but at a much slower rate. Sometimes countless years will pass before they notice any signs of decay. Sometimes they remain infants for centuries, and then one day they simply wake up old and withered. It is different for everyone." He yawned again and licked a paw. "But, no, human. Mortals cannot live forever. Nothing lives forever, not even the immortal Fey."

"And don't forget time is screwy here," I added, frowning at the contradiction but deciding to ignore it. "You might spend a year in Faery and go home to find twenty years have passed, or a hundred years. We don't want to stay here any longer than we have to."

"Relax, Ethan. I wasn't suggesting we buy a vacation home in the wyldwood." Kenzie's voice was light, but her gaze was suddenly far away. "I was just...wondering."

Grimalkin sniffed. "Well. Now, I am bored."

He stood, arched his tail over his back as he stretched, and trotted off down the hall. Even before he turned the corner, he vanished from sight.

I eyed the guards stationed very close to the "guest suites," and resentment simmered. "Guess these are our rooms, then," I said, crossing the hall and nudging a door open. It swung back to reveal a large room with a bed against one wall, a fireplace on the other and two giant glass doors leading to a balcony outside. "Fancy," I muttered, letting the door creak shut. "Nicest jail cell I've ever been in."

Kenzie didn't answer. She still stood in the same spot, gazing down the corridor where Grimalkin had vanished, her expression remote. I walked back, but she didn't look at me.

"Hey." I reached out and touched her elbow, and she started. "You all right?"

She took a breath and nodded. "Yeah," she said, a little too brightly. "I'm fine, just tired." She sighed heavily, rubbing her eyes. "I think I'm gonna crash for a bit. Wake me up when they announce dinner or something, okay?"

"Sure."

As I watched her walk toward her room, amazement and guilt clawed at me, fighting an equal battle within. Kenzie was still here. *Why* was she still here? She could've gone home, back to her family and friends and a normal life. Back to the real world. Instead, she'd chosen to stay in this crazy, upside-down nightmare where nothing made sense. I only hoped she would live to regret it.

"Ethan," Kenzie said as I turned away. I looked back, and she smiled from across the hall. "If you need to talk," she said softly, "about anything...I'm here. I'm willing to listen."

My heart gave a weird little lurch. No one had ever told me that, not with any real knowledge of what they were getting into. *Oh, Kenzie. I wish I could. I wish I could...tell you everything, but I won't do that to you. The less you know about Them—and me—the better.*

"To my whining?" I snorted, forcing a half grin. "Very generous of you, but I think I'll be fine. Besides, this is just another way of wheedling an interview out of me, right?"

"Darn, I've become predictable." Kenzie rolled her eyes and pushed her door open. "Well, if you change your mind, the offer still stands. Just knock first, okay?"

I nodded, and her door swung shut, leaving me alone in the hall.

For a moment, I thought about exploring the palace, seeing what my sister's home looked like, maybe checking for possible escape routes. But I had the feeling Meghan was keeping a close eye on me. She was probably expecting me to try something. I caught the impassive gaze of an Iron knight, watching me from the end of the hall, heard the gremlins snickering at me from the ceiling, and resentment boiled. She had no right to keep me here, especially after she was the one who'd left. She had no say in my life.

But they were watching me, a whole realm of Iron fey, making sure I wouldn't do anything against their queen's wishes. I didn't want a pack of gremlins trailing me through the palace, ready to scamper off to warn Meghan. And truthfully, I was exhausted. If I *was* going to pull something off, I needed to be awake and alert to do it.

Ignoring the buzz and snickers of the gremlins, I pushed my door open again. Thankfully, they didn't follow.

The room seemed even larger from inside, the high windows and arched balcony doors filling the air with sunlight. I spared a quick glance outside, confirming that the garden was several stories down and crawling with fey, before flopping back on the bed. My rattan dropped to the carpet, and I left them there, still within easy reach. Lacing my hands behind my head, I stared blankly at the ceiling.

Wonder what Mom and Dad are doing right now? I thought, watching the lines in the plaster blur together, forming strange creatures and leering faces. *They'll probably stick an ankle bracelet on me after this. I wonder if they've called the police yet, or if Mom suspects that I'm here.* I remembered my last words to Mom, snapped out in frustration and anger, and closed my eyes. *Dammit, I have to get back to the real world. Meghan isn't going to look hard for Todd. I'm the only one who has a chance of finding him.*

But there'd be no getting out today. Beyond this room, Meghan's Iron fey would be watching my every move. And I didn't know any trods from the Iron Court back to the real world.

My eyes grew heavy, and the faces in the ceiling blurred and floated off the plaster. I closed my eyes, feeling relatively safe for the first time since coming to the Nevernever, and let myself drift off.

★ ★ ★

A faint tapping sound had me bolting upright.

The room was dark. Silvery light filtered in from the windows, throwing long shadows over the floor. Beyond the glass, the sky was twilight-blue, dotted with stars that sparkled like diamonds. I gazed around blearily, noting that someone had left a tray of food on the table on the opposite wall. The moonlight gleamed off the metallic plate covers.

Swinging myself off the bed, I rubbed my eyes, wondering what had woken me. Maybe it was just a lingering nightmare, or I'd just imagined I'd heard the tap of something against the window....

Looking through the glass, my skin prickled, and I snatched a rattan from the side of the bed. Something crouched on the balcony railing, silhouetted against the sky, peering through the glass with the moonlight blazing down on him. It glimmered off his silver hair and threw his shadow across the balcony and into the room. I saw the gleam of a too-bright eye, the flash of perfectly white teeth as he grinned at me.

It was the faery from the courtyard, the gentry who had been practicing with the knight this afternoon. He was dressed in loose clothing of blue and white, with a leather strap across his chest, the hilt of a sword poking up behind one shoulder. Intense, ice-blue eyes glowed in the darkness as he peered through the glass and waved.

Gripping my weapon, I walked to the balcony doors and yanked them open, letting in the breeze and the sharp scent of metal. The faery still crouched on the railing, perfectly balanced, his elbows resting on his knees and a faint smile on his face. The wind tossed his loose hair, revealing the tips of the pointed ears knifing away from his head. I raised my stick and gave him a hard smile.

"Let me guess," I said, sliding through the door onto the

balcony. "You heard about the human in the castle, so you decided to come by and have a little fun? Maybe give him nightmares or put centipedes in his pillowcase?

The faery grinned. "That wasn't very friendly of me," he said in a surprisingly soft, clear voice. "And here I thought I was dropping by to introduce myself." He stood, easily balancing on the rails, still smiling. "But if you're so sold on me putting centipedes in your bed, I'm sure I can find a few."

"Don't bother," I growled at him, narrowing my eyes. "What do you want?"

"You're Ethan Chase, right? The queen's brother?"

"Who's asking?"

The faery shook his head. "They said you were hostile. I see they weren't exaggerating." He hopped off the railing, landing soundlessly on the veranda. "My name is Keirran," he continued in a solemn voice. "And I was hoping we could talk."

"I have nothing to say to you." Alarm flickered. If this faery had come by to propose a deal, I was beyond not interested. "Let me save you some time," I continued, staring him down. "If the next sentence out of your mouth includes the words *deal, bargain, contract, favor* or anything of the sort, you can leave right now. I don't make deals with your kind."

"Not even if I'm offering a way out of the Iron Realm? Back to the mortal world?"

My heart jumped to my throat. *Back to the mortal world. If I can go home…if I can get Kenzie home, and find Todd… I'd accomplished what I'd come here to do; I'd alerted Meghan to the threat of these new fey, and I doubted she was going to bring me into her inner circle anytime soon, not with her being so adamant about keeping me "safe." I had to get home. If this faery knew a way…*

Shaking my head, I took a step back. *No.* The fey always offered what you wanted the most, tied up in a pretty, sparkling package, and it always came at a high, high price. Too high a price. "No," I said out loud, firmly banishing any temptation to hear him out. "Forget it. Like I said, I don't make deals with you people. Not for anything. I have nothing to offer you, so go away."

"You misunderstand me." The faery smiled, holding up a hand. "I'm not here to bargain, or make a deal or a trade, or anything like that. I simply know a way out of the Iron Realm. And I'm offering to lead you there, free of charge. No obligation whatsoever."

I didn't trust him. Everything I knew was telling me this was some sort of trap, or riddle or faery word game. "Why would you do that?" I asked cautiously.

He shrugged, looking distinctly fey, and leaped onto the railing again. "Truthfully? Mostly because I'm *bored,* and this seems as good a reason to get out of here as any. Besides—" he grinned, and his eyes sparkled with mischief "—you're looking for a half-breed, right? And you said the exiles and half-breeds are disappearing from the mortal realm." I narrowed my eyes, and he made a placating gesture. "Gremlins talk. I listened. You want to find your friend? I know someone who might be able to help."

"Who?"

"Sorry." Keirran crossed his arms, still smiling. "I can't tell you until you've agreed you're coming along. You might go to the queen otherwise, and that would ruin it." He hopped onto one of the posts, inhumanly graceful, and beamed down at me. "Not to brag, but I'm sort of an expert at getting into and out of places unseen. But if we're going to leave, it should be soon. So, what's your answer? Are you coming, or not?"

This still seemed like a bad idea. I didn't trust him, and despite what he said, no faery did anything for free. Still, who knew how long it would take Meghan to figure out what was going on, how long before she would let me go? I might not get another chance.

"All right," I muttered, glaring up at him. "I'll trust you for now. But I'm not leaving Kenzie behind. She's coming with us, no matter what you say."

"I'd already planned for it." Keirran grinned more widely and crouched down on the pole. "Go on and get her, then," he said, looking perfectly comfortable, balanced on the top. "I'll wait for you here."

I drew back, grabbed my other stick from under the bed, and walked to the door, feeling his piercing eyes on me the whole way.

I half expected to find my door locked, despite Meghan's assurances that I was a guest in the palace. But it opened easily, and I slipped into the obscenely bright hallway, lit by glowing lanterns and metallic chandeliers. The guards were still there, pretending not to notice me as I crossed the hall to Kenzie's room.

Her door was closed, but as I lifted my knuckles to tap on it, I paused. Beyond the wood, I could hear faint noises coming from inside. Soft, sniffling, gasping noises. Worried, I reached down and quietly turned the handle. Her door was also unlocked, and it swung slowly inward.

Kenzie sat on the bed with her back to me, head bowed, her delicate shoulders heaving as she sobbed into the pillow held to her chest. Her curtains had been drawn, except for one, and a thin strand of moonlight eased through the crack and fell over her, outlining the small, shaking body.

"Kenzie." Quickly, I shut the door and crossed the room, coming to stand beside her. "Are you all right?" I asked, feeling completely stupid and awkward. Of course she wasn't all right; she was crying her eyes out into her pillow. I fully expected her to tell me to leave, or make some snarky comment that I totally deserved. But she wiped her eyes and took a deep breath, trying to compose herself.

"Yeah," she whispered, hastily rubbing a palm over her cheeks. "Sorry. I'm fine. Just…feeling a little overwhelmed, I guess. I think it's finally caught up to me."

I noticed her keys then, glinting on the mattress, and a small photograph encased in a plastic keychain. Looking to her for permission, I picked it up, making the keys jingle softly, and examined the picture. Kenzie and a small, dark-haired girl of maybe ten smiled up at me, faces close together. Kenzie's arm was raised slightly as if she was holding a camera up in front of them.

"My sister," she explained as I glanced back at her. "Alex. Or Alexandria. I'm not the only one in my family with a long, complicated name." She smiled, but I could see her trying to be brave, to not burst into tears again. "Actually, she's my stepsister. My mom died three years ago, and a year after that Dad remarried. I…I always wanted a sibling…." Her eyes glimmered in the darkness, and her voice caught. "We were supposed to go to the lake house this weekend. But…I don't know what's happening to them now. I don't know if they think I'm dead, or kidnapped or if Alex is waiting up for me to come home—" She buried her face in her pillow again, muffling her sobs, and I couldn't watch any longer.

Putting down the keys, I sat beside her and pulled her into my arms. She leaned against me and I held her quietly as she cried herself out. Dammit, here I was again, thinking only of myself. Why had it come to this before I realized Kenzie had a family, too? That she was just as worried for them as I was for mine?

"You never said anything," I murmured as her trembling subsided, trying not to make it sound like an accusation. "You didn't tell me you had a sister."

A shaky little laugh. "You didn't seem particularly open to listening, tough guy," she whispered back. "Besides, what could we do about it? You were already trying to get us out as fast as you could. Me whining about my home life wasn't going to speed anything up."

"Why didn't you go back this afternoon?" I pulled back to look at her. "Meghan offered to take you home. You could've gone back to your family."

"I know." Kenzie sniffed, wiping her eyes. "And I wanted to. But…we came here together, and I wouldn't have gotten this far…without you." She dropped her head, speaking quietly, almost a whisper. "I'm fully aware that you've saved my life on more than one occasion. With all the weirdness and faery cats and bloodthirsty snake monsters and everything else, I would've been dead if I had to do this by myself. It wouldn't be right, going back alone. And besides, I still have a lot to see here." She looked up at me then, her eyes wide and luminous in the shadows of the room. Her cheeks were tinged with color, though she still spoke clearly. "So, either we get out of here together, or not at all. I'm not leaving without you."

We stared at each other. Time seemed to slow around us, the moonlight freezing everything into a cold, silent portrait. Kenzie's face still glimmered with tears, but she didn't move. Heart pounding, I gently brushed a bright blue strand from her eyes, and she slid a cool hand up to my neck, soft fingers tracing my hairline. I shivered, unsure if I liked this strange, alien sensation twisting the pit of my stomach, but I didn't want it to stop, either.

What are you doing, Ethan? a voice whispered in my head, but I ignored it. Kenzie was watching me with those huge, trusting brown eyes, solemn and serious now, waiting. My heart contracted painfully. I didn't deserve that trust; I knew I should pull away, walk out, before this went too far.

A loud tap on the window made us both jump apart. Rising, I glared out the one open window, where a silver-headed face peered in curiously.

Kenzie yelped, leaping up, and I grabbed her arm. "It's all right!" I told her, as she looked at me in shock. "I know him. He's…here to help."

"Help?" Kenzie repeated, glaring at the fey boy, who waved at her through the glass. "Looks more like spying to me. What does he want?"

"I'll tell you in a second."

I opened the balcony doors, and Keirran ducked into the room. "So," the faery said, smiling as he came in, "Here we all are. I thought something might've happened to you, but if I'd known what was going on, I wouldn't have interrupted." His gaze slid to Kenzie, and his smile widened. "And you must be Kenzie," he said, walking over and taking her hand. But instead of shaking it, he brought her fingers to his lips, and she blushed. I stiffened, tempted to stride over and yank him away, but he dropped her hand before I could move. "My name's Keirran," he said in that soft, confident voice, and I noticed Kenzie gazing up at him with a slightly dazed look on her face. "Has Ethan told you the plan yet?"

Kenzie blinked, then glanced at me, confused. "What plan?"

I stepped between them, and the faery retreated with a faintly amused look. "We're leaving," I told her in a low voice. "Now. We don't have time for Meghan to decide to send us home—we have to find Todd now. Keirran says he knows a way out of the Nevernever. He's taking us back to the mortal world."

"Really?" Kenzie shot the fey boy a look, but it was more of curiosity than distrust. "Are you sure?"

The faery bowed. "I swear on my pointed ears," he said, before straightening with a grin. "But, like you said, we should leave now. While most of the castle is asleep." He gestured out the window. "The trod isn't far. We'll just have to get to it without anyone seeing us. Come on."

I snatched my weapons, gave Kenzie a reassuring nod, and together we followed the faery out the balcony doors onto the veranda. The night air was cool, and the silver moon seemed enormous, hovering so close I could practically see craters and ridges lining the surface. Below us, the garden was quiet, though the moonlight still glinted off the armor of several knights stationed throughout the perimeter.

Kenzie peered over the ledge, then drew back quickly. "There are so many guards," she whispered, looking back at Keirran. "How are we going to make it through without anyone seeing us?"

"We're not going that way," Keirran replied, hopping lightly onto the railing. He gazed up at the roof of the palace, at the great spires and towers lancing toward the sky. Putting two fingers to his lips, he blew out a soft whistle.

A knotted rope flew down from one of the towers, uncoiling in midair, dropping toward us with a faint hiss. Keirran glanced back at me and grinned.

"Hope you're not afraid of heights."

Even with a rope, it was difficult to scale the walls of the Iron Queen's palace. This high up, most of them were sheer metal or glass, making it hard to get a foothold. Keirran, unsurprisingly, moved like a squirrel or a spider, scrambling from ledge to ledge with the obnoxious natural grace of his kind. I had a hard time keeping up, and Kenzie struggled badly, though she never made a sound of complaint. We rested when we could, perched on narrow shelves that gave a stunning view of the city at night. Mag Tuiredh sparkled below us, a glittering carpet of lights and polished edges that reflected the moon. Even I had to admit, Meghan's kingdom was strangely beautiful under the stars.

"Come on," Keirran said encouragingly from a ledge above us. "We're almost there."

Heaving myself up the last wall, I turned and reached over the edge, pulling Kenzie up behind me. Her arms trembled as she took my hand and dragged herself onward, but as she reached the top, her legs gave out and she collapsed.

I caught her as she sagged against me, backing away from the edge. She shivered in my arms, her heart beating way too fast, her skin pale and cold. Wrapping my arms around her, I turned so that my body was between her and the slicing wind, feeling her delicate frame pressed against mine. Her fingers tangled in my shirt, and I wondered if she could feel the pounding beneath her palm.

"Sorry," Kenzie whispered, pulling away, standing on her own. She still kept a slender hand on my chest to steady herself, a tiny spot of warmth in the cold. "I guess a career in rock climbing isn't in my future."

"You don't have to do this," I told her gently, and she gave me a warning look. "You can stay here, and Meghan will send you back home—"

"Don't make me push you off this roof, tough guy."

Shaking my head, I followed her across a narrow rooftop flanked by a pair of towers, the wind whipping at our hair and clothes. Keirran stood a few feet away, talking to what looked like three huge copper and brass insects. Their "wings" looked like the sails on a hang glider, and their long dragonfly bodies were carried on six shiny jointed legs that gleamed in the cold light. As we stared, the creatures' heads turned in our direction, their eyes huge and multifaceted. They buzzed softly.

"These," Keirran said, smiling as he turned back to us,

"are gliders. They're the quickest and easiest way to get out of Mag Tuiredh without being seen. You just have to know how to avoid the air patrols, and luckily, I'm an expert." He scratched one glider on the head as if it was a favorite dog, and the thing cooed in response.

Standing beside me, Kenzie shuddered. "We're flying out of here on giant bugs?" she asked, eyeing the gliders as if they might swarm her any second.

"Be nice," Keirran warned. "They get their feelings hurt easily."

"Master!"

A different sort of buzz went through the air then, and a second later, something small, dark and fast zipped by us, leaping at Keirran with a shrill cry. Keirran winced but didn't move, and the tiny creature landed on his chest, a spindly, bat-eared monster with eyes that flashed electric green. Kenzie jumped and pressed closer to me, whispering: "What is *that?*"

"That's a gremlin," I answered, and she stared at me. "Yeah, it's exactly what you think it is. You know those sudden, un-explainable glitches when something just breaks, or when your computer decides to crash? Say hello to what causes it."

"Not all of them," Keirran said mildly, as the tiny fey scrab-bled to his shoulders, buzzing madly. "Give some credit to the bugs and the worms, too." He held up a hand. "Razor, calm down. Say hi to our new friends."

The gremlin, now perched on Keirran's arm, turned to stare at us with blazing green eyes and started crackling like a bad radio station.

"They can't understand you, Razor," Keirran said mildly. "English."

"Oh," said the gremlin. "Right." It grinned widely, baring a mouthful of sharp teeth that glowed neon-blue. "Hiiiiiiii."

"He knows French and Gaelic, too," Keirran said, as Razor

cackled and bounced on his shoulder. "It's surprisingly sim-ple to teach a gremlin. People just underestimate what they're capable of."

Before we could say anything about this bizarre situation, Keirran plucked the gremlin off his shoulder and tossed it on the glider, where it scrambled to the front and peered out ea-gerly. "Shall we get going?" he asked, and the glider's wings fluttered in response. "Gliders are easy to control," he con-tinued with absolute confidence, while I gave him a look that implied the exact opposite. "Steer them by pulling on their front legs and shifting your weight from side to side. They'll basically do the rest. Just watch me and do what I do."

He stepped to the edge of the roof and spread his arms. In-stantly, the glider picked its way across the roof and crawled up his back, curling its legs around his chest and stomach. He glanced back at us and winked.

"Your turn."

A cry of alarm echoed from somewhere below, making me jump. I peered down and saw a packrat on the balcony of Kenzie's room, looking around wildly.

"Uh-oh," Keirran muttered, sounding remarkably calm. "You've been discovered. If we're going to do this, we need to do it now, before Glitch and the entire air squad is up here looking for us. Hurry!"

Without waiting for an answer, he dove off the building. Kenzie gasped, watching him plunge toward the ground, a streak of silver and gold. Then the glider's wings caught the breeze, and it swooped into the air again, circling the tower. I heard the gremlin's howl of glee, and Keirran waved to us as he soared by.

I glanced at Kenzie. "Can you do this? It's probably just going to get more dangerous from here on out."

Her eyes flashed, and she shook her head. "I already told

you," she said, her voice firm. "We go home together, or not at all. What, you think I'm scared of a couple giant bugs?"

I shrugged. She did look pale and a bit creeped out, but I wasn't going to comment on it. Kenzie frowned and stalked forward, her lips pressed into that tight line again. I watched her walk to the edge of the roof, hesitate just a moment, and spread her arms as Keirran had done. She shook a little as the glider crawled up her back, but she didn't shy away, which was remarkable considering she had a monstrous insect perching on her shoulders. Peering off the roof, she took a deep breath and closed her eyes.

"Just like Splash Mountain at Disneyland," I heard her whisper. Then she launched herself into empty space. She plummeted rapidly, and a shriek tore free, nearly ripped away by the wind, but then the current caught her glider and she rose into the air after Keirran.

My turn. I stepped forward, toward the last glider, but a shout from below made me pause.

"Prince Ethan!" Glitch's head appeared as the First Lieutenant hauled himself up the rope and onto the roof. His hair sparked green and purple lightning as he held out his hand. "Your highness, no!" he cried, as I quickly raised my arms. The glider inched over and crawled up my back, achingly slow. "You can't leave. The queen ordered you to stay. Did Keirran talk you into this? Where is he?"

Glitch knows Keirran, does he? "I'm not staying, Glitch," I called, backing up as the First Lieutenant eased forward. The glider gave an annoyed buzz, hastily wrapping its legs around my middle as I overbalanced it. "Tell Meghan I'm sorry, but I have to go. I can't stay here any longer."

"Ethan!"

I turned and threw myself off the roof, clutching the glider's legs as it plunged toward the ground. For a second, I thought we would smash headfirst into the garden below, but then the glider swooped upward, climbing in a lazy arc, the wind whipping at my face.

Keirran dropped beside me, wearing his careless grin, as Glitch's shouts faded away behind us. "Not bad, for your first time," he said, nodding as Kenzie swooped down to join us. Razor cackled and bounced on his shoulder, huge ears flapping in the wind. "We need to hurry, though," the faery said, glancing behind us. "Glitch will go straight to the queen, and she is *not* going to be happy. With either of us. And if Ash decides to pursue..." For the first time, a worried look crossed his face. He shook it off. "The trod isn't far, but we'll have to cross into the wyldwood to get to it. Follow me."

The gliders were surprisingly fast, and from this height, the Iron Realm stretched out before us, beautiful and bizarre. Far below, the railroad cut through the grassy plateau, snaking between huge iron monoliths that speared up toward the sky and around bubbling pools of lava, churning red and gold in the darkness. We passed mountains of junk, metal parts glinting under the stars, and flew over a swamp where strands of lightning flickered and crawled over oily pools of water, mesmerizing and deadly.

Finally, we soared over a familiar canopy, where the trees grew so close together they looked like a lumpy carpet. Keirran's glider dropped down so that it was nearly brushing the tops of the branches.

"This way," I heard him call, and he dropped from sight, vanishing into the leaves. Hoping Kenzie and I wouldn't fly headfirst into the branches, I followed, passing through the canopy into an open clearing. Darkness closed on us instantly as the light of the moon and stars disappeared and the gloom of the wyldwood rose up to replace it.

I could just make out the bright gleam of Keirran's hair

through the shadows, and spiraled down, dodging branches, until my feet lightly touched the forest floor. As soon as I landed, the glider uncurled its legs and pulled itself up to an overhanging limb, clinging there like a huge dragonfly.

"Well," Keirran said, as Kenzie landed and her glider did the same, hanging next to mine. "Here we are."

An ancient ruin rose up before us, so covered in vines, moss and fungi it was nearly impossible to see the stones beneath. Huge gnarled trees grew from the walls and collapsed ceiling, thick roots snaking around the stones.

"The trod to the mortal realm is inside," Keirran explained, as Kenzie pressed close to me, staring at the ruins in amazement. I was tempted to reach down and take her hand, but I was glad I hadn't when Keirran abruptly drew his sword with a soft rasping sound. I glared at him and drew my weapons as well, putting myself between her and the faery. He glanced over his shoulder with a faintly apologetic look.

"Forgot to tell you," he said, gesturing to the ruin, "this place is normally unoccupied, but it is right in the middle of goblin territory. So, we might run into a few locals who won't be happy to see us. Nothing you can't handle, right?"

"You couldn't have told us earlier?" I growled as we started toward the ruins. Keirran shrugged, his curved steel blade cutting a bright path through the darkness. Razor chattered on his shoulder, only his eyes and neon grin visible in the gloom.

"It's just a few goblins. Nothing to—whoops."

He ducked, and a spear flew overhead, striking a nearby tree. Kenzie yelped, and Razor blipped out of sight like an image on a television screen as a chorus of raucous voices erupted from the ruins ahead. Glowing eyes appeared in the stones and among the roots. Pointed teeth, claws and spear tips flashed in the shadows, as about a dozen short, evil fey poured from the ruins and shook their weapons at us.

"A *few* goblins, huh?" I glared at Keirran and backed away. He grinned weakly and shrugged.

The goblins started forward, cackling and jabbing the air with their spears. I quickly turned to Kenzie and pressed one of my sticks into her hands.

"Take this," I told her. "I'll try to keep them off us, but if any gets too close, smack it as hard as you can. Aim for the eyes, the nose, whatever you can reach. Just don't let them hurt you, okay?"

She nodded, her face pale but determined. "Tennis lessons, don't fail me now." I started to turn, but she caught my wrist, holding it tightly as she gazed up at me. "You be careful, too, Ethan. We're going home together, okay? Just remember that."

I squeezed her hand and turned back to the approaching horde. Keirran was waiting for them calmly, sword in hand.

I joined him, and he gave me a curious look from the corner of his eye. "Interesting," he mused, smiling even as the horde prepared to attack. "I've never seen anyone fight goblins with half a broom handle."

I resisted the impulse to crack him in the head. "Just worry about yourself," I told him, twirling my weapon in a slow arc. "And I'll do the same."

A bigger, uglier goblin suddenly leaped onto a rock and leered at us. "Humans," he rasped with a flash of yellow teeth. "I thought I smelled something strange. You sure picked the wrong spot to stumble into. Trying to get home, are we?" He snickered, running a tongue along his jagged fangs. "We'll save you the trouble."

"We don't have to do this," Keirran said mildly, seemingly unconcerned about the approaching horde. "Surely there are other travelers you can accost."

The goblins edged closer, and I eased into a ready stance, feeling an almost savage glee as they surrounded us. No rules now; no teachers, principals or instructors to stop me. I felt the old anger rise up, the hatred for all of Faery bubbling to the surface, and grinned viciously. There was nothing to hold me back now; I didn't have to worry about hurting anyone. I could take my anger out on the goblins' ugly, warty skulls, and there would be no consequences.

"And miss out on three tasty humans, wandering through my territory?" The goblin chief snorted, shaking his head. "I don't think so. We eat well tonight, boys! Dibs on the liver!"

Cheering, the goblins surged forward.

One charged me with its spear raised, and I swung my rattan, felt my weapon connect beneath the goblin's jaw. It flew back with a shriek, and I instantly slashed down again, cracking another's lumpy green skull. A third goblin scuttled in from the other side, stabbing its spear up toward my face. I dodged, snaked my free arm around the spear, and yanked it out of the faery's grasp. It had a split second to gape in surprise before I bashed the side of its head with its own weapon and hurled it away.

Beside me, Keirran was moving, too, spinning and twirling like a dancer, his sword flashing in deadly circles. Though I couldn't see exactly what he was doing, he was inhumanly fast. Goblin body parts flew through the air, horrific and disgusting, before turning into mud, snails or other unpleasant things.

Three more goblins came at me, one of them the big goblin who'd spoken before, the chief. I shuffled away, blocking their attacks, whipping my rattan from one spear to the next. The frantic clacking of wood echoed in my ears as I waited for an opening, a chance to strike. The goblin's size was actually a handicap for me; they were so short, it was hard to hit them. A spear tip got through my defenses and tore through my sleeve, making me grit my teeth as I twisted away. Too close.

Suddenly, Kenzie was behind them, bringing her stick

smashing down on a goblin's head. It met with a satisfying crack, and the goblin dropped like a stone. Kenzie gave a triumphant yell, but then the chief whirled with a snarl of rage, swinging his spear at her legs. It struck her knee, and she crumpled to the dirt with a gasp.

The chief lunged forward, raising his spear, but before either of us could do anything, a tiny black form landed on his head from nowhere. Razor buzzed like a furious wasp, hissing and snarling as the goblin flailed.

"Bad goblin!" the gremlin howled, clinging like a leech. "Not hurt pretty girl! Bad!" He sank his teeth into the goblin's ear, and the chief roared. Reaching up, the goblin managed to grab the tiny Iron fey, tear him off, and hurl him into the brush.

With a snarl, I kicked a goblin into a stone wall, snatched Kenzie's rattan from the ground, and attacked the chief. I didn't see the other fey. I didn't see Keirran. I forgot everything Guro taught me about fighting multiple opponents. All I knew was that this thing had hurt Kenzie, had tried to kill her, and it was going to pay.

The goblin scuttled backward under my assault, frantically waving his spear, but I knocked it from his claws and landed a solid blow between his ears. As he staggered back, dazed, I pressed my advantage, feeling the crack of flesh and bone under my sticks. My rattan hissed through the air, striking arms, teeth, face, neck. The goblin fell, cringing, in the dirt, and I raised my weapons to finish it off.

"Ethan!"

Keirran's voice brought me up short. Panting, I stopped beating on the goblin and looked up to see that the rest of the tribe had run off with the fall of their chief. Keirran had already sheathed his weapon and was watching me with a half amused, half concerned expression. Kenzie still sat where she had fallen, clutching her leg.

"It's over," Keirran said, nodding to the empty forest around us. "They're gone."

I glanced at my sticks, and saw that my weapons, as well as my hands, were spattered with black goblin blood. With a shiver, I looked back at the chief, saw him curled around himself in the dirt, moaning through bloody lips, his teeth shattered and broken. My gut heaved, and I staggered away.

What am I doing?

The chief groaned and crawled away, and I let him go, watching the faery haul itself into the bushes. Through the horror and disgust of what I'd just done, I still felt a nasty glow of vindication. Maybe next time, they would think twice about assaulting three "tasty" humans.

Keirran watched it go as well, then walked over to Kenzie, holding out a hand. "Are you all right?" he asked, drawing her to her feet, holding her steady. I clenched my fists, wanting to stalk over there and shove him away from her. Kenzie grimaced, her face tightening with pain, but she nodded.

"Yeah." Her cheeks were pale as she gingerly put weight on her injured leg, wincing. "I don't think anything's broken. Though my knee might swell up like a watermelon."

"You're very lucky," Keirran went on, and all traces of amusement had fled his voice. "Goblins poison the tips of their weapons. If you'd gotten cut at all…well, let's just say a watermelon knee is better than the alternative."

Anger and fear still buzzed through me, making me stupid, wanting to hit something, though there was nothing left to fight. I turned my rage on Keirran, instead.

"What the hell is wrong with you?" I snarled, stalking forward, wanting him farther away from Kenzie. He flinched, and I swung my rattan around the clearing, at the disintegrating piles of goblin. "You knew there were goblins here, you knew we would have to fight our way out, and you still brought us this way. You could've gotten us killed! You could've gotten *Kenzie* killed! Or was that your plan all along? Bring the stupid humans along as bait, so the goblins will be distracted? I should've known never to trust a faery."

"Ethan!" Kenzie scowled at me, but Keirran held up a hand. "No, he's right," he murmured, and a flicker of surprise filtered through my anger. "I shouldn't have brought you this way. I thought I could deal with the goblins. If you had been seriously hurt, it would've been on my head. You have every reason to be angry." Turning to Kenzie, he bowed deeply, his gaze on the ground between them. "Forgive me, Mackenzie," he said in that clear, quiet voice. "I allowed pride to cloud my judgment, and you were injured because of it. I'm sorry. It won't happen again."

He sounded sincere, and I frowned as Kenzie quickly assured him it was all right. What kind of faery was he, anyway? The fey had no conscience, no real feelings of regret, no morals to get in the way of their decisions. Either Keirran was an exception or a very good actor.

Which reminded me…

"The chief said he smelled *three* humans," I told Keirran, who gave me a resigned look. "He didn't think you were fey. He thought you were human, too."

"Yeah." Keirran shrugged, offering a small grin. "I get that a lot."

Razor appeared on his shoulder with a buzzing laugh. "Stupid goblins," he crowed, bouncing up and down, making Keirran sigh. "Funny, stupid goblins think master is funny elf. Ha!" He buzzed once more and sat down, grinning like a psychotic piranha.

"You're a half-breed," I guessed, wondering how I hadn't

seen it earlier. He didn't look like any of the other Iron fey, but he couldn't be part of the Summer or Winter courts, either; normal fey couldn't enter the Iron Realm without harming themselves. (I was still trying to figure out how *Grimalkin* did it, but everything about that cat was a mystery.) But if Keirran was a half-breed, he didn't have the fey's deathly allergy to iron; his human blood would protect him from the ill effects of Meghan's court.

"I guess you could say that." Keirran sighed again and looked toward the trees, where most of the goblins had scattered. "More like three-quarters human, really. Can't blame them for thinking I was the real thing."

I stared at him. "Who are you?" I asked, but then the bushes snapped, and Keirran winced.

"I'll tell you later. Come on, let's get out of here. The goblins are coming back, probably with reinforcements."

I started to reach for Kenzie, but then I saw my hands, streaked with blood past my wrists, and let them drop. Keirran took her arm instead, helping her along, and she gave me an unreadable look as she limped past. I followed them up the stairs and ducked through the crumbling archway as furious cries echoed from the trees around us. The angry sounds faded as soon as I crossed the threshold, and everything went black.

GHOSTS OF THE FAIRGROUND

I emerged, squinting in the darkness, trying to see where I was. For a second, it didn't seem as if we'd left the Nevernever at all. Trees surrounded us, hissing in the wind, but I looked closer and saw they were regular, normal trees. A few yards away, three strands of barbed wire glinted in the moonlight, and beyond the wires, a scattering of fluffy white creatures peered at us curiously.

"Are those sheep?" Kenzie asked, sounding weary but delighted. Razor gave an excited buzz from Keirran's shoulder, leaped to the top of the first wire, and darted into the pasture. Sheep baaed in terror and fled, looking like clouds blowing across the field, and Keirran sighed.

"I keep telling him not to do that. They lose enough to the goblins as is."

"Where are we?" I asked, relieved to be back in the real world again, but not liking that I didn't know where we were. The wind here was cool, and the wooded hills beyond the pasture seemed to go on forever. Keirran watched Razor, buzzing happily from the back of a terrified sheep, and shook his head.

"Somewhere in rural Maryland."

"Maryland," I echoed in disbelief.

He grinned. "What, you think all trods lead to Louisiana?"

I took a breath to answer, but paused. *Wait. How does he know where I live?*

"Where to now?" Kenzie asked, grimacing as she leaned against a fencepost. "I don't think I'll be able to walk very fast with this knee. Someone might need to give me a piggyback ride later on."

"Don't worry." Keirran gestured over the rolling hills. "There's an abandoned fairground a couple miles from here. It's a hangout for the local fey, most of them exiled. The trod there will take us to where we need to go."

"And where is that?" I asked, but Keirran had moved up to the fence, peering over the wire at Razor, still tormenting the flock of sheep. "Razor!" he called over the bleating animals. "Come on, stop scaring the poor things. You're going to give them a heart attack."

The gremlin ignored him. I could just barely see him in the darkness, his electric-green eyes and glowing smile bouncing among the flock. I was about to suggest we just leave and let him catch up, when Kenzie stepped up to the fence, her expression puzzled.

"Where is he?" she asked, staring out over the field. "The sheep are going nuts, but I don't see Razor at all."

Oh, yeah. We were back in the real world now. Which meant Kenzie couldn't see the fey; they were invisible to humans unless they made a conscious effort to un-glamour themselves. I told her as much.

"Huh," she said in a neutral voice, then looked out over the pasture again, at the sheep racing through the grass like frantic clouds. A defiant expression crossed her face, and she took a breath.

"Razor!" she barked, making Keirran jump. "No! Bad gremlin! You stop that, right now!"

The gremlin, shockingly, looked up from where he was

bouncing on a rock, sheep scattering around him. He blinked and cocked his head, looking confused. Kenzie pointed to the ground in front of her.

"I want to see you. Come here, Razor. Now!"

And, he did. Blipping into sight at her feet, he gazed up expectantly, looking like a mutant Chihuahua awaiting commands. Keirran blinked in astonishment as she snapped her fingers and pointed at him, and Razor scurried up his arm to perch on his shoulder. She smiled, giving us both a smug look, and crossed her arms.

"Dog training classes," she explained.

The road stretched before us in the moonlight, a narrow strip of pavement that wove gently over and between the hills. Keirran led us on silently, Razor humming a raspy tune on his shoulder. No cars passed us; except for an owl and the flocks of sheep, snoozing in their pastures, we were alone.

"Wish I had my camera." Kenzie sighed as a black-faced ewe watched us from the side of the road, blinking sleepily. It snorted and trotted off, and Kenzie gazed after it, smiling. "Then again, maybe not. It might be weird, explaining how I could take pictures of the Maryland countryside when I never left Louisiana." She shivered, rubbing her arms as a cold breeze blew across the pasture, smelling of sheep and wet grass. I wished I had my jacket so I could offer it to her.

"What do you do?" Kenzie went on, her gaze still roaming the woods beyond the hills. "When you get home, I mean? We've been to Faeryland—we've seen things no one else has. What happens when you finally get home, knowing what you do, that no one else will ever understand?"

"You go back to what you were doing before," I replied. "You try to get on with your life and pretend it didn't happen. It'll be easier for you," I continued as she turned to me, frowning. "You have friends. Your life is fairly normal. You're not a freak who can see Them everywhere you go. Just try to forget about it. Forget the fey, forget the Nevernever, forget everything weird or strange or unnatural. Eventually, the nightmares will stop, and you might even convince yourself that everything you saw was a bad dream. That's the easiest way."

"Hey, tough guy, your bitterness is showing." Kenzie gave me an exasperated look. "I don't want to forget. Just burying my head in the sand isn't going to change anything. They'll still be out there, whether I believe in them or not. I can't pretend it never happened."

"But you won't ever see them," I said. "And that will either make you paranoid or drive you completely crazy."

"I'll still be able to talk to you, though, right?"

I sighed, not wanting to say it, but knowing I had to. "No. You won't."

"Why?"

"Because my life is too screwed up to drag you into it."

"Why don't you let me decide what's best for my life," Kenzie said softly, not quite able to mask her anger, the first I'd ever heard from her, "and who I want to be friends with?"

"What do you think is going to happen once we go home?" I asked, not meeting her stare. "You think I can be normal and hang out with you and your friends, just like that? You think your parents and your teachers will want you hanging around someone like me?"

"No," Kenzie said in that same low, quiet voice. "They won't. And you know what? I don't care. Because they haven't seen you like I have. They haven't seen the Nevernever, or the fey, or the Iron Queen, and they won't ever understand. *I* didn't understand." She paused, seeming to struggle with her next words. "The first time I saw you," she said, pushing her bangs from her eyes, "when we first talked, I thought you were this brooding, unfriendly, hostile, um..." She paused.

"Jerk," I finished for her.

"Well, yeah," Kenzie admitted slowly. "A pretty handsome jerk, I might add, but a huge, colossal megajerk nonetheless." She gave me a quick glance to see how I was taking this. I shrugged.

Not going to argue with that.

And then, a second later:

She thought I was handsome?

"At first, I just wanted to know what you were thinking." Kenzie pushed back her hair, the blue-and-black strands fluttering around her face. "It was more of a challenge, I guess, to get you to see me, to talk to me. You're the only one, in a very long time anyway, who talked to me like a real person, who treated me the same as everyone else. My friends, my family, even my teachers, they all tiptoe around me like I'm made of glass. They never say what they're really thinking if they feel it might upset me." She sighed, looking out over the fields. "No one is ever real with me anymore, and I'm sick and tired of it."

I held my breath, suddenly aware that I was very close to that dark thing Kenzie was hiding from me. *Tread softly, Ethan. Don't sound too eager or she might change her mind.* "Why is that?" I asked, trying to keep my voice light, like I didn't care. Wrong move.

"Um, because of my dad," Kenzie said quickly, and I swore under my breath, knowing I had screwed up. "He's this bigshot lawyer and everyone is terrified of him, so they pussyfoot around me, too. Whatever." She shrugged. "I don't want to talk about my dad. We were talking about you."

"The huge, colossal megajerk," I reminded her.

"Exactly. I don't know if you realize this, Ethan, but you're

a good-looking guy. People are going to notice you, bad-boy
reputation or not." I gave her a dubious look, and she nodded. "I'm serious. You didn't see the way Regan and the others were staring the first time you came into the classroom.
Chelsea even dared me to go up and ask if you had a girlfriend." One corner of her mouth curled in a wry grin. "I'm
sure you remember how *that* turned out."

I grimaced and looked away. *Yeah, I was a total jackass, wasn't
I? Believe me, if I could take back everything I said, I would. But it
wouldn't stop the fey.*

"But then, we came to the Nevernever," Kenzie went on,
gazing a few yards up the road, where Keirran's bright form
glided down the pavement. "And things started making a lot
more sense. It must be hard, seeing all these things, knowing
they're out there, and not being able to talk about it to anyone. It must be lonely."

Very lightly, she took my hand, sending electric tingles up
my arm, and my breath caught. "But you have me now," she
said in a near whisper. "You can talk to me…about Them.
And I won't tease or make fun or call you crazy, and you don't
have to worry about it frightening me. I *want* to know everything I can. I want to know about faeries and Mag Tuiredh
and the Nevernever, and you're my only connection to them
now." Her voice grew defiant. "So, if you think you can shut
me out of your life, tough guy, and keep me in the dark, then
you don't know me at all. I can be just as stubborn as you."

"Don't." I couldn't look at her, couldn't face the quiet sin-
cerity in her voice. Fear stirred, the knowledge that she was
only putting herself in danger the longer she stayed with me.
"There is no connection, Kenzie," I said, pulling my hand
from hers. "And I won't be telling you anything about the
fey. Not now, not ever. Just forget that you ever saw them,
and leave me alone."

Her stunned, hurt silence ate into me, and I sighed, stabbing my fingers through my hair. "You think I want to keep pushing people away?" I asked softly. "I don't enjoy being the freak, the one everyone avoids. I really, truly do not take pleasure in being a complete asshole." My voice dropped even lower. "Especially to people like you."

"Then why do it?"

"Because people who get close to me get hurt!" I snapped, finally whirling to face her. She blinked, and the memory of another girl swam through my head, red ponytail bobbing behind her, a spray of freckles across her nose. "Every time," I continued in a softer voice. "I can't stop it. I can't stop Them from following me. If it was just me that the fey picked on, I'd be okay with that. But someone else always pays for my Sight. Someone else always gets hurt instead of me." Tearing my gaze from hers, I looked out over the fields. "I'd rather be alone," I muttered, "than to have to watch that again."

"Again?"

"Hey," Keirran called from somewhere up ahead. "We're here."

Grateful for the interruption, I hurried to where the faery waited for us beneath the branches of a large pine by the side of the road. Striding through weeds, I followed Keirran's gaze to where the top of a Ferris wheel, yellow and spotted with rust, poked above the distant trees. Lights flickered through the branches.

"Come on," Keirran encouraged, sounding eager, and jogged forward. We followed, trailing him under branches, through knee-high grass and across an empty, weed-choked parking lot. Past a wooden fence covered in vines and ivy, the trees fell away, and we were staring at the remains of an abandoned fairground.

Though the park seemed empty, lanterns and torchlight

flickered erratically, lighting the way between empty booths, some still draped with the limp, moldy forms of stuffed animals. A popcorn cart lay overturned in the weeds a few yards away, the glass smashed, the innards picked clean by scavengers. We passed the bumper cars, sitting empty and silent on their tracks, and walked beneath a swing ride, the chains creaking softly in the wind. The carousel sat in the distance, peeling and rusted, dozens of once-colorful horses now flaking away with age and time.

Keirran skidded to a halt in front of a darkened funnel cake booth, his face grave. "Something is wrong," he muttered, turning slowly. "This place should be crawling with exiles. There's supposed to be a goblin market here year-round. Where is everyone?"

"Looks like your friend might not be here," I said, switching my sticks to both hands, just in case there was trouble. He didn't seem to hear me and abruptly broke into a sprint that took him between the midway aisles. Kenzie and I hurried after him.

"Annwyl!" he called, jogging up to a booth that at one point had featured a basketball game, as several nets dangled from the back wall. The booth was dark and empty, though flowers were scattered everywhere inside, dried stems and petals fluttering across the counter.

"Annwyl," Keirran said again, leaping easily over the wall, into the booth. "Are you here? Where are you?"

No one answered him. Breathing hard, the faery gazed around the empty stall for a moment, then turned and slammed his fist into the counter, making the whole structure shake. Razor squeaked, and Kenzie and I stared at him.

"Gone," he whispered, bowing his head, as the gremlin buzzed worriedly and patted his neck. "Where is she? Where is everyone? Are they all with *her?*"

"What's going on?" I leaned against the counter, brushing away drifts of petals and leaves. They had a rotten, sickly sweet smell, and I tried not to breathe in. "Who's with her? Who is Annwyl? Why—?"

I trailed off, my blood turning cold. Was it my imagination, or had I just seen a white shimmer float between the booths farther down the aisle? Carefully, I straightened, gripping my weapons, my skin starting to prickle with goose bumps. "Keirran, we have to get out of here now."

He looked up warily, reaching back for his weapon. And then, something slipped from the booths onto the dusty path, and we both froze.

At first, it looked like a giant cat. It had a sleek, muscular body, short fur and a long, thin tail that lashed its hindquarters. But when it turned its head, its face wasn't a cat's but an old, wrinkled woman's, her hair hanging limply around her neck, her eyes beady and cruel. She turned toward us, and I ducked behind the stall, pulling Kenzie down with me, as Keirran vanished behind the counter. I saw that the cat-thing's front paws were actually bony hands with long, crooked nails, but worst of all, her body flickered and shimmered in the air like heat waves. Like the creepy fey that had chased me and Kenzie into the Nevernever. Except this one seemed a bit more solid than the others. Not nearly so transparent.

I suddenly had a sinking suspicion of what had happened to the exiles.

Keirran squeezed through a crack in the cloth walls and crouched down beside us. "What is that?" he whispered, gripping his sword. "I've never seen anything like it before."

"I have." I peeked around the corner. The cat-thing was turning in slow circles, as if she knew something was there but couldn't see it. "Something similar took my friend and chased us—" I gestured to Kenzie and myself "—into the

Nevernever. I think they're the ones that have been kidnapping exiles and half-breeds."

Keirran's gaze darkened, and he suddenly looked extremely dangerous, eyes glowing with an icy light as he stood slowly. "Then perhaps we should make sure it doesn't hurt anyone else."

"You sure that's a good idea?"

"Ethan." Kenzie squeezed my arm, looking frightened but trying not to let it show. "I don't see it," she whispered. "I don't see anything."

"But the little boys can," hissed a voice behind us, and another cat-thing padded out of the darkness between the stalls.

I jumped to my feet, pulling Kenzie up with me. The cat-fey's wizened face creased in a smile, showing sharp feline teeth. "Little humans," she purred, as the other faery came around the corner, boxing us in. I shivered as the air around us grew cold. "You can see us and hear us. How encouraging."

"Who are you?" Keirran demanded, and raised his sword, pointing it at the nearest cat-thing. On his shoulder, Razor growled and buzzed at the faeries, baring his teeth. "What did you do to the exiles here?"

The cat-fey hissed and drew back at the sight of the iron weapon. "Not human," rasped the other behind us. "The bright one is not completely human. I can feel his glamour. He is strong." She growled, taking a step forward. "We should bring him to the lady."

I raised my sticks and eased back, closer to Keirran, trapping Kenzie between us. She glanced around wildly, trying to see the invisible threats, but it was obvious that she didn't even hear them.

The second cat-thing blinked slowly, running a tongue along her thin mouth. "Yes," she agreed, flexing her nails. "We will bring the half-breed to the lady, but it would be a shame to waste all that lovely glamour. Perhaps we will just take a little."

Her mouth opened, stretching impossibly wide, a gaping hole in her wrinkled face. I felt a ripple around us, a pulling sensation, as if the cat-fey was sucking the air into itself. I braced myself for something nasty, pressing close to Kenzie, but except for a faint sluggish feeling, nothing happened.

But Keirran staggered and fell to one knee, putting a hand against the booth to catch himself. As I stared, he seemed to fade a bit, his brightness getting dimmer, the color leeched from his hair and clothes. Razor screeched and flickered from sight, going in and out like a bad television station. The other faery cackled, and I glared at it, torn between helping Keirran and protecting the girl.

Suddenly, the cat-thing choked, convulsed and hurled itself back from Keirran. "Poison!" she screeched, gagging and heaving, as if she wanted to cough up a hairball. "Poison! Murder!" She spasmed again, curling in on herself as her body began to break apart, to dissolve like sugar in water. "Iron!" she wailed, clawing at the ground, at herself, her beady eyes wild. "He's an Iron abomination! Kill him, sister! Kill them all!"

She vanished then, blowing away in the breeze, as the other cat-thing screamed its fury and pounced.

I brought my rattan down, smashing it over the faery's skull, then sliding away to land a few solid blows on its shoulder. It screeched in pain and whirled on me, favoring its right leg. "So, you're real enough to hit, after all." I grinned. Snarling, it lunged, clawing at me, and I sidestepped again, angling out like Guro had taught me, whipping my rattan several times across the wizened face.

Shaking its head, the faery backed up, hissing furiously, one eye squeezed shut. Pale, silvery blood dripped from its mouth and jaw, writhing away as soon as it touched the ground. I

twirled my sticks and stepped closer, forcing it back. Kenzie
had retreated a few steps and was crouched next to Keirran; I
could hear her asking if he was all right, and his quiet assurance that he was fine.

"Boy," the cat-faery hissed, her lips pulled back in a snarl
of hate, "you will pay for this. You all will. When we return,
there will be nothing that will save you from our wrath."

Turning, the cat-thing bounded into the darkness between
the stalls and vanished from sight.

I breathed a sigh of relief and turned to Keirran, who was
struggling upright, one hand still on the booth wall. Razor
made angry, garbled noises on his shoulder, punctuated with
the words "Bad kitty!"

"You okay?" I asked, and he nodded wearily. "What just
happened there?"

"I don't know." He gave Kenzie a grateful smile and took a
step forward, standing on his own. "When that thing turned
on me, it felt like everything—my strength, my emotions,
even my memory—was being sucked out. It was...awful." He
shuddered, rubbing a forearm. "I feel like there are pieces of
me missing now, and I'll never get them back."

I remembered the dead piskie, the way she'd looked right
before she died, like all her color had been drained away. "It
was draining your magic," I said, and Keirran nodded. "So,
these things, whatever they are, they eat the glamour of regular fey, suck them dry until there's nothing left."

"Like vampires," Kenzie put in. "Vampire fey that hunt
their own kind." She wrinkled her nose. "That's creepy. Why
would they do that?"

I shook my head. "I have no idea."

"It got more than it bargained for, though," Keirran went
on, gazing at the spot where the cat-faery had died. "Whatever they are, it looks like they're still deathly allergic to iron."

"So they're not Iron fey, at least."

"No." Keirran shivered and dropped his hands. "Though I have no idea *what* they are."

"Keirran!"

The shout echoed down the rows, making Keirran jerk his head up, hope flaring in his eyes. A moment later, a willowy girl in a green-and-brown dress turned a corner and sprinted toward us. Keirran smiled, and Razor gave a welcoming buzz, waving his arms.

I tensed. The girl was fey, I could see that easily. The tips of her ears peeked up through her golden-brown hair, which was braided with vines and flowers and hung several inches past her waist. She had that unnatural grace of all fey, that perfect beauty where it was tempting to stare at her and completely forget to eat, sleep, breathe or anything else.

Keirran stepped forward, forgetting Kenzie and me completely, his eyes only for the faery approaching us. The fey girl halted just shy of touching him, as if she'd intended to fling herself into his arms but thought better of it at the last moment.

"Annwyl." Keirran hesitated, as if he, too, wanted to pull her close, only to decide against it. His gaze never left the Summer faery, though, and she didn't seem to notice the two humans standing behind him.

There was a moment of awkward silence, broken only by Razor, chattering on Keirran's shoulder, before the faery girl shook her head.

"You shouldn't be here, Keirran," she said, her voice lilting and soft, like water over a rock bed. "It's going to get you in trouble. Why did you come?"

"I heard what was happening in the mortal realm," Keirran replied, stepping forward and reaching for her hand. "I heard the rumor that something is out here, killing off exiles and half-breeds." His other hand rose as if to brush her cheek. "I had to come see you, to make sure you were all right."

Annwyl hesitated. Longing showed on her face, but she stepped back before Keirran could touch her. His eyes closed, briefly, and he let his arm drop. "You shouldn't be here," the girl insisted. "It isn't safe, especially now. There are...creatures."

"We saw," Keirran replied, and Annwyl gave him a frightened look. His gaze hardened, ice-blue eyes glinting dangerously. "Those things," he went on. "Is *she* aware of them? Is that why the market has been disbanded?"

The fey girl nodded. "She knows you're here," she replied in her soft, rippling voice. "She's waiting for you. I'm supposed to bring you to her. But..."

Her gaze finally slid to mine, and the large, moss-green eyes widened. "You brought mortals here?" she asked, sounding confused. "Who...?"

"Ah. Yes, where are my manners?" Keirran glanced back, as well, as if just remembering us. "I'm sorry. Ethan, this is Annwyl, formerly of the Summer Court. Annwyl, may I introduce...Ethan Chase."

The faery gasped. "Chase? The queen's brother?"

"Yes," Keirran said, and nodded to Kenzie. "Also, Kenzie St. James. They're both friends of mine."

I glanced at Keirran, surprised by the casual way he threw out the word *friends*. We'd only just met and were virtually strangers, but Keirran acted as if he'd known us far longer. But that was crazy; I'd never seen him before tonight.

Solemnly, the Summer faery pulled back and dropped into a deep curtsy, directed at me, I realized. "Don't," I muttered, waving it off. "I'm not a prince. You don't have to do that with me."

Annwyl blinked large, moss-green eyes. "But...you are,"

she said in her rippling voice. "You're the queen's brother. Even if you're not one of us, we—"

"I said it's fine." Briefly, I wondered what would happen if all faeries knew who I was. Would they treat me with respect and leave me alone? Or would my life get even more chaotic and dangerous, as they saw me as a weak link that could be exploited? I had a feeling it would be the latter. "I'm not anyone special," I told the Summer girl, who still looked unconvinced. "Don't treat me any different than you would Keirran."

I couldn't be sure, but I was almost positive Keirran hid a small grin behind Annwyl's hair. The Summer girl blinked again, and seemed about to say something, when Kenzie spoke up.

"Um, Ethan? Sorry to be a normal human and all, but... who are we talking to?"

Keirran chuckled. "Oh, right." To Annwyl, he said, "I'm afraid Mackenzie can't see you right now. She's only human."

"What?" Annwyl glanced at Kenzie, and her eyes widened. "Oh, of course. Please excuse me." A shiver went through the air around her, and Kenzie jumped as the faery girl materialized in front of us. "Is this better?"

Kenzie sighed. "I'll never get used to that."

The Summer faery smiled, but then her eyes darkened and she drew back. "Come," she urged, glancing around the fairgrounds. "We can't stay out here. It's gotten dangerous." Her gaze swept the aisles like a wary deer's. "I'm supposed to bring you to the mistress. This way."

We followed Annwyl across the dead amusement park, through the silent fairway, past the Ferris wheel, creaking softly in the wind, until we came to the House of Mirrors in the shadow of a wooden roller coaster. Walking past weird, distorted reflections of ourselves—fat, short, tall with gorilla-like arms—we finally came to a narrow mirror in a shadowy corner, and Annwyl looked back at Keirran.

"It's a bit...crowded," she warned, her gaze flicking to me and Kenzie. "No one wants to be on this side of the Veil, not with those *things* out there." She shuddered, and I saw Keirran wince, too. "Fair warning," she continued, watching Keirran with undeniable affection. "The mistress is a little...cranky these days. She might not appreciate you showing up now, especially with two humans."

"I'll risk it," Keirran said softly, holding her gaze. Annwyl smiled at him, then put her hand to the mirror in front of us. It shimmered, growing even more distorted, and the fey girl stepped through the glass, vanishing from sight.

Keirran looked at us and smiled. "After you."

Taking Kenzie's hand, I stepped through the shifting glass, and the real world faded behind us once more.

We stepped through the doorway into a dark, underground room, a basement maybe, or even a dungeon. The Summer girl beckoned us forward, down the shadowy halls. Torches flickered in brackets as we followed Annwyl down the damp corridors, and gargoyles watched us from stone columns, sneering as we went by.

Fey also walked these halls: boggarts and bogies and a couple of goblins, fey that preferred the dank and damp and shadows, avoiding the light. They eyed us with hungry curiosity, and Kenzie eyed them back, able to See again now that we were back in Faery. They kept their distance, though, and we walked up a flight of long wooden steps, where a pair of crimson doors perched at the top. Annwyl pushed them open.

Noise and light flooded the stairway. The doors opened into an enormous, red-walled foyer, and the foyer was filled with fey.

Faeries stood or sat on the carpeted floors, talking in low murmurs. Goblins muttered amongst themselves, clumped in small groups, glancing around warily. Brownies, satyrs and piskies hovered through the room, looking lost. A couple red-caps stood in a corner, baring their fangs at whoever got too close. One of them noticed me and nudged his companion, jerking his chin in our direction. The other grinned, running a pale tongue over his teeth, and I glared stonily back, daring it to try something. The redcap sneered, made a rude gesture, and went back to threatening the crowd.

More fey clustered along the walls, some of them standing guard over tables and boxes of weird stuff. In one corner, a faery in a white cloak straightened a stand of feather masks, while near the fireplace, a crooked hag plucked a skewer of mice from the flames and set it, still smoking, next to a plate of frogs and what looked like a cooked cat. The stench of burning fur drifted to me across the room, and Kenzie made a tiny gagging noise.

But even with all the weird, unearthly and dangerous fa-eries in the room, there was only one that really mattered.

In the center of all the chaos, a cigarette wand in one hand and a peeved look on her face, was the most striking faery I'd ever seen. Copper-gold hair floated around her like a mane, and a gown hugged her slender body, the long slit up the side showing impossibly graceful legs. She was tall, regal and obvi-ously annoyed, for she kept pursing her lips and blowing blue smoke into snarling wolves that ripped each other to pieces as they thrashed through the air. A black-bearded dwarf stood beneath her glare, a wooden box sitting beside him. The box had been draped with a dark cloth, and growling, hissing noises came from within as it shook back and forth.

"I don't care if the beast was already paid for, darling." The faery's high, clear voice rang out over the crowd. "You're not keeping that thing here." Her tone was hypnotic, exasperated as it was. "I will not have my human pets turned into stone because the Duchess of Thorns has an unnatural craving for cockatrice eggs."

"Please." The dwarf, held up his thick hands, pleading. "Leanansidhe, please, be reasonable."

I sucked in a breath, and my blood turned to ice.

Leanansidhe? Leanansidhe, the freaking Exile Queen? I leveled a piercing glare at Keirran, who offered a weak grin. Everyone in Faery knew who Leanansidhe was, myself included. Meghan had mentioned her name a few times, but beyond that, you couldn't meet an exiled fey who hadn't heard of the dangerous Dark Muse and wasn't terrified of her.

"Get it out of my house, Feddic." The Exile Queen pointed to the door we'd come through. "I don't care what you do with it, but I want it gone. Or would you like to be barred from my home permanently? Take your chances with the life-sucking monsters out in the real world?"

"No!" The dwarf shrank back, eyes wide. "I'll...I'll get rid of it, Leanansidhe," he stammered. "Right now."

"Be sure that you do, pet." Leanansidhe pursed her lips, sucking on her cigarette flute. She sighed, and the smoke image of a rooster went scurrying away over our heads. "If I find one more creature in this house turned to stone..." She trailed off, but the terrifying look in her eyes spoke louder than words.

The dwarf grabbed the hissing, cloth-covered box and hurried away, muttering under his breath. We stepped aside as he passed and continued down the stairs without glancing at us, then disappeared into the shadows.

Leanansidhe pinched the bridge of her nose, then straightened and looked right at us. "Well, well," she purred, smiling in a way I did not like at all, "Keirran, darling. Here you are again. To what do I owe the pleasure?" She gave me a cursory glance before turning back to Keirran. "And you brought a pair of humans with you, I see. More strays, darling?" She shook her head. "Your concern for hopeless waifs is very touching, but if you think you're going to dump them here, dove, I'm afraid I just don't have the room."

Keirran bowed. "Leanansidhe." He nodded, looking around at the crowd of fey. "Looks like you have a full house."

"Noticed that, did you, pet?" The Exile Queen sighed and puffed out a cougar. "Yes, I have been reduced to running the Goblin Market from my own living room, which makes it very difficult to concentrate on other things. Not to mention it's driving my human pets even more crazy than usual. They can barely strum a note or hold a tune with all the chaos around." She touched two elegant fingers to her temple, as if she had a headache. Keirran looked unimpressed.

The Exile Queen sniffed. "Sadly, I'm very busy at the moment, darling, so if you want to make yourself useful, why don't you be a good boy and take a message home? Tell the Iron Queen that something is going on in the real world, and she might want to know about it. If you're here just to make googly-eyes at Annwyl, my darling prince, I'm afraid I don't have time for you."

Prince? Wait. "Wait." I turned, very slowly, to stare at Keirran, ignoring the Exile Queen for the moment. Keirran grimaced and didn't look at me. "Care to say that again?" I asked, disbelief making my stomach knot. My mouth was suddenly dry. "You're a prince—of the Iron Realm? Then, you…you're Meghan's…" I couldn't even finish the thought.

From the corner of my eye, Leanansidhe straightened. "Ethan Chase." Her voice was low and dangerous, as if she'd just figured out who was standing in her living room.

I couldn't look at her now, though. My attention was riveted to Keirran.

He shot me a pained, embarrassed wince. "Yeah. I was going to tell you…sooner or later. There just wasn't a good time." He paused, his voice going very soft. "I'm sorry… Uncle."

Razor let out a high-pitched, buzzing laugh. "Uncle!" he howled, oblivious to the looks of horror and disgust he was getting from every faery in the room. "Uncle, uncle! Uncle Ethan!"

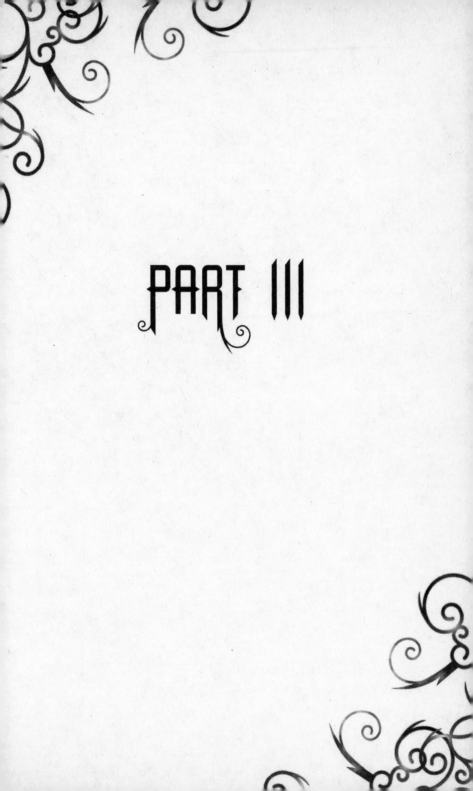

PART III

LEANANSIDHE'S PRICE

I felt numb. And slightly sick.

Keirran—this faery before me—was Ash and Meghan's *son*. How had I not figured it out before? Everything fit together: his human blood, his Iron glamour, even the familiar expressions on his face. They were familiar because I'd seen them before. On Meghan. I could see the resemblance now; his eyes, hair and facial features—they were all my sister's. But Ash's shadow hovered there as well, in his jaw, his stance, the way he moved.

For a second, I hated him.

Before either of us could say anything, the exiled fey in the room gasped and snarled, surging away from Keirran as if he had a disease. Murmurs of "the Iron prince," spread through the crowd, and the circle of fey seemed to hover between bowing down or fleeing the room. Leanansidhe gave us both an extremely exasperated glare, as if we were the cause of her headaches, and snapped her fingers at us.

"Annwyl, darling." The Exile Queen's tone made the fey girl cringe, and Keirran moved to stand protectively beside her. "Wait here, would you, dove? Try to keep the masses in check while I deal with this little bump. You three." She shifted that cold gaze to us, her tone brooking no argument. "Follow me, pets. And, Keirran, keep that wretched gremlin under control this time, or I'll be forced to do something drastic."

Kenzie, forgotten beside us all, shot me a worried glance, and I shrugged, trying to look unconcerned. We started to follow Leanansidhe, but Annwyl and Keirran lingered for a moment. Leanansidhe rolled her eyes. "Sometime today, pets." She sighed, as Annwyl finally turned away and Keirran looked dejected. "While I'm still in a reasonable enough mood not to turn anyone into a cello."

Turning in a swirl of blue smoke, the Exile Queen led us out of the room, down several long, red-carpeted hallways, and into a library. Huge shelves of books lined the walls, and a lively tune swam through the air, played by a human with a violin in the far corner.

"Out, Charles," Leanansidhe announced as she swept into the room, and the human quickly packed up his instrument and fled through another door.

The Exile Queen spun on us. "Well!" she exclaimed, gazing down at me, her hair writhing around her. "Ethan Chase. This *is* a surprise. The son and the brother of the Iron Queen, come to visit at the same time, what an occasion. How is your darling older sister, pet?" she asked me. "I assume you've been to see her recently?"

"Meghan's fine," I muttered, feeling self-conscious with Keirran standing there. Now that I knew we were…related… it felt weird, talking about Meghan in front of him.

Screw that. You want weird? Weird is having a nephew the same age as you. Weird is your sister having a kid, and not telling your family about him. Weird is being an uncle to a freaking half-faery! Forget weird, you are so beyond weird that it's not funny.

Leanansidhe *tsked* and looked at Keirran, and a slow smile crossed her lips. "And Keirran, you devious boy," she purred. "You didn't tell him, did you?" She laughed then, shaking her head. "Well, this is an unexpected family drama, isn't it? I wonder what the Iron Queen would say if she could be here now?"

"Wait a second." Kenzie's voice broke in, bewildered and incredulous. "Keirran is *your nephew?* He's the Iron Queen's son? But...you're the same age!" She gestured wildly. "How in the world does that work?"

"Ah, well." Keirran shrugged, looking embarrassed. "Remember the screwy time differences in Faery? That's part of it. Also, the fey mature at a faster rate than mortals—comes with living in a place as dangerous as the Nevernever, I guess. We grow up quickly until we hit a certain point, then we just... stop." He gave another sheepish grin. "Trust me, you're not the only ones to be shocked. It was a big surprise for Mom, too."

I glared at Keirran, forgetting Kenzie and Leanansidhe for the moment. "Why didn't you say anything?" I demanded.

Keirran sighed. "How?" he asked, lifting his hands away from his sides, before letting them drop. "When would it have come up? *Oh, by the way, I'm the prince of the Iron Realm, and your nephew. Surprise!*" He shrugged again, made a hopeless gesture. "It would've been weird. And...awkward. And I'm pretty sure you wouldn't have wanted anything to do with me if you knew."

"Why didn't Meghan say anything? That's kind of a big thing to keep from your family."

"I don't know, Ethan." Keirran shook his head. "She never talks about you, never speaks about her human life. I didn't even know I had another family until a few years ago." He paused, ran his fingers through his silver hair. "I was shocked when I heard that the queen had a brother living in the mortal world. But when I asked her about it, she told me that we had to live separate lives, that mingling the two families would only bring trouble to us both. I disagreed—I wanted to meet you, but she forbade me to come and see you at all."

He sounded sincere and genuinely sorry, that he hadn't been able to introduce himself. My anger with him dissolved a little, only to switch to another target. *Meghan,* I thought, furious. *How could you? How could you not tell us? What was the point?*

"When I heard you were at the palace," Keirran went on, his face earnest, as if he was willing me to believe him, "I couldn't believe it. I had to see for myself. But when Razor told me what you said—that something was killing off exiles and half-breeds—I knew I had to get to Annwyl, make sure she was safe. So I thought, *two birds with one stone, why not?*" He offered a shrug and a wry grin, before sobering once more. "I didn't tell you everything, and I'm sorry for that. But I had to make certain you would follow me out of the Iron Realm."

My head was still reeling. Meghan's son. My nephew. I could barely wrap my mind around it. I didn't know if I should be disgusted, horrified, ecstatic or completely weirded out. I *did* know that I was going to have to talk to Meghan about this, ask why she felt it was important to keep us in the dark. Screw this "living separate lives" crap. She had a kid! Half-faery or no, you did not keep that sort of thing from your family.

"Well," Leanansidhe interjected with a wave of her cigarette flute, "much as I'm enjoying this little drama, pets, I'm afraid we cannot sit around and argue the whole day. I have larger problems to attend to. I assume you boys did not see the abominations lurking around the fairgrounds?"

"We did, actually."

It wasn't Keirran who answered the Exile Queen. It was Kenzie. I grimaced and turned away from the Iron prince, vowing to deal with this later, when I had time to think it through. Right now, the Dark Muse had turned her attention on the girl who, up until this point, had been standing off to the side, watching the drama play out. Truthfully, I was happy for that; it was probably best that she avoid Leanansidhe's notice as much as she could. But, of course, Kenzie could never stay silent for long.

"We did see them," she repeated, and the Dark Muse blinked at her in surprise. "Well, *they* did," she continued, jerking her head at me and Keirran. "I couldn't see anything. But I do know something attacked us. They're the ones killing off your people, right?"

"And, who are you again, dove?"

"Oh, sorry," Kenzie went on, as Leanansidhe continued to stare as if she was seeing the girl for the first time. "I'm Mackenzie, Ethan's classmate. We sort of got pulled into the Nevernever together."

"How...tenacious," Leanansidhe mused after a moment. And I didn't know if she found Kenzie amusing or offensive. I hoped it was the former. "Well, if you must know, darling, yes, something out there is making exiles disappear. As you can see from the state of my living room, the exiled fey are practically tearing down my walls trying to get in. I haven't had this much trouble since the war with the Iron fey." She paused and leveled a piercing glare at Razor, humming on Keirran's shoulder. The gremlin seemed happily oblivious.

"Any idea what's causing it?" Kenzie asked, slipping into reporter mode like she had at the tournament. If she'd had a notebook, it would have been flipped open right now, pencil scribbling furiously. Leanansidhe sighed.

"Vague ideas, darling. Rumors of horrible monsters sucking the glamour out of their victims until they are lifeless husks. I've never seen the horrid things, of course, but there have been several disappearances from the fairgrounds, as well as all over the world."

"All over the world?" I broke in. "Is it really that wide-spread?"

Leanansidhe gave me an eerie stare. "You have no idea, darling," she said softly. "And neither do the courts. Your sister remains happily ignorant to the threat in the mortal realm, and Summer and Winter do not even care. But…let me show you something."

She strode to a table in the corner of the room, where a huge map of the world lay spread across the wood. Red dots marked the surface, some isolated, some clumped together. There were a fair number spread across North America, but also a bunch in England, Ireland and Great Britain. Scattered, perhaps. It wasn't as though a whole area was covered with red. No continent was unmarked, however. North America, Europe, Africa, Australia, Asia, South America. They all had their share of red dots.

"I've been tracking disappearances," Leanansidhe said into the stunned silence. "Exiles and half-breeds alike. As you can see, darlings, it's quite widespread. And each time I send someone out to investigate, they do not return. It's becoming—" Leanansidhe pursed her lips "—annoying."

I gazed at the map, my fingers hovering over a spot in the United States. Two bright red dots in the state of Louisiana, near my home town.

Todd.

Keirran scanned the table, his expression grave. "And the other courts do nothing?" he murmured. "Mab and Oberon and Titania don't know what's going on?"

"They've been informed, darling," Leanansidhe said, waving her cigarette flute in a dismissive manner. "However, the Summer and Winter courts do not think it important enough to intervene. What do they care about the lives of a few exiles and half-breeds? As long as the problem remains in the mortal realm, they are content to do nothing."

"Why didn't you tell Meghan?" I broke in. "She would've done something. She's trying to do something now."

Leanansidhe frowned at me. "That might be true, pet. But sadly, I have no way to get a message to the Iron Queen without my informants dropping dead from iron sickness. It is very difficult to contact the Iron Realm when no one is willing to set foot there. In fact, I was waiting for this one—" she waved her flute at Keirran "—to come sniffing around after Annwyl again, so that I could give him a message to bring back to Mag Tuiredh."

Keirran blushed slightly but didn't reply. Razor giggled on his shoulder.

I looked down at the map again, my thoughts whirling. So many gone. A part of me said not to care, that the fey were finally getting what they deserved after centuries of making humans disappear.

But there was more at stake now. Todd was still missing, and I'd promised to find him. Meghan would be getting involved soon. And now, there was Keirran.

I didn't want to think about Keirran right now.

"Then," I muttered, continuing to gaze at the map, "you're going to need someone who can investigate these things, someone who isn't a half-breed or an exile, who doesn't have any glamour they can suck dry." *Someone who's human.*

"Exactly, darling." Leanansidhe stared down with a chilling gleam in her eyes. I could feel it on the back of my neck without even seeing her. "So...are *you* volunteering, pet?"

I sighed.

"Yeah," I muttered and straightened to face her. "I am. I have a friend I've got to find, but this has become even bigger than that. I don't know what freaks are out there, and I don't

like it. If these glamour-sucking things are so widespread, it's
only a matter of time before all the exiles are gone, and then
they might start on the Nevernever."

Where Meghan is.

"Excellent, darling, excellent." Leanansidhe beamed, looking pleased. "And what about you two?" she asked, gesturing
to Kenzie and Keirran, on opposite ends of the table. "What
will the son of the Iron Queen do, now that he's aware of the
danger? You can always go home, you know, warn the kingdom. Though I can't imagine the Iron Queen will be pleased
when she finds out what you've been doing."

"I'm going with Ethan," Keirran said softly. "I have to.
Whatever these things are, I won't stand by while they kill
off any more of our kind, exiled or not."

"Including Annwyl, is that right, pet?"

Keirran faced the Exile Queen directly, raising his chin.
"Especially her."

"I'm going, too," Kenzie piped in, and frowned at me, as
if guessing I was just about to suggest she go home. Which I
was, but she didn't need to know.

"Kenzie, this isn't your fight anymore." I looked at Keirran,
hoping he would back me on this. He just shrugged unhelp-
fully. "You don't have a stake in this," I continued, trying to
be reasonable. "You have no family or siblings or—" I looked
at Keirran "—girlfriends to worry about. You didn't even
know Todd very well. We're closer to the mortal world than
we've ever been now, and you can go home anytime. Why
are you still here?"

"Because I want to be!" she snapped, like that was the end
of it. We glared at each other, and she threw up her hands.
"Jeez, Ethan, we've been over this already. Get it through your
stubborn head, okay? Do you think, with everything I've seen,
I can just go home and forget it all? I'm not here because of

family or siblings or friends—I'm here because of you! And because I *want* to see this! I want to know what's out there."

"You can't even see them," I argued. "These things exist in the real world, remember? You don't have the Sight, so how are you going to help us when you won't even know where they are?"

She pursed her lips. "I'll...think of something."

"*I* may be able to help with that, darling," Leanansidhe broke in. We looked up, and the Exile Queen smiled at Kenzie, twiddling her cigarette holder. "You are a spunky little thing, aren't you, pet? I rather like you. With all the riffraff from the Goblin Market hanging out in my living room, I'm certain we'll be able to find something that will help you with your nonexistent Sight. However..." She raised one perfectly manicured nail. "A warning, my dove. This is not a simple request, nor does it come cheap. To grant a human the Sight is not something I take lightly. I will have something from you in return, if you agree."

"No!" My outburst made Kenzie start, though Leanansidhe blinked calmly, looking irritated and amused at the same time. "Kenzie, no," I said, taking a step toward her. "Never make a deal with the fey. The price is always too high."

Kenzie regarded me briefly, then turned back to the Exile Queen, her expression thoughtful. "What kind of price are we talking about?" she asked softly.

"Kenzie!"

"Ethan." Her voice was quiet but firm as she looked over her shoulder. "It's my decision."

"The hell it is! I'm not going to let you do this—"

"Ethan, darling," Leanansidhe ordered, and brought her finger and thumb together. "Shush."

And suddenly, I couldn't speak. I couldn't make a sound. My mouth opened, vocal chords straining to say something, but I had gone as mute as the paint on the wall. "This is my home," the Dark Muse continued, and the lights flickered on and off as she stared at me. "And here you will obey my rules. If you don't like it, pet, you're welcome to leave. But the girl and I have business to conduct now, so sit down and be a good boy, won't you? Don't make me turn you into a very whiny guitar."

I clenched my fists, wanting to hit something, wanting to grab Kenzie and get us both out of there. But even if I left, Leanansidhe wouldn't let Kenzie go, not without completing the bargain. Attacking someone as powerful as the Exile Queen was a very stupid idea, even for me. I wanted to protect Kenzie, but I couldn't do that if Leanansidhe turned me into a guitar. So I could only stand there, clenching and unclenching my fists, as Kenzie prepared to deal with the Exile Queen. Keirran watched me, his gaze apologetic, and I resisted the urge to hit him, too.

"Ethan." Kenzie looked back at me, horror crossing her face as she realized what had happened, then whirled on Leanansidhe. "Whatever you just did to him," she demanded, bristling, "stop it right now."

"Oh, pish, darling. He's just a little tongue-tied at the moment. Nothing he won't recover from. Eventually." The Exile Queen gave me a dismissive wave. "Now, my dove. I believe we have some business to conclude. You want to be able to see the Hidden World, and I want something from you, as well. The question is, what are you willing to pay?"

Kenzie stared at me a moment longer, then slowly turned back to the Dark Muse. "I take it we're not talking about money."

Leanansidhe laughed. "Oh, no, my pet. Nothing so crude as that." She strolled forward until Kenzie was just a foot away, gazing up at the Exile Queen looming over her. "You have something else that I'm interested in."

I started forward, but Keirran grabbed my arm.

"Ethan, don't," he whispered as I glared at him, wondering if I shouldn't lock his elbow out and force him to his knees. "She'll do something nasty if you try to interfere. I've seen it. Even if it's not on you, she could take it out on others. I can't let you hurt yourself...or Annwyl."

"I can feel the creative energy in you, pet," the Exile Queen mused, lightly stroking Kenzie's long black hair, and Keirran had to tighten his grip on my arm. "You are an artist, aren't you, darling? A smith of words, one might say."

"I'm a journalist," Kenzie replied cautiously.

"Exactly so, darling," said Leanansidhe, moving a few steps back. "You create music with words and sentences, not notes. Well, here is my bargain, my pet—I will offer you a little of my...shall we say 'divine inspiration,' for a very special piece I'm willing to commission."

"And...what do you want me to write about?"

"I want you to publish something about me, darling," Leanansidhe said, as if that were obvious. "That's not such a horrible price, is it, pet? Oh, but here is the real kicker—every word you put down on paper will practically sing from the page. It will touch everyone who reads it, in one form or another. The words will be yours, the thoughts will be yours. I will just add a little inspiration to make the work truly magnificent. Let me do this, and I will give you the ability to see the fey."

Kenzie, no! I wanted to shout. *If you let her do this, you'll be giving a piece of yourself to Leanansidhe. She'll take a bit of your life in exchange for the inspiration, that's how the Dark Muse works!*

Kenzie hesitated, considering. "One piece?" she said at last, as I turned desperately to Keirran, grabbing his collar. "That's all?"

Say something, I thought, beseeching the faery with my gaze. *Dammit, Keirran, you know what's going on. You can't let her agree without the full knowledge of what she's getting into. Say something!*

"Of course, darling," Leanansidhe said. "Just one tiny piece, written by you. With my help, of course.

"Please," I mouthed, and Keirran sighed.

"That's not all, Leanansidhe," he said, releasing my arm and stepping forward. "You're not telling her everything. She deserves to know the real price of your inspiration."

"Keirran, darling," Leanansidhe said, a definite note of irritation beneath the cheerful facade, "if I lose this deal because of you, I'm going to be very unhappy. And when I am unhappy, pet, *everyone* in my home is unhappy." She glowered at Keirran, and the lights on the walls flickered. "I did you a favor by taking the Summer girl in, darling. Remember that."

Keirran backed off, giving me a dark look, but it was enough. "What does he mean?" Kenzie asked as the Exile Queen huffed in frustration. "What's the 'real price'?"

"Nothing much, darling," Leanansidhe soothed, switching tones as she turned back to the girl. "Just…in the terms of the contract, you will agree to forfeit a tiny bit of your life to me, in exchange for the inspiration. Not much, mind you," she added, as Kenzie's mouth dropped open. "A month or two, give or take. Of course, this is your natural lifespan only—it does not count for fatal accidents, sickness, disease or other untimely demises. But that is my offer for the Sight, my pet. It really is one of my more generous offers. What say you?"

No, I thought at Kenzie. *Say no. That's the only thing you can say to an offer like that.*

"Sure," Kenzie said immediately, and I gaped at her. "Why not? A month of my life, in exchange for a lifetime of seeing the fey?" She shrugged. "That's not too bad, in the long run."

What? Stunned, I could only stare at the girl in horror. *Do you know what you just did? You gave away a month of your existence to a faery queen! You let her shorten your life for nothing.*

Leanansidhe blinked. "Well," she mused after a moment. "That was easy. How fortunate for me. Humans are usually extraordinarily attached to their lives, I've found. But, if that is your decision, then we have a deal, my pet. And I will get you the things you need to acquire the Sight." She smiled, terribly pleased with herself, and looked at me and Keirran. If she saw how I was staring at Kenzie, dumbstruck, she didn't comment. "I will fetch Annwyl to show you your rooms. Meet me here tomorrow, darlings, and we will discuss where you will go next. Until then, the mansion is yours."

My voice finally returned a few hours later.

I hadn't seen Annwyl or Keirran for a while, not since the Summer girl had brought us to Leanansidhe's guest rooms and quickly vanished, saying she had work to do. Keirran didn't wait very long before following her down the hall. Kenzie, I think, was avoiding me, for she disappeared into her room and didn't answer the door when I knocked a few minutes later.

So I prowled the mansion, which was huge, wandering its endless corridors, hoping some exiled fey would try to pick a fight with me. Nobody did, leaving me to brood without any distractions.

Keirran. Meghan's son...and my nephew, disturbing as that was. The whole situation was completely screwed up. I knew time flowed differently in Faery, but still. Keirran was *my* age, as were Meghan and Ash...

I shook my head, veering away from that train of thought. My family had just gotten a whole lot weirder. I wondered what Mom would say, if she knew about Keirran. She'd probably freak out.

Maybe that's why Meghan didn't tell us, I thought, glaring at a bogey crouched under a low shelf like a huge spider, daring it to do something. It took one look at me and vanished into the shadows. *Maybe she knew Mom wouldn't be able to handle it. Maybe she was scared of what I would think…but, no, that's not an excuse! She still should've told us. That's not something you can just hide away and hope no one finds out.*

Meghan had a reason for not telling us about Keirran, and for trying to keep him away from us, as well. What was it? As far as I could tell, Keirran had no prejudice against humans; he was polite, soft-spoken, respectful. *The complete opposite of me,* I thought, rolling my eyes. *Mom would absolutely love him.* But Meghan never wanted us to meet, which seemed really odd for her, as well. What could possibly be so horrible that you would have a child and keep it a secret from the rest of your family?

What wasn't she telling us about Keirran?

Voices drifted down the corridor from somewhere up ahead, the soft, garbled buzz of a conversation. I heard Annwyl's lyrical tone through an archway at the end of the hall, and Keirran's quiet voice echo it. Not wanting to disturb…whatever they were doing, I turned to leave, when Kenzie's name filtered through the conversation and caught my attention.

Wary now, I crept down the corridor until it ended at a large, circular room filled with vegetation. An enormous tree loomed up from the center, extending gnarled branches skyward, which was easy because the room had no ceiling. Bright sunlight slanted through the leaves, spotting the carpet of grass and wildflowers surrounding the trunk. Birds twittered overhead and butterflies danced through the flowers, adding to the dazzling array of color and light.

It wasn't real, of course. Leanansidhe's mansion, according to rumors, existed in a place called the Between, the veil that separated Faery from the mortal world. Supposedly, when using a trod, you passed very briefly through the Between, then into the other realm. How Leanansidhe managed to set up an entire mansion in the space between worlds was baffling, something you just shouldn't wonder about. No one knew what the outside of the mansion looked like, but I was pretty sure it didn't have sunlight and birdsong. This room was all faery glamour. A really good illusion—I could smell the wildflowers, hear the bees buzzing past my ear and feel the warmth of the sun—but an illusion nonetheless. I hadn't come here to smell the flowers, I was here to discover why two faeries were talking about Kenzie.

Keirran sat beneath the trunk, one knee drawn up to his chest, watching Annwyl as she moved gracefully through the flowers. Every so often, the Summer faery would pause, brushing her fingers over a petal or fern, and the plant would immediately straighten, unfurling new and brighter leaves. Butterflies danced around her, perching on her hair and clothes, as if she was an enormous blossom drifting through the field.

I eased closer, skirting the edges of the room, keeping a row of giant ferns between myself and the two fey. Peering through the fronds, feeling slightly ridiculous that I would stoop this low, I strained my ears in the direction of the tree.

"Leanansidhe wants the ceremony done tonight," Annwyl was saying, raising an arm to touch a low-hanging branch. It stirred, and several withered leaves grew full and green again. "I think it would be better if you performed the ritual, Keirran. She knows you, and the boy might object if I go anywhere near her."

"I know." Keirran exhaled, resting his chin on his knee. "I just hope Ethan doesn't hate me for my part in giving Kenzie the Sight. He's probably still reeling from that last load of bricks I dropped on his head."

"You mean that you're his nephew?" Annwyl asked mildly, and my gut twisted. I still wasn't used to the idea. "But, surely he understands how time works in both worlds. He had to realize that his sister would start her own family, even if she wasn't in the mortal realm, right?"

"How could he?" Keirran muttered. "She never told him. She never told *me*." He sighed again, and though I couldn't see his face very well, his tone was morose, almost angry. "She's hiding something, Annwyl. I think they all are. Oberon, Titania, Mab—they all know something. And no one will tell me what it is." His voice lowered, frustrated and confused. "Why don't they trust me?"

Annwyl turned, giving him a strange look. Snapping a twig from the nearest branch, she knelt in front of Keirran and held up the stick. "Here. Take this for a moment."

Looking bewildered, Keirran did.

"Do what I was doing just now," she ordered. "Make it grow."

His brow furrowed, but he shrugged and glanced down at the bare stick. It shivered, and tiny buds appeared along the length of the wood, before unfurling into leaves. A butterfly floated down from Annwyl's hair to perch on the end.

"Now, kill it," Annwyl said.

She received another puzzled look, but a second later frost crept over the leaves, turning them black, before the entire twig was coated in ice. The butterfly dropped away and spiraled toward the ground, lifeless in an instant. Annwyl flicked the branch with her fingers, and it snapped, one half of the stick spinning away into the flowers.

"Do you see what I'm getting at, Prince Keirran?"

He hung his head. "Yes."

"You're the Iron prince," Annwyl went on in a gentle voice. "But you're not simply an Iron faery. You have the glamour of all three courts and can use them seamlessly, without fail. No one else in Faery has that ability, not even the Iron Queen." She put a hand on his knee, and he looked down at it. "They fear you, Keirran. They're afraid of what you can become, what your existence might mean for them. It's the nature of the courts, sadly. They don't react well to change."

"Are you afraid of me?" Keirran asked, his voice nearly lost in the sighing leaves.

"No." Annwyl pulled her hand away and rose, gazing down at him. "Not when you were kind to me, and risked so much to bring me here. But I know the courts far better than you do, Keirran. I was just a humble servant to Titania, but you are the Iron prince." She took a step back, her voice mournful but resolved. "I know my place. I will not drag you into exile with me."

As Annwyl turned away, Keirran rose swiftly, not touching her but very close. "I'm not afraid of exile," he said quietly, and the Summer girl closed her eyes. "And I don't care what the courts say. My own parents defied those laws, and look where they are now." His hand rose, gently brushing her braid, causing several butterflies to flit skyward. "I would do the same for you, if you just gave me the chance—"

"No, Prince Keirran." Annwyl spun, her eyes glassy. "I won't do that, not to you. I wish things were different, but we can't... The courts would... I'm sorry."

She whirled and fled the room, leaving Keirran standing alone under the great tree. He scrubbed a hand over his eyes, then wandered back to lean against the trunk, staring out at nothing.

Feeling like an intruder who had just witnessed something he shouldn't have, I eased back into the corridor. My suspicions had been confirmed; Meghan *was* hiding something from us. I was definitely going to have to talk to her about that, demand why she thought it was so important to keep her family in the dark.

First, however, I had to find Kenzie, before this ritual was supposed to begin. She needed to know what having the Sight really meant, what the fey did to those who could See them. If she'd really understood the consequences, she never would have made that bargain.

Although, deep down, I knew that was a lie. Kenzie had known *exactly* what she was getting into and chose to do it anyway.

I finally found her in the library, hidden between towering shelves of books, leaning against the wall. She glanced up as I came into the aisle, the massive tome in her hands making her look even smaller. That strange, unfamiliar sensation twisted my stomach again, but I ignored it.

"Hey." She gave me a hesitant smile, as if she wasn't sure if I was mad at her or not. "Has your voice come back yet?"

"Yeah." It came out harsher than I'd wanted, but I plunged on. "I need to talk to you."

"I suppose you do." She sighed, pushing a strand of hair behind her ear. For a moment, she stared at the pages in front of her. "I guess...you want to know why I agreed to that bargain."

"Why?" I took a step forward, into the narrow space. "Why would you think your life was an acceptable trade for something that you have no business seeing in the first place?" Anger flickered again, but I couldn't tell if it was directed at Kenzie, Leanansidhe, Keirran or something else. "This isn't a game, Kenzie. You just shortened your life by trading it away to a faery. Don't think she won't collect. They always do."

"It's a month, Ethan. Two at the most. It won't matter in the long run."

"It's your life!" I stabbed my fingers through my hair, frustrated that she refused to see. "What would've been 'too much,' Kenzie? A year? Two? Would you have become her 'apprentice'? Giving away bits of your life for the inspiration she offers? That's what she does, you know. And every single person she helps dies an early death. Or becomes trapped in this crazy between-worlds house, entertaining her for eternity." I paused, fisting my hand against the shelf. "I can't watch that happen to you."

We both fell silent. Kenzie hesitated, picking at the pages of the book. "Look," she began, "I realize you know almost everything about the fey, but there are things you don't know about me. I don't like talking about it, because I don't want to be a burden on anyone, but…" She chewed her lip, her face tightening. "Let's just say I view things a little differently than most people. I want to learn everything I can, I want to *see* everything I can. That's why I want to become a reporter—to travel the world, to discover what's out there." Her voice wavered, and her eyes went distant. "I just don't want to miss anything."

I sighed. "Promise me you won't make any more deals," I said, taking another step toward her. "No matter what you see, no matter what they offer you, promise that you won't agree to it."

She watched me over the edge of the book, brown eyes solemn. "I can't make that promise," she said quietly.

"Why?"

"Why do you care?" she shot back, defiant. "You told me to leave you alone, to forget about you when we went back, because you're going to do the same. Those were your words, Ethan. You don't want me around and you don't care."

I huffed and closed the last few steps. Taking the book from her hands, I snapped it shut, replaced it on the shelf, and grabbed her shoulders, forcing her to look at me. She stiffened, raising her chin, glaring at me with wounded eyes.

"I care, all right?" I said in a low voice. "I know I come off as a bastard sometimes, and I'm sorry for that. But I do care about…what happens to you here. I don't want to see you get hurt because of Them. Because of me."

Kenzie met my gaze and stepped forward, so close that I could see my reflection in her dark eyes. "I want to see Them, Ethan," she said, firm and unshakable. "I'm not afraid."

"I know, that's what scares me." I released her, kicking myself for acting so roughly, yet reluctant to let her go. "You're going to have the Sight now," I said, feeling raw apprehension spread through my insides. "That means the fey will hound you relentlessly, wanting to bargain, or make a deal, or just make your life hell. You've seen it. You know what they're capable of."

"Yes," Kenzie agreed, and suddenly took my hand, sending a shiver up my arm. "But I've also spoken with a talking cat, fought a dragon, and watched the Iron Realm light up at night. I've seen a faery queen, climbed the towers of a huge castle, flown on a giant metal insect, and made a deal with a legend. How many people can say that? Can you blame me for not wanting to let it go?"

"And if it gets you killed?"

She shrugged and looked away. "No one lives forever."

I had no answer for that. There *was* no answer for that.

"Hey." Keirran appeared at the end of the aisle, and we jumped apart. His gremlin grinned manically from his shoulder, lighting the shelves with a blue-white glow. "What are you two doing?"

He gave me a half wary, half hopeful look, unsure of where we stood, if we were cool. I shrugged, not smiling, but not glaring at him, either. It was the best I could offer for now.

"Nothing," I said, and nodded to Kenzie. "Futilely trying to convince stubborn reporters not to go through with this." She snorted. "Hi, Mr. Pot. Meet Mr. Kettle."

"Kenzie." Annwyl stepped forward. Her hair was loose, falling down her back in golden-brown waves, petals and leaves scattered throughout. Keirran watched her, his face blank, but he didn't say anything. A tiny glass vial gleamed from her fingertips as she held it up. "Leanansidhe told me to give this to you."

I clenched my fists to keep from dashing the vial to the floor. Kenzie reached out and plucked it from her hand, holding it up to the light. It sparkled dully, half-full with amber liquid, throwing tiny slivers of gold over the carpet.

"So," she mused after a moment, "is it 'down the hatch' right now and, *poof,* I'll be able to see the fey? Is that how this works?"

"Not yet," Annwyl said solemnly. "There is a ritual involved. To gain the Sight, you must stand in the middle of a faery ring at midnight, spill a few drops of your blood onto the ground, and then drink that. The Veil will lift, and you'll be able to see the Hidden World for the rest of your life."

"Doesn't sound too hard." Kenzie gave the vial a small shake, dislodging a few black specks that swirled around the glass. "What's in here, anyway?"

Keirran smiled. "Probably best you don't know," he warned. "In any case, Leanansidhe has a trod that will take us to a faery ring. There's a catch, though. When the full moon shines down on a faery ring, the local fey can't resist. We'll probably run into a few of them, dancing under the moonlight. You know, like they do."

"Well, then it's a good thing I'll have you two around to protect me." She glanced my way, a shadow of uncertainty crossing her face. "You'll be there, right?"

"Yeah." I gave her a resigned look. *I'd say what a stupid idea this is, but you won't listen to me. I only hope the cost will be worth it.*

"So," I muttered, looking at Keirran, "where is this faery ring?"

He grinned, reminding me suddenly of Meghan, and my stomach clenched. "Not far by trod, but probably farther than you've ever been," he said mysteriously. "This particular ring is several thousand years old, which is vital to the ritual tonight—the older the ring, the more power it holds. It's somewhere deep in the moors of Ireland."

Kenzie's head jerked up, her eyes brightening. "Ireland?"

"Yay!" Razor crowed, bouncing up and down on his shoulder. "Sheep!"

CHAPTER SEVENTEEN

THE FAERY RING

"Better hurry, darlings," Leanansidhe announced, walking into the dining room with a swooshing of fabric and smoke. "The witching hour is fast approaching, at least where you're headed. And it will be a full moon tonight, so you really don't want to miss your window." She glanced at me, wandering back to the corner of the room, and sighed. "Ethan, darling, why don't you sit down and eat? You're making my brownies very nervous with all that pacing."

Too bad for them, I thought, chewing a roll I'd snagged from the dining-room table in the middle of the room. The table was enormous and covered with enough food to feed an army, but I couldn't sit still. Keirran and Kenzie sat opposite each other, talking quietly and occasionally giving me worried looks as I paced around them, while Razor cavorted among the plates, scattering food and making small messes. Several redcaps, dressed in butler suits with pink bow ties, skulked back and forth, cleaning up and looking like they really wanted to bite the gremlin's head off. I kept a wary eye on them every time they approached Kenzie, tensing to jump in if they so much as looked at her. They reminded me of the motley that had chased me into the library and set it on fire, leading to my expulsion. If they made any threatening moves toward Kenzie, even a leer, they were going to get an expensive china plate to the back of the skull.

"Ethan," Leanansidhe warned, "you're wearing a hole through my carpet, darling. *Sit down*." She pointed to a chair with her cigarette holder, pursing her lips. "The minions aren't going to bite anyone's knees off, and I'd hate to have to turn you into a harp for the rest of the evening. Sit."

I pulled out a chair beside Kenzie and sat, still glaring at the biggest redcap, the guy with the fishhook through his nose. He sneered and bared his teeth, but then Razor knocked over a platter of fruit, and he hurried off with a curse. Leanansidhe threw up her hands.

"Keirran, dove. Your gremlin. *Please* keep it under control." The Exile Queen pinched the bridge of her nose and sighed heavily. "Worse than having Robin Goodfellow in my house," she murmured, as Kenzie clapped her hands, and Razor bounced happily into her lap. Leanansidhe shook her head. "Anyway, darlings, when you are finished here, I will have Annwyl show you the way to the trod. Meet her in the main hall, and she will take you out through the basement. If you have any questions about the ritual, I'm sure she can answer them for you." At the mention of Annwyl's name, Keirran glanced up, and Leanansidhe smiled at him. "I'm not a compete soulless harpy all the time, darling. Besides, you two remind me of another pair, and I just *adore* the irony." She snapped her fingers and handed her cigarette flute to the redcap who scurried up. "Now, I'm off to meet a jinn about another disappearance, so don't wait up for me, darlings. Oh, and, Kenzie, pet, when you finish the ritual, you might feel a bit odd for a moment."

"Odd?"

"Nothing to worry about, dove." The Exile Queen waved her hand. "Merely the completion of our bargain. I will see you three again soon, but not too soon, I hope." She looked directly at me when she said this, before turning away in a swirl of glitter and lights. "*Ciao,* darlings!"

And she was gone.

As soon as she left, Annwyl came into the room, not looking at any of us. "Leanansidhe has bid me to show you to the faery ring tonight," she said in her musical voice, gazing straight ahead. "We can leave whenever you are ready, but the ritual takes place at midnight, so we should depart soon—"

She paused as Keirran pushed back his chair and walked up to her. Taking her hand, the prince drew her to the table and pulled out the chair next to his, while Razor giggled and waved at her from Kenzie's lap.

"I really shouldn't be here," Annwyl said, perching gingerly on the seat. Her green eyes darted around the room, as if the Exile Queen was hiding somewhere, listening to her. "If Leanansidhe finds out—"

"She can take it up with me," Keirran broke in, sliding into his own chair. "Just because you have to be here doesn't mean Leanansidhe should treat you like a servant." He sighed, and for a second, his expression darkened. "I'm sorry. I know you miss Arcadia. I wish there was another place you could go."

"I'm fine, Keirran." Annwyl smiled at him, though her expression was wistful. "Avoiding Leanansidhe isn't much different than avoiding Queen Titania in one of her moods. I worry most for you. I don't want you to accede to Leanansidhe's every whim and favor because of me."

Keirran stared down at his plate. "If Leanansidhe asked me to fight a dragon," he said in his quiet, sincere voice, "if it meant keeping you safe, I would go into the depths of the Deep Wyld and fight Tiamat herself."

"How long have you two known each other?" Kenzie asked, as I gagged silently into a coffee mug. These two just needed to admit defeat and get on with it already.

Keirran spared her a quick glance and a smile. "I'm not sure," he admitted, shrugging. "It's hard to say exactly, especially in human years."

"We met at Elysium," Annwyl put in. "Midsummer's Eve. When Oberon was hosting. I was chosen to perform a dance for the rulers of the courts. And when it started, I noticed that the son of the Iron Queen couldn't stop staring at me the whole time."

"I remember that dance," Keirran said. "You were beautiful. But when I tried to talk to you, you ran away." He gave me and Kenzie a wry grin. "No one from Summer or Winter wants to talk to the Prince of the Iron Realm. I'd poison their blood or shoot toxic vapors from my nose or something. Annwyl even sicced a school of undine on me once when I was visiting Arcadia. I very nearly drowned."

Annwyl blushed. "But that didn't deter you, did it?"

"So, how did you end up here?" I asked. And Keirran's eyes narrowed.

"Summer Court politics," he said, frowning. "One of the minor nobles was jealous about Annwyl's proximity to Titania, that she was a personal favorite, so she started the rumor that Annwyl was more beautiful and graceful and gifted than even the Summer Queen, and that Oberon would be blind not to see her."

I winced. "That didn't go over well, I'm sure."

"Titania heard of it, of course." Annwyl sighed. "By then, the rumor had spread so far there was no telling who first mentioned such a thing. The Queen was furious, and even though I denied it, she still feared I would steal her husband's attention away."

"So she banished you," I muttered. "Yeah, that sounds like her."

"She banished you?" Kenzie repeated, sounding outraged,

"because someone said you were prettier? That's totally unfair! Can't any of the other rulers do something about it? You're the prince of the Iron Realm," she said, looking at Keirran. "Can't you get the Iron Queen to help?"

Keirran grimaced. "Ah, I'm not really supposed to be here," he said with a half embarrassed, half defiant smile. "If the other courts knew I was hanging around the Exile Queen, they wouldn't approve. They're afraid she'll put treasonous thoughts in my head, or use me to overthrow the other rulers. But..." And his eyes hardened, the shadow of his father creeping over him, making him look more fey than before. "I don't care what the courts dictate. Annwyl shouldn't suffer because Titania is a jealous shrew. So, I asked Leanansidhe to do me a favor, to let her stay here, with the rest of the exiles. It's not ideal, but it's better than being out in the real world."

"Why?" asked Kenzie.

"Because faeries banished to the real world, with no way to get home, eventually fade away into nothing," Annwyl said solemnly. "That's why exile is so terrifying. Cut off from the Nevernever, surrounded by iron and technology and humans that no longer believe in magic, we slowly lose ourselves, until we cease to exist at all."

"Except the Iron fey," I put in, glancing at Keirran. "So, you'd be in no danger."

"Well, that and I'm partly human," he replied, shrugging. "You're right—iron has no effect on me. But for a Summer fey..." He glanced at Annwyl, worry shining from his eyes. No explanation was needed.

The Summer girl sniffed. "I'm not as delicate as that, Prince Keirran," Annwyl said, giving him a wry smile. "You make me sound as fragile as a butterfly wing. I watched the druids perform their rites under the full moon long before your ancestors ever set foot on the land. I'm not going to blow away in the first strong wind that comes through the mortal world. Speaking of which," she went on, rising from the table, "we should get going. Midnight isn't far now, not where we're headed. I'll show you the way."

I followed Annwyl, Keirran and Kenzie back through Leanansidhe's huge basement—or dungeon, I guess—trailing a few steps behind to glare at the things skulking in the shadows. Annwyl had warned us that it might be cold once we emerged from the trod, and Kenzie wore a "borrowed" wool jacket that was two sizes too big for her. The Summer girl offered to find one for me, claiming Leanansidhe had tons of human clothes lying around that she'd never miss, but I didn't want to put myself into her or Leanansidhe's debt any more than I had to, so I refused. As usual, I carried my rattan sticks, in case we were jumped by anything nasty. They were starting to fray a little, though, and I found myself wishing more and more for the solid, steel blade in my room at home.

Was I ready for this? Or, more important, was *Kenzie* ready for this? I'd always considered my Sight a curse, something that I feared and hated and wished I didn't have. It had brought me nothing but trouble.

But to hear Kenzie talk about it, she considered the Sight a gift, something that she was willing to bargain for, something that was worth a tiny piece of her life. It staggered me; the fey were manipulative, untrustworthy and dangerous, that was something I'd always known. How could we see them so differently? And how was I going to protect her, once they realized she had the Sight, as well?

Wait. Why are you even thinking about that? What happened to your promise to not get involved? I felt a stab of annoyance with myself for bringing that up, but my thoughts continued ruthlessly. *You can't protect her. Once you find Todd and get home, she'll go back to her world, and you'll go back to yours. Everyone who hangs around you gets hurt, remember? The best protection you can give anyone is staying the hell away from them.*

Yeah, but it was different now. Kenzie was going to have the Sight. She'd be drawn even more heavily into my crazy, screwed-up world, and she was going to need someone to show her the ins and outs of Faery.

Don't kid yourself, Ethan. That's an excuse. You just want to see her. Admit it; you don't want to let her go.

So…what if I didn't?

"We're here," Annwyl said quietly, stopping at a large stone arch flanked by torch-holding gargoyles. "The ring isn't far. Past this doorway are woods, and then a stretch of moor, with the faery ring in the center of a small grove. It shouldn't be long now." She started forward, but Keirran caught her wrist.

"Annwyl, wait," he said, and she turned back. "Maybe you should stay here," he suggested, looking down at her hand. "We can find the ring on our own."

"Keirran…"

"If those things are anywhere nearby—"

"I'm sure you'll protect me. And I'm not entirely defense-less, either."

"But—"

"Keirran." Stepping close, Annwyl, placed a palm on his cheek. "I can't hide out at Leanansidhe's forever."

He sighed, covering the hand with his own. "I know. I just…worry." Releasing her, he gestured to the arch. "All right then, after you."

Annwyl ducked through the arch, disappearing into the black, Keirran close behind her. I looked at Kenzie, and she smiled back.

"Are you absolutely sure this is what you want?"

She nodded. "I'm sure."

"You know I'm probably going to hover around you for the rest of your life, now. I'll be that creepy stalker guy, always watching you through the fence or following you down the hallway, making sure you're all right."

"Oh?" She laughed. "Is that all it takes to get you to stick around? I should've done the whole bargain-your-life-away-to-the-faeries thing sooner."

I didn't see how she could joke about it, but I half smiled. "I'll be sure to wear a hockey mask, then. So you know it's me."

We went through the arch.

And emerged between two giant, rectangular-shaped rocks standing in the middle of an open field. As Annwyl had warned, the air on this side of the trod was icy. It swept across the rolling moors and sliced through my T-shirt, making my skin prickle. Above us, the sky was crystal clear, with a huge white moon blazing down directly overhead, turning everything black and silver. From where we stood, atop a small rise that sloped gently away into the moors, you could see for miles.

"Wow." Kenzie sighed. "Now I really, really wish I had my camera."

Annwyl pointed a graceful finger down the slope to a cluster of trees at the foot of a rocky hill. "The ring is there," she said quietly with a brief glance toward the sky. "And the moon is nearly right overhead. We must hurry. But remember," she warned, "when the full moon shines down on a faery ring, the fey will appear to dance. We will not be alone."

We started down the slope, picking our way over rocks and bramble, as the wind moaned softly around us and made me shiver with more than the cold. As we drew closer to the trees, I could hear faint strands of music on the wind, the whispers of many voices rising in song. My heart pounded, and I clenched my fists, ignoring the voices and the sudden urge to follow them, the pull that drew me steadily toward the dark clump of trees.

Movement flashed between the trunks, and the whispered song grew clearer, more insistent. I noticed Kenzie, tilting her head with a puzzled expression, as if she could just barely hear something on the wind.

Afraid that she might slip off without me, lured away by the intoxicating faery music, I reached for her hand, trapping it in mine. She blinked at me, startled, before giving me a smile and squeezing my palm. I kept a tight hold of her as we slipped through the forest, walking toward the music and lights, until the trees opened up and we stood at the edge of a clearing full of fey.

Music swirled around the clearing, dark and haunting and compelling. It took all my willpower not to walk toward the circle of unearthly dancers in the center of the glade. Summer sidhe, tall, gorgeous and elegant, swayed and danced in the moonlight, their movements hypnotic and graceful. Piskies and faery lights bobbed in the air, winking in and out like enormous fireflies.

"Ethan," Kenzie whispered, staring at the clearing. Her voice sounded dazed. "There is something here, right? I keep thinking I hear music, and…" Her fingers tightened around mine. "I really want to go stand in that ring over there."

I followed her gaze. Surrounding the dancers, seeming to glow in the darkness, a ring of enormous white toadstools stood in a perfect circle in the center of the glade. The ring was huge, nearly thirty feet across, the mushrooms forming a complete, unbroken circle. Strands of moonlight slanted in through the branches overhead, dappling the ground inside the circle, and even I could feel that this was a place of old, powerful magic.

"It's calling me," Kenzie whispered, as the circle of dancing fey suddenly stopped, their inhuman eyes trained on us. Smiling, they held out their hands, and the urge to join them returned, powerful and compelling. I clamped down on my will to stay where I was and squeezed Kenzie's hand in a death grip.

Keirran lifted his arm to let Razor scurry to an overhead branch. "I hope they don't mind us interrupting their dancing," he murmured. "Wait here. I'll explain what's going on."

I watched him walk confidently up to the observing sidhe, who waited for him with varying degrees of curiosity and alarm. They knew who he was, I realized. The son of the Iron Queen, the prince of the Iron Court, was probably someone you would remember, especially if his glamour was essentially fatal to you.

Keirran spoke quietly to the circle of dancers, who glanced up at us, smiled knowingly, and bowed.

Keirran stepped into the circle, turned and held out his hand. "All right, Kenzie," he called. "It's almost time. Are you ready?"

She gave me a brave smile, released my hand, and stepped forward. Crossing the line of mushrooms, not seeing the dancers that parted for her, she walked steadily toward Keirran, waiting in the center.

I started to follow, but Annwyl stopped me at the edge, putting out her arm.

"You cannot be there with her."

"The hell I can't," I shot back. "I'm not leaving her alone with them."

"Only the mortal who wishes the Sight is allowed in the ring," Annwyl continued calmly. "Otherwise the ritual will fail. Your girl must do this by herself." She smiled, giving me a soothing look. "She will be fine. As long as Keirran is there, nothing will harm her."

Worried, hating the barrier separating us now, I stood at

the edge of the toadstools and watched Kenzie walk up to the figure waiting in the center of the ring. It might've been the moonlight, the strangeness of the surroundings, or the unearthly dancers, but Keirran didn't look remotely human anymore. He looked like a bright, glowing faery, his silver hair reflecting the pale light streaming around him, his ice-blue eyes shining in the darkness. I clenched my fist around my rattan as Kenzie approached him, looking small and very mortal in comparison.

The faery prince smiled at her and suddenly drew a dagger, the deadly blade flashing in the shadows like a fang. I tensed, but he held it between them, point up, though the deadly cutting edge was still turned toward the girl.

"Blood must be spilled for the recipient to gain the Sight," Annwyl murmured as Keirran's lips moved, probably reciting the same thing to Kenzie. "For something to be given, something must be taken. A few drops are all that is needed."

Kenzie paused just a moment, then reached a hand out to the blade. Keirran kept the weapon perfectly still. I saw her brace herself, then quickly run her thumb along the sharp edge, wincing. Drops of blood fell from the blade and her hand, sparkling as they caught the light. A collective sigh went through the circle of fey around them as the crimson drops hit the earth, and I shivered.

"Now only one thing remains," Annwyl whispered, and there was a glint of amber as Kenzie pulled out the vial. "But be warned," she continued, speaking almost to herself, though I had the suspicion she was doing this for my benefit, letting me hear what was going on. "The Sight goes both ways. Not only will you be aware of the fey, they will be aware of you, as well. The Hidden Ones always know whose gazes can pierce the mist and the glamour, who can see through the Veil into the heart of Faery." Keirran stepped back a pace, raising his hand, as if calling her forward. "If you are prepared to embrace this world, to stand between them and be a part of neither, then complete your final task, and join us."

Kenzie looked back at me, blood slowly dripping from her cut fingers to spatter in the grass. I don't know if she expected me to leap in and try to stop her, or if she was just checking to see my reaction. Maybe she was asking, hoping, for my consent, my approval. I couldn't give her that; I'd be lying if I said I could, but I wasn't going to stop her. She had made up her mind for reasons of her own; all I could do now was watch over and try to keep her safe.

I managed a tiny nod, and that was all she needed. Tipping her head back, she put the vial to her lips, and the contents were gone in a heartbeat.

A breeze hissed through the clearing, rattling the branches and making the grass sway. I thought I heard tiny, whispering voices on the wind, a tangle of words spoken too fast to understand, but they were gone before I had the chance to listen. In the center of the ring, Kenzie stumbled, as if she was being battered by gale force winds, and fell to her knees.

I leaped across the toadstools, through the watching fey, who paid me no attention, and dropped beside her as she knelt in the grass. One hand clutched her heart, gasping. Her face was very pale, and I thought she was going to faint.

"Kenzie!" I caught her as she doubled over, gasping soundlessly. "Are you all right? What's happening?" I glared at Keirran, who hadn't moved from where he stood, and gestured sharply. "Keirran, what's going on? Get over here and help!"

"It's all right," Kenzie said, gripping my arm and slowly sitting up. She took a deep breath, and color returned to her cheeks and lips, easing my panic. "It's fine, Ethan. I'm fine. I just…couldn't catch my breath for a second. What happened?"

"Leanansidhe," Annwyl said, joining Keirran a few feet

away. Their gazes were solemn as they watched us, beautiful and inhuman under the moon. "The Dark Muse has taken her price."

Dread gripped my stomach with a cold hand. But Kenzie wasn't looking at me, or any of us, anymore. Her mouth was open in a small *O,* as she slowly stood up, staring at the ring of fey surrounding us. "Have...have they been here the whole time?" she whispered.

Keirran gave her a small, faintly sad smile. "Welcome to our world."

One of the Summer sidhe came forward, tall and elegant in a cloak of leaves, golden hair braided down his back. "Come," he said, holding out a long-fingered hand. "A mortal gaining the Sight is cause for celebration. One more to see us, one more to remember. Tonight, we will dance for you. Prince Keirran...." He turned and bowed his head to the silver haired fey across from me. "With your permission..."

Keirran nodded solemnly. And the music rose up once more, eerily compelling, haunting and beautiful. The fey began to dance, swirling around us, flashes of color and graceful limbs. And suddenly, Kenzie was in that crowd, swept from my side before I could stop it, eyes bright as she danced among the fey.

I started forward, heart pounding, but Keirran held out his arm. "It's all right," he said. I turned to glare at him, but his face was calm. "Let her have this. Nothing will harm her tonight. I promise."

The promise thing threw me. If you were a faery and you said the word *promise,* you were bound to carry it through, no matter what. And if they couldn't keep that promise, they would die, so it was a pretty serious thing. I didn't know if Keirran's human side protected him from that particular rule, or if he really meant it, but I forced myself to relax, watching Kenzie twirl and spin among the unearthly dancers.

Resentment bubbled. A part of me, a large part, actually, wanted to grab Kenzie and pull her back, away from the faeries and their world and the things that wanted to hurt her. I couldn't help it. The fey had tormented me all my life; nothing good had come out of knowing them, seeing them. My sister had ventured into their world, become their queen, and they'd taken her from me.

And now, Kenzie was a part of that world, too.

"Hey."

I turned. Kenzie had broken away from the circle and now stood behind me, the moonlight shining off her raven hair. She'd dropped her coat and looked like some kind of faery herself, graceful and slight, smiling at me. My breath caught as she extended a hand. "Come and dance," she urged.

I took a step back. "No thanks."

"Ethan."

"I don't want to dance with the faeries," I protested, still backing away. "It breaks my Things-Your-Classmates-Won't-Beat-You-Up-For rule."

Kenzie wasn't impressed. She rolled her eyes, grabbed my hand and tugged me forward even as I half resisted.

"You're not dancing with the faeries," she said, as I made one last attempt to stop, to hang on to my dignity. "You're dancing with me."

"Kenzie..."

"Tough guy," she answered, pulling me close. My heart stuttered, looking into her eyes. "Live a little. For me."

I sighed in defeat, let go of my resolve.

And danced with the fey.

It was easy, once you actually let yourself go. The faery music made it nearly impossible not to lose yourself, to close your eyes and let it consume you. I still kept a tiny hold on my willpower as I swayed with Kenzie, back and forth in the center of the ring, while beautifully inhuman Summer fey twirled around us.

Kenzie moved closer, leaning her head on my chest while her arms snaked around my waist. "You're actually really good at this," she murmured, while my heartbeat started thudding loudly in her ear. "Did they teach dancing in kali?"

I snorted. "Only the kind with sticks and knives," I muttered, trying to ignore the warmth spreading through my stomach, making it hard to think. "Though my old school did make us take a class in ballroom dancing. For our final grade, we had to wear formal attire and waltz around the gym in front of the whole school."

"Ouch." Kenzie giggled.

"That's not the worst of it. Half the class played sick that day, and I was one of the only guys to show up, so of course they made me dance with everyone. My mom still has the pictures." I looked down at the top of her head. "And if you tell anyone about that, I may have to kill you."

She giggled again, muffling her laughter in my shirt. I kept my hands on her slim hips, feeling her body sway against mine. As the eerie music swirled around us, I knew that if I remembered anything about this night, it would be this moment, right now. With Kenzie less than a breath away, the moonlight spilling down on her as she danced, graceful as any faery.

"Ethan?"

"Yeah?"

She paused, tracing the fabric along my ribs, not knowing how crazy it was making me. "How 'bout that interview now?"

I let out a long breath. "What do you want to know?"

"You said people around you get hurt, that I wasn't the only one the fey targeted because of you," she continued, and my stomach dropped. "Will you... Can you tell me what happened? Who was the other person?"

Groaning, I closed my eyes. "It's not something I like to talk about," I muttered. "It took years for the nightmares to finally stop. I haven't told anyone about it, ever..."

"It might help," Kenzie said quietly. "Getting it off your chest, I mean. But if you don't want to, I understand."

I held her, listening to the music, to the faeries spinning around us. I remembered that day; the horror and fear that people would find out, the crushing guilt because I knew I couldn't tell anyone. Would Kenzie hate me if I told her? Would she finally understand why I kept my distance? Maybe it *was* time...to tell someone. It would be a relief, perhaps. To voice the secret that had been hanging over me for years. To finally let it go.

All right, then. I'll...try.

"It was about six years ago," I began, swallowing the dryness in my throat. "We—my parents and I—had just moved into the city from our little backwater farm. My parents raised pigs, you know, before we came here. There's an interesting freebie for your interview. The tough guy's parents were pig farmers."

Kenzie was quiet, and I instantly regretted the cynical jab. "Anyway—" I sighed, squeezing her hand in apology "—I met this girl, Samantha. She lived on my block, and we went to the same school, so we became friends pretty quick. I was really shy back then—" Kenzie snorted, making me smile "—and Sam was pretty bossy, much like someone else whose name I won't mention." She pinched my ribs, and I grunted. "So, I usually ended up following her wherever she wanted to go."

"I'm having a hard time picturing that," Kenzie murmured with a faint smile. "I keep seeing this scowling little kid, stomping around and glaring at everyone."

"Believe what you want, I was actually pretty docile back then. The scowling and setting things on fire came later."

Kenzie shook her head, feathery black strands brushing my cheek. "So, what happened?" she asked softly.

I sobered. "Sam was horse crazy," I continued, seeing the red-haired girl in the back of my mind, wearing her cowboy hat. "Her room was full of horse posters and model ponies. She went to equestrian camp every summer, and the only thing she ever wanted for her birthday was an Appaloosa filly. We lived in the suburbs, so it was impossible for her to keep a horse in her backyard, but she was saving up for one just the same."

Kenzie's palm lingered on my chest, right over my heart, which was pounding against her fingers. "And then, one day," I continued, swallowing hard, "we were at the park, for her birthday, and this small black horse came wandering out of the trees. I knew what it was, of course. It had un-glamoured itself, so that Sam could see it, too, and didn't run away when she walked up to it."

"It was a faery?" Kenzie whispered.

"A phouka," I muttered darkly. "And it knew what it was doing, the way it kept staring at me. I was terrified. I wanted to leave, to go back and find the grown-ups, but Sam wouldn't listen to me. She kept rubbing its neck and feeding it bread crumbs, and the thing acted so friendly and tame that she was convinced it was just someone's pony that had gotten loose. Of course, that's what it wanted her to think."

"Phoukas," Kenzie muttered, her voice thoughtful. "I think I read about them. They disguise themselves as horses or ponies, to lure people onto their backs." She drew in a sharp breath. "Did Sam try to ride it?"

I closed my eyes. "I told her not to." My voice came out shaky at the end. "I begged her not to ride it, but she threatened she would make me sorry if I went and blabbed. And I didn't do anything. I watched her lead it to a picnic bench and swing up like she did with every horse in her summer camp. I knew what it was, and I didn't stop her." A familiar chill ran up my spine as I remembered, just before Sam hopped on, the phouka turned its head and gave me a grin that was more demonic than anything I'd ever seen. "As soon as she was on its back," I whispered, "it was gone. It took off through the trees, and I could hear her screaming the whole way."

Kenzie clenched her fingers in my shirt. "Did she—"

"They found her later in the woods," I interrupted. "Maybe a mile from where we had first seen the phouka. She was still alive but..." I stopped, took a careful breath to clear my throat. "But her back was broken. She was paralyzed from the waist down."

"Oh, Ethan."

"Her parents moved after that." My voice sounded flat in my ears, like a stranger's. "Sam didn't remember the black pony—that's another quirk about the fey. The memory fades, and people usually forget about them. No one blamed me, of course. It was a freak accident, only...I knew it wasn't. I knew if I had said more, argued more, I could have saved her. Sam would've been angry with me, but she would still be okay."

"It—"

"Don't say 'it's not your fault,'" I whispered harshly. There was a stinging sensation in my throat, and my eyes were suddenly blurry. Releasing her, I turned away, not wanting her to see me fall apart. "I knew what that thing was," I gritted out. "It was there because of me, not Sam. I could have physically stopped her from getting on, but I didn't, because I was afraid she wouldn't like me. All her dreams of riding her own horse, of competing in rodeos, she lost it all. Because I was too scared to do anything."

Kenzie was silent, though I could feel her watching me.

Around us, the faery dancers twirled in the moonlight, graceful and hypnotic, but I couldn't see their beauty anymore. All I
could see was Sam, the way she laughed, the way she bounced
from place to place, never still. She would never run again,
or go hiking through the woods, or ride her beloved horses.
Because of me.

"That's why I can't get let anyone get close," I rasped. "If
Sam taught me anything, it's that I can't afford to have friends.
I can't take that chance. I don't care if the fey come after me—
I've dodged them all my life. But they're not satisfied with just
hurting me. They'll go after anyone I care about. That's what
they do. And I can't stop them. I can't protect anyone but myself and my family, so it's better if people leave me alone. No
one gets hurt that way."

"Except you."

"Yeah." I sighed, scrubbing a hand over my face. "Just me.
I can handle that." A heaviness was spreading through me,
gathering in my chest, that same feeling of helpless despair,
the knowledge that I couldn't do anything, not really. That
I could only watch as the people around me became targets,
victims. "But, now...you're here. And..."

Her arms slipped around my waist from behind, making
my heart jump. I drew in a sharp breath as she pressed her
cheek to my back. "And you're scared I'm going to end up
like Sam," she whispered.

"Kenzie, if something happened to you because of me—"

"Stop it." She gave me a little shake. "Ethan, you can't control what they do," she said firmly. "Stop blaming yourself.
Faeries will play their nasty tricks and games whether you can
see them or not. The fey have always tormented humans, isn't
that what you told me?"

"Yeah, but—"

"No buts." She shook me again, her voice firm. "You didn't

make that girl get on that phouka. You tried to warn her. Ethan, you were a little kid facing down a faery. You did nothing wrong."

"What about you?" My voice came out husky, ragged. "I pulled you into this mess. You wouldn't even be here if I hadn't—"

"I'm here because I want to be," Kenzie said in that soft, calm voice. "You said it yourself—I could've gone home anytime I wanted. But I stayed. And you're not going to cut me out of your life. Not now. Because no matter what you think, no matter how much you say you want to be alone, that it's better for everyone if you keep your distance, you can't go through this all by yourself." Her arms tightened around me, her voice dropping to a murmur. "I'm staying. I'm right here, and I'm not going anywhere."

I couldn't say anything for a few seconds, because I was pretty sure if I opened my mouth I would break down. Kenzie didn't say anything, either, and we just stood there for a little while, her arms wrapped around my waist, her slim body against mine. The fey danced and twirled their eerie patterns around us, but they were distant mirages, now. The only thing that was real was the girl behind me.

Slowly, I turned in her arms. She gazed up at me, her fingers still locked against the small of my back, holding me captive. I was suddenly positive that I didn't want to move, that I was content to stay like this, trapped in the middle of a faery ring, until the sun rose and the Fair Folk disappeared, taking their music and glamour with them. As long as she was here.

I slipped my hand into her hair, brushing a thumb over her cheek, and she closed her eyes. My heart was pounding, and a tiny voice inside was warning me not to do it, not to get close. If I did, They would only hurt her, make her a target, use her to get to me. But I couldn't fight this anymore, and I was tired of trying. Kenzie had been brave enough to stand with me against the fey and hadn't left my side once. Maybe it was time to stop living in fear…and just live.

Cupping her face with my other hand, I lowered my head…

And my nerves jangled a warning, that cold chill spreading over the back of my neck and down my spine. I tried not to listen, but years of vigilant paranoia, developing an almost unnatural sixth sense that told me I was being watched, could not be ignored so easily.

Growling a curse, I raised my head and scanned the clearing, trying to see past the unearthly dancers into the shadows of the trees. From the edge of the woods, high in the branches above the swirling fey, a pair of familiar golden eyes gleamed in the darkness, watching us.

I blinked, and the eyes vanished.

I swore again, cursing the rotten timing. Kenzie opened her eyes and raised her head, turning to glance at the now empty spot.

"Did you see something?"

I sighed. "Yeah." Reluctantly, I pulled back, determined to finish what we'd started—later. Kenzie looked disappointed but let me go. "Come on, then. Before he finds the others." Taking her hand, I strode out of the ring, parting ranks of fey as I did. Just inside the tree line, Keirran and Annwyl waited at the edge of the shadows, their backs to us.

"Keirran!" I called, breaking into a jog, Kenzie sprinting to keep up. Keirran didn't turn, and I tapped his shoulder as I stopped beside him. "Hey, we've got company—oh."

"So nice to see you, human," a voice purred from an overhead branch. Grimalkin sniffed, looking from me to Keirran, and smiled. "How amusing that you are both here. The queen is not at all happy with either of you."

THE FEY OF CENTRAL PARK

Keirran visibly winced.

"What are you doing here, cat?" I demanded, and Grimalkin turned a slow, bored gaze on me. "If you're here to take us back to Meghan, you can forget it. We're not going anywhere."

He yawned, sitting up to scratch an ear. "As if I have nothing better to do than play nursemaid to a pair of wayward mortals," he sniffed. "No, the Iron Queen simply asked me to find you, to see if you were still alive. And to make sure that you did not wander into a dragon's lair or fall down a dark hole, as you humans are so prone to doing."

"So she sent you to babysit us." I crossed my arms. "We don't need your help. We're doing fine on our own."

"Oh?" Grimalkin curled his whiskers at me. "And where will you go after this, human? Back to Leanansidhe's? I have already been there, and she will tell you the same thing I am about to." He yawned again and stretched on the branch, arching his tail over his back, making us wait. Sitting back down, he raised a paw and gave it a few slow licks. I tapped my fingers impatiently on my arm. From the few stories Meghan had told me about the cait sith, I'd thought she might be exaggerating. Now I knew she was not.

"Leanansidhe has a lead she wishes you to follow up on,"

he finally announced, when I was just about ready to throw a rock at him. "There have been a great many disappearances around Central Park in New York. She thinks it would be prudent to search the area, see what you can turn up. If you are able to turn up anything."

"New York?" Kenzie furrowed her brow. "Why there? I thought New York would be a place the fey avoid, you know, because it's so crowded and, um...iron-y."

"It is indeed," the cat said, nodding. "However, Central Park has one of the highest populations of exiled fey in the world. Many half-breeds also come from that area. It is a small oasis in the middle of a vast population of humans. Also, there are more trods to and from Central Park than you would ever guess."

"So, how are we supposed to get to New York from Ireland?"

Grimalkin sighed. "One would think I would not have to explain how this works to mortals, again and again and again," he mused. "Worry not, human. Leanansidhe and I have already discussed it. I will lead you there, and then you can flounder aimlessly about to your heart's content."

Razor suddenly blipped onto Keirran's shoulder with a hiss, glaring at Grimalkin. "Bad kitty!" he screeched, making Keirran flinch and jerk his head to the side. "Evil, evil, sneaky kitty! Bite his tail off! Pull his toes out! Burn, burn!" He bounced furiously on Keirran's shoulder, and the prince put a hand over his head to stop him.

"What about the queen?" he asked over Razor's muffled hisses and occasional "bad kitties." "Doesn't she want you to return to the Iron Court?"

"The queen asked me to find you, and I did." Grimalkin scratched an ear, not the least bit concerned with the raging gremlin threatening to set him on fire. "Beyond that, I am afraid I cannot be expected to drag you back if you do not wish to go. Though…the prince consort did mention the phrase, *throw away the key,* at one point."

I couldn't be sure, but I thought I saw Keirran gulp. Razor gave a buzz that sounded almost worried.

"So, if we are done asking useless questions…" Grimalkin hopped to a lower branch, waving his tail and watching us with amusement. "And if you are all quite finished dancing under the moon, I will lead you to your destination. We will have to cut back through Leanansidhe's basement, but she has several trods to New York due to the amount of business she conducts there. And she is not exactly pleased with all the disappearances in her favorite city, so I suggest you hurry."

"Right now?"

"I do not see the point in repeating myself, human," Grimalkin said with a disdainful glance in my direction. "Follow along or not. It makes no difference to me."

I'd never been to New York City or Central Park, though I had seen images of them both online. As seen from above, the park was pretty amazing: an enormous, perfectly rectangular strip of nature surrounded by buildings, roads, skyscrapers and millions of people. It had woodlands, meadows, even a couple of huge lakes, smack-dab in the middle of one of the largest cities in the world. Pretty damn impressive.

It was no wonder that it was a haven for the fey.

It was early twilight when we went through yet another archway in Leanansidhe's dungeon and came out beneath a rough stone bridge surrounded by trees. At first, it was hard to believe we stood at the heart of a city of millions. Everything seemed quiet and peaceful, with the sun setting in the west and the birds still chirping in the branches. A few seconds later, however, it became clear that this wasn't the wil-

derness. The Irish moors had been completely silent; stand in
one place long enough, and it felt as if you were the only person in the entire world. Here, though, the air held the quiet
stillness of approaching night, you could still catch the faint
sounds of horns and street traffic, filtering through the trees.

"Okay," I muttered, looking at Grimalkin, who strutted to a
nearby log and hopped up on it. "We're here. Where to now?"

The cat sat down and licked dew off his paw. "That is up
to you, human," he stated calmly. "I cannot look over your
shoulder every step of the way. I brought you to your destination—what you do next is no concern of mine." He drew
the paw over his ears and licked his whiskers before continuing. "According to Leanansidhe, there have been several disappearances in Central Park. So you are in the right place to
start looking for…whatever it is that you are looking for."

"You do realize Central Park is over eight *hundred* acres.
How are we supposed to find anything?"

"Certainly not by standing about and whining at me." Grimalkin yawned and stretched, curling his tail over his back.
"I have business to attend to," he stated, hopping off the log.
"So this is where we must part. If you find anything, return
to this bridge—it will take you back to Leanansidhe's. Do try
not to get lost, humans. It is becoming rather tedious hunting you down."

With a flick of his bushy tail, Grimalkin trotted away,
leaped up an embankment, and vanished into the brush.

I looked at Kenzie and the others. "Any ideas? Other than
wandering around a giant-ass park without a clue, that is."

Surprisingly, it was Annwyl that spoke. "I remember coming here a few times in the past," she said. "There are several
places that are hot spots for the local fey. We could start there."

"Good enough." I nodded and gestured down the path.
"Lead the way."

Yep, Central Park was enormous, a whole world unto it-self, it seemed. We followed Annwyl down twisty forest paths, over wider cement roads lined with trees, across a huge flat lawn that still had people milling about, tossing footballs or lying together on blankets, watching the stars.

"Strange," Annwyl murmured as we crossed the gigantic field, passing a couple making out on a quilt. "There's always a few of us on the lawn at twilight—it's one of our favorite dancing spots. But this place feels completely empty." A breeze whispered across the lawn, and she shivered, hugging herself. Keirran put his hands on her shoulders. "I'm afraid of what we might find here."

"We haven't found anything yet, Annwyl," Keirran said, and she nodded.

"I know."

We continued past the lawn, walking by a large, open-air stage on the banks of a lake. A statue of two lovers embrac-ing sat just outside the theater, together for all time. Again, Annwyl paused, gazing at the structure as if she expected to see someone there.

"Shakespeare in the park." She sighed, sounding wistful. "I watched *A Midsummer Night's Dream* here once. It was in-credible—the Veil was the thinnest I'd ever seen at that point. So many humans were almost ready to believe in us." She shook her head, her face dark. "Something is very wrong. We haven't seen a single exile, half-blood or anyone. What has happened here?"

"We have to keep looking," Kenzie said. "There has to be someone who knows what's going on. Is there another place we could search?"

Annwyl nodded. "One more place," she murmured. "And if we don't find anyone there, then there's no one to be found. Follow me."

She took us down another path that turned into a rocky trail, winding its way through a serene landscape of flowers and plants. Rustic wooden railings and benches lined the path, and a few late-blooming flowers still poked up from the vegetation. *Quaint* was the word that came to mind as we trailed Annwyl through the lush gardens. Quaint and picturesque, though I didn't voice my opinion out loud. Keirran and Annwyl were faeries, and Kenzie was a girl, so it was okay for them to notice such things. As a card-carrying member of the guy club, I wasn't going to comment on the floral arrangements.

"Where are we?" I asked instead. "What is this place?"

Annwyl stopped at the base of a tree, fenced in by wooden railings and in full bloom despite the cool weather. "This," she said, gazing up at the branches, "is Shakespeare's Garden. The most famous human of our world. We come to this place to pay tribute to the great Bard, the mortal who opened people's minds again to magic. Who made humans remember us once more." She reached out to the tree and gently touched a withered leaf with her finger. The branch shuddered, and the leaf uncurled, green and alive again. "The fact that it's empty now, that no one is here, is terrifying."

I craned my neck to look up at the tree. It was empty, except for a lone black bird near the top branches, preening its feathers. Annwyl was right; it was strange that we hadn't run into any fey, especially in a place like this. Central Park had everything they could ask for: art and imagination, huge swaths of nature, a never-ending source of glamour from all the humans who passed through. This place should be teeming with faeries.

"Aren't there other places we could check?" Kenzie asked. "Other...faery hangouts?"

"Yes," Annwyl said, but she didn't sound confident. "There are other places. Sheep Meadow—"

"Sheep!" Razor buzzed.

"—Tavern on the Green and Strawberry Fields. But if we didn't run into anyone by now, I doubt we're going to have much luck."

"Well, we can't give up," Kenzie insisted. "It's a big park. There have to be other places we can—"

A cry shattered the silence then, causing us all to jerk up. It was faint, echoing over the trees, but a few seconds later it came again, desperate and terrified.

Keirran drew his sword. "Come on!"

We charged back down the path, following the echo of the scream, hoping we were going in the right direction. As we left Shakespeare's Garden, the path split before us, and I paused a second, panting and looking around. I could just see the top of the theater off to the left, but directly ahead of us...

"Is that...a castle?" I asked, staring at the stone towers rising over the trees.

"Belvedere Castle," Annwyl said, coming up behind me. "Not really a castle, either. More of an observatory and sightseeing spot."

"Is that why it's so small?"

"Look!" Kenzie gasped, grabbing my arm and pointing to the towers.

Ghostly figures, white and pale in the moonlight, swarmed the top of the stone castle, crawling over its walls like ants. Another scream rang out, and a small, dark figure appeared in the midst of the swarm, scrambling for the top of the tower.

"Hurry!" Keirran ordered and took off, the rest of us close behind.

Reaching the base of the castle steps, I whirled, stopping Kenzie from following me up. "Stay here," I told her, as she took a breath to protest. "Kenzie, you can't go charging up there! There're too many of them, and you don't have anything to fight with."

"Screw that," Kenzie retorted, and grabbed a rattan stick from my hand. "I do now!"

"Ethan," Keirran called before I could argue. The faery prince stood a few steps up, glaring at the top of the staircase. "They're coming!"

Ghostly fey swarmed over the walls and hurled themselves down the steps toward us. They were small faeries, gnome- or goblin-sized, but their hands were huge, twice as big as mine. As they drew closer, I saw that they had no mouths, just two giant, bulging eyes and a pair of slits for a nose. They dropped from the walls, crawling down like lizards or spiders, and flowed silently down the steps toward us.

At the head of our group, Keirran raised his hand, eyes half-closed in concentration. For a second, the air around him turned cold, and then he swept his arm down toward the approaching fey. Ice shards flew before him in a vicious arc, ripping into the swarm like an explosion of shrapnel. Wide-eyed, several of them jerked, twisted into fog and disappeared.

Damn. Where have I seen that *before?*

Brandishing his weapon, Keirran charged up the steps with me close behind him. The evil, mouthless gnomes scuttled toward us, eyes hard and furious, raising their hands as they lunged. One of them clawed at my arm as I jerked back. Its palm opened up—or rather, a gaping, tooth-lined mouth opened up on its palm, hissing and chomping as it snatched for me.

"Aagh!" I yelped, kicking the gnome away. "That is not cool! Keirran!"

"I saw." Keirran's sword flashed, and an arm went hurtling away, mouth shrieking. The ghostly fey pressed in, raising their horrible hands. Surrounded by tiny, gnashing teeth, Keirran stood his ground, cutting at any faery that got too close. "Are the others all right?" he panted without looking back.

I spared a split-second glance at Kenzie and Annwyl. Keirran and I were blocking the lower half of the steps, so the gnomes were focused on us, but Kenzie stood in front of Annwyl, her rattan stick raised to defend the Summer girl if needed.

I almost missed the gnome that ducked through Keirran's guard and leaped at me, both hands aiming for my throat. I stumbled back, raising my stick, but a vine suddenly whipped over the stair rail and coiled around the faery in midair, hurling it away. I looked back and saw Annwyl, one hand outstretched, the plants around her writhing angrily. I nodded my thanks and lunged forward to join Keirran.

Gradually, we fought our way up the steps until we reached the open courtyard at the base of the towers. The ugly gnomes fell back, swiping at us with their toothy hands as we pressed forward. One managed to latch onto my belt; I felt the razor-sharp teeth slice through the leather as easily as paper before I smashed the hilt of my weapon into its head with a curse. We fought our way across the deck, battling gnomes that swarmed us from all directions, until we stood in the shadow of the miniature castle itself. Kenzie and Annwyl hung back near the top of the steps, Annwyl using Summer magic to choke and entangle her opponents, while Kenzie whapped them with her stick once they were trapped.

But more kept coming, scaling the walls, rushing us with arms raised. A cry behind us made me look back. Several gnomes stood in a loose circle around Kenzie and Annwyl. They weren't attacking, but the faery's hands were stretched toward the Summer girl, the horrible mouths opened wide. Annwyl had fallen to her hands and knees, her slender form fraying around the edges as if she was made of mist and the wind was blowing her away. Kenzie rushed forward and swung at one gnome, striking it in the shoulder. It turned with a hiss and grabbed the stick in both hands. There was a splintering crack, and the rattan shredded, breaking apart, as the faery's teeth made short work of the wood.

"Annwyl!" Keirran turned back, rushing forward to defend the Summer girl and Kenzie, and in that moment of distraction a wrinkled, gnarled hand landed on my arm. Jagged teeth sank into my wrist, and I cried out, shaking my arm to dislodge it, but the thing clung to me like a leech, biting and chewing. Gritting my teeth, I slammed my arm into the wall several times, ignoring the burst of agony with every hit, and the gnome finally dropped away.

The gnomes pressed forward, sensing blood. My wrist and forearm were soaked red and felt as if I'd just stuck my arm into a meat grinder. As I staggered back, half-blind with pain, a big raven swooped down and landed on the wall across from me. And, maybe it was the delirium from the pain and loss of blood, but I was almost sure it winked.

There was a burst of cold from Keirran's direction, and the bird took off. Several shrieks of pain showed the Iron prince was taking revenge for the Summer faery, but that didn't really help me, backed against a wall, dripping blood all over the flagstones. I braced myself as the swarm tensed to attack.

"You really do meet the strangest people in New York," called a new voice somewhere overhead.

I looked up. A lean figure stood atop one of the towers, arms crossed, gazing down with a smirk. He shook his head, dislodging several feathers from his crimson hair, giving me a split-second glance of his pointed ears.

"For example," he continued, still grinning widely, "you look *exactly* like the brother of a good friend of mine. I mean, what are the odds? Of course, he's supposed to be safely home in Louisiana, so I have no idea what he's doing in New York City. Oh, well."

The gnomes whirled, hissing and confused, looking from me to the intruder and back again. Sensing he was the bigger threat, they started edging toward the tower, raising their hands to snarl at him.

"Huh, that's kinda disturbing. I bet none of you have pets, do you?"

A dagger came flying through the air from his direction, striking a gnome as it rushed forward, turning it into mist. A second later, the stranger landed next to me, still grinning, pulling a second dagger from his belt. "Hey there, Ethan Chase," he said, looking as smug and irreverent as I remembered. "Fancy meeting you here."

The pack lifted their arms again, mouths opening, and I felt that strange, sluggish pull. The faery beside me snorted. "I don't think so," he scoffed, and lunged into their midst.

Pushing myself off the wall, I started to follow, but he really didn't need much help. Even with the gnomes sucking away at his glamour, he danced and whirled among them with no problem, his dagger cutting a misty path through their ranks. "Oy, human, go help your friends!" he called, dodging as a piranha-gnome leaped at him. "I can finish up here!"

I nodded and ran to the foot of the stairs where Keirran had drawn back, placing himself between the gnomes, Annwyl and Kenzie, his eyes flashing as he dared anything to come close. Annwyl slumped against the ground, and Kenzie stood protectively beside her, still holding one half of the broken rattan. A few gnomes surrounded them, arms outstretched and glaring at Keirran; one was doubled over a few feet away as if sick.

Leaping from the stairs, I dropped behind one of the faeries with a yell, bringing my stick crashing down on its skull.

It dropped like a stone, fading into nothing, and I quickly stepped to the side, kicking another in the head, flinging it away.

Hissing, the rest of the pack scattered. Screeching and jabbering through their nasty hand-mouths, they scuttled into the bushes and up the walls, leaving us alone at the foot of the stairs.

Panting, I looked toward the others. "Everyone okay?"

Keirran wasn't listening. As soon as the gnomes had gone, he sheathed his weapon and immediately turned to Annwyl, dropping down beside her. I heard them talking in low murmurs, Keirran's worried voice asking if she was all right, the Summer girl insisting she was fine. I sighed and turned to Kenzie; they would probably be unreachable for a while.

Kenzie approached sheepishly, one half of the broken rattan in her hand. "Sorry," she said, holding up the ruined weapon with a helpless gesture. "It…uh…died a noble death. I can only hope it gave that thing a wicked tongue splinter."

I took the broken stick from her hand, tossed it into the bushes, and drew her into a brief, one-armed hug.

"Better the stick than you," I muttered, feeling her heart speed up, her arms circling my waist to cling to me. "Are you all right?"

She nodded. "They were doing something to Annwyl when Keirran came leaping in. He killed several, but they backed off and started doing that creepy thing with their hands, and Annwyl…" She shivered, looking back at the Summer faery in concern. "It was a good thing you came and chased them off. Annwyl wasn't looking so good…and you're bleeding again!"

"Yeah." I gritted my teeth as she stepped away and gently took my arm. "One of them mistook my arm for the stick. Ow!" I flinched as she drew back the torn sleeve, revealing a mess of blood and sliced skin. "You can thank Keirran for this," I muttered as Kenzie gave me a horrified, apologetic look. "He went swooping in to rescue his girlfriend and left me alone with a half dozen piranha fey."

And speaking of swooping...

"Hey," came a familiar, slightly annoyed voice from the top of the stairs, "not to rain on your little reunion or anything, but did you forget something back there? Like, oh, I don't know...me?"

I heard a gasp from Annwyl as the redheaded faery came sauntering down the steps, lips pulled into a smirk.

"Remember me?" he said, hopping down the last step to face us, still grinning. Kenzie eyed him curiously, but he looked past her to Keirran and Annwyl. "Oh, hey, and the princeling is here, too! Small world! And what, may I ask, are you doing way out here with the queen's brother?"

"What are *you* doing here?" I growled, as Keirran and Annwyl finally joined us. Keirran had on a wide, relieved smile, and the other faery grinned back at him; obviously they knew each other. Annwyl, on the other hand, looked faintly star-struck. I guess you couldn't blame her, considering who this was.

"Me?" The faery laced his hands behind his skull. "I was supposed to meet a certain obnoxious furball near Shakespeare's Garden, but then I heard a racket so I decided to investigate." He shook his head, giving me a bemused look. "Jeez, you're just as much trouble as your sister, you know that? It must run in the family."

"Um, excuse me," Kenzie put in, and we stared at her. "Sorry," she continued, looking around at each of us, "but do you all know each other? And if you do, would you mind letting me in on the secret?"

The Great Prankster grinned at me. "You wanna tell her? Or should I?"

I ignored him. "Kenzie," I sighed, "this is Robin Goodfellow, a friend of my sister's." Her eyes went wide, and I nodded. "You might know him better as—"

"Puck," she finished for me in a whisper. She was staring at him now, awe and amazement written across her face. "Puck, like from *A Midsummer Night's Dream?* Love potions and Nick Bottom and donkey heads? That Puck?"

"The one and only." Puck grinned. Pulling a green hankie from his pocket, he wadded it up and tossed it in my direction. I caught it with my good hand. "Here. Looks like those things chewed on you pretty good. Wrap that up, and then someone can tell me what the heck is going on here."

"That's what we were trying to figure out," Keirran explained, as Kenzie took the handkerchief and started wrapping my mangled wrist. The slashes weren't deep, but they were extremely painful. Damn piranha-faery. I clenched my teeth and endured, as Keirran went on. "Leanansidhe sent us here to see what was happening with the exiles and half-breeds. We were trying to find them when you showed up."

Razor abruptly winked into sight on Keirran's shoulder. Seeing Puck, the gremlin gave a trill that wasn't quite welcoming, making Puck wrinkle his nose. "Oh, hey, Buzzsaw. Still hanging around, are you?" He sighed. "So, let me get this straight. Scary Dark Muse has got you tromping all over Central Park on some sort of crazy secret mission, and she didn't tell *me* about it? Well, I'm kinda hurt." Crossing his arms, he gave Keirran and me a scrutinizing look, and his green eyes narrowed sharply. "How did you two get involved in this, anyway?"

Something in his voice made the hairs rise along my arm. Me and Keirran. Not Kenzie or Annwyl; he wasn't even looking at them. Puck knew something. Just like Meghan. It was as if he'd confirmed that Keirran and I were never supposed to meet, that seeing us together was definitely a bad thing.

I couldn't think about that now, though. Puck was certainly not going to tell me anything. "My friend Todd was kidnapped," I said, and he arched an eyebrow at me. "He's a half-breed, and was taken by the same type of creatures that suck out the glamour of normal fey."

"I *thought* that's what they were doing. Ugh." Puck gave an exaggerated shiver and brushed at his arms. "Nasty creepy things. I'm feeling very violated right now." He shook himself, then frowned at me. "So, you just decided to go look for him? Just like that? Without telling anyone about it? Wow, you *are* just like your sister."

"We had to do something, Puck," Keirran broke in. "Exiles and half-breeds all over the world are disappearing. And these…glamour-eaters…are making them disappear. Summer and Winter weren't offering any help. I could go to Oberon, but he won't listen to me."

Kenzie finished wrapping my arm, tying it off as gently as she could. I nodded my thanks and turned to the Summer faery. "But he'll listen to you," I told Puck. "Someone has to tell the courts about this."

"And you think *I* should be messenger boy?" Puck crossed his arms. "What do I look like, a carrier pigeon? What about you? What are you four planning?" He looked at all of us, Keirran especially, and smiled. "Whatever it is, I think I should stick around for it."

"What about Grimalkin?"

"Furball?" Puck snorted. "He probably set this whole thing up. If he wants to see me, he'll find me. Besides, this sounds much more exciting."

"We've got this."

"Really? Your arm begs to differ, kid. What would Meghan

say if she knew you were out here? *Both* of you?" he added, glancing at Keirran.

"We'll be fine," I insisted. "I don't need Meghan's help. I survived without her for years. She never bothered to keep tabs on me until now."

Puck narrowed his eyes to glowing slits, looking rather dangerous now, and I quickly switched tactics. "And we're just going back to Leanansidhe, to let her know what we found. There's nothing here, anyway."

"But the courts have to know what's going on," Keirran added. "You felt what those things were doing. How long before they kill all the exiles in the real world and start eyeing the Nevernever?"

"You have to go to them," I said. "You have to let them know what's going on. If you tell Oberon—"

"He might not listen to me, either." Puck sighed, scratching the back of his neck. "But...I see your point. Fine, then." He blew out a noisy breath. "Looks like the next stop on my list is Arcadia." That grin crept up again, eager and malicious. "I guess it's about time I went home. Titania is going to be *so* happy to see me."

At the mention of Titania, Annwyl shivered and wrapped her arms around herself. The longing on the Summer girl's face was plain; it was obvious that she wanted to go home, back to the Summer Court. Keirran didn't touch her but leaned in and whispered something in her ear, and she smiled at him gratefully.

They didn't see the way Puck stared at them, his eyes hooded and troubled, a shadow darkening his face. They didn't see the way his gaze narrowed, his mouth set into a grim line. It caused a chill to skitter up my back, but before I could say anything, the Summer Prankster yawned noisily and stretched, raising long limbs over his head, and the scary look on his face vanished.

"Well," he mused, dusting off his hands, "I guess I'm off to the Summer Court, then. You sure you four don't need any help? I feel a little left out of the action."

"We'll be fine, Puck," Keirran said. "If you see my parents, tell them I'm sorry, but I had to go."

Puck winced. "Yeah, that's going to go over so well for me," he muttered. "I can already hear what ice-boy is going to say about this." Shaking his head, he backed up, leaves and dust starting to swirl around him. "You two remind me of a certain pair." He grinned, looking from me to Keirran. "Maybe that's why I like you so much. So be careful, okay? If you get into trouble, I'll probably get blamed for it."

The whirlwind of dust and leaves whipped into a frenzy, and Puck twisted into himself, growing smaller and darker, until a huge black raven rose from the cyclone and flapped away over the trees.

"Wow," murmured Kenzie, uncharacteristically quiet until now. "I actually met Robin Goodfellow."

"Yeah," I said, cradling my arm. My wrist hurt like hell, and the mention of my sister was making me moody. "He's a lot less insufferable in the plays."

For some reason, Razor found that hilarious and cackled with laughter, bouncing up and down on Keirran's back. The prince sighed. "He won't go back to Arcadia," he said grimly, staring at the spot where the raven had disappeared. "Not immediately. He'll go to Mag Tuiredh, or he'll at least try to get a message there. He's going back to tell my parents where we are."

"Great," I muttered. "So we don't have a lot of time, whatever we do."

Keirran shook his head. "What now?" he asked. "Should

we go back to Leanansidhe and tell her the park is basically a dead zone?"

"My vote is yes," I said. I shifted my arm to a more comfortable position, gritting my teeth as pain stabbed through my wrist. "If we run into any more of those things, I'm not going to be able to fight very well."

"Back to the bridge, then?"

"Wait," Kenzie said suddenly. She was staring back toward the castle, her gaze turned toward one of the towers, dark and hazy in the moonlight. "I thought I saw something move."

I turned, following her gaze, just as a head poked up from one of the observation platforms, looking around wildly. Its eyes glowed orange in the shadows.

PASSING DOWN THE SWORDS

"Todd!" I called, rushing forward.

The dark figure jerked its head toward me, eyes going wide. I leaped up the steps, taking them two at a time, the others close behind. "Hey!" I barked, as the shadowy figure scrambled over the edge of the wall, landing on the deck with a grunt. "Todd, wait!"

I put on a burst of speed, but the figure raced across the courtyard, leaped over the edge and plummeted into the pond at the bottom with a splash.

"Annwyl," Keirran said as we reached the spot the half-breed went over. He was swimming for the edge of the pond, drawing rapidly away. "Can you stop him?"

The Summer girl nodded. Waiting until the half-breed reached the shore, she immediately flung out a hand, and coils of vegetation erupted from the ground, snaking around him. There was a yelp of fear and dismay and the sound of wild thrashing as Annwyl continued to wrap him in vines.

"Got him," Keirran muttered, and leaped onto the wall. He crouched there for a split second, balanced gracefully on the edge, then dropped the long way down to the ground, landing on a sliver of solid ground below us as lightly as a cat. Sheathing his sword, he started across the pond.

I scowled at the back of his head, as I, being a mere mortal, had to retrace my steps back down the stairs and around the pond. Kenzie followed. By the time we reached the place the half-breed was trapped, Keirran stood a few feet from the writhing lump of vegetation, hands outstretched as he tried to quiet him.

"Easy, there." Keirran's quiet, soothing voice drifted over the rocks. "Calm down. I'm not going to hurt you."

The half-breed responded by howling and swiping at him with a claw-tipped hand. Keirran dodged easily. I saw his eyes half close in concentration and felt a slow pulse of magic extend out from where he stood, turning the air thick, making me feel sluggish and sleepy. The half-breed's wild struggles slowed, then stilled, until a loud snore came from the vegetation lump.

Keirran looked up almost guiltily as I joined him, staring at the tangle of vines, weeds, flowers and half-breed. "He was going to hurt himself," he murmured, stepping back as I knelt beside the unconscious form. "I figured this was the easiest way to calm him down."

"No complaints here," I muttered, using my uninjured hand to peel back the tangle of vines. A face emerged within the vegetation, an older, bearded face, with short tusks curling up from his jaw.

I slumped. "It's not Todd," I said, standing back up. Disappointment flickered, which surprised me. What had I been expecting? Todd's last known location was Louisiana. There was no reason he would show up in New York.

Kenzie leaned over my shoulder. "Not Todd," she agreed, blinking at the thick, bearded face, the blunt yellow teeth poking from his jaw. "What is he, then?"

"Half-troll," Keirran supplied. "Homeless, by the looks of it. He probably made part of Central Park his territory."

I stared at the half-troll, annoyed that he wasn't Todd, and frowned. "So, what do we do with him?"

"Hold on," Kenzie said, stepping around me. Kneeling down, she pushed aside weeds and vines, grunting in concentration, until she emerged with a small square item in her hand.

"Wallet," she said, waving it at us, before flipping it open and squinting at it. "Shoot, it's too dark to see anything. Anyone have a minilight?"

Keirran gestured. A small globe of heatless fire appeared overhead, making her jump. "Oh, well, that's handy," she said with a wry grin. "I bet you're fun on camping trips."

The prince smiled faintly. "I can also open cans and make your drinks cold."

"What does the license say?" I asked, trying not to sound impatient. "Who is this guy?"

Kenzie peered at the card. "Thomas Bend," she read, holding the driver's license underneath the pulsing faery light. "He's from…Ohio."

We all stared at him. "Then what the heck is he doing here?" I muttered.

"Oh, you're back, darlings," Leanansidhe said, sounding faintly resigned. "And *what,* may I ask, is *that?*"

"We found him in the park," I said, as Thomas the half-troll stumbled in behind us, shedding mud and leaves and gaping at his surroundings. After he'd woken up, he'd seemed to calm down, remaining passive and quiet when we spoke to him. He'd followed us here without complaint. "He's not from New York. We thought he might be one of yours."

"Not mine, darlings." Leanansidhe wrinkled her nose as the troll blinked at her, orange eyes huge and round. "And why did you feel the need to bring the creature here, pets? You could have asked him yourself and spared my poor carpets."

"Lady," whispered the half-troll, cringing back from the Exile Queen. "Lady. Big Dark. Lady."

"That's all he'll say," Kenzie said, looking worriedly back at the troll. "We tried talking to him. He doesn't remember anything. I don't even think he knows who he is."

"He was being chased through Central Park by our ghostly friends," Keirran added, sounding grim and protective. He hadn't let Annwyl out of his sight the entire way back to Leanansidhe's, and now stood between her and Leanansidhe, watching both the Exile Queen and the half-troll. Razor peeked down from the back of his neck, muttering nonsense. "We fought them off with Goodfellow's help, but we didn't see anyone else there."

"Goodfellow?" The Exile Queen pulled a face. "Ah, so that's what Grimalkin was talking about, devious creature. Where is our darling Puck now?"

"He went back to the Seelie Court to warn Oberon."

"Well, that is something, at least." Leanansidhe regarded the half-breed with cool disinterest. "And what of the park locals, darlings?" she asked without looking up. "Did they mention anything about ladies and dark places?"

"There weren't any others," I told her, and she did look at me then, raising her eyebrows in surprise. "He's the only one we could find."

"The park is a dead zone," Annwyl said. I could see she was shivering. "They're all gone. No one is left. Just those horrible glamour-eaters. I think...I think they killed them all."

Glamour-eaters. The term was catching on, though that was a good name for them. They couldn't hurt me or Kenzie that way, because we had no magic. And Keirran was the son of the Iron Queen; his glamour was poison to them. But everyone else, including Annwyl, the exiles and the rest of Summer and Winter, were at risk.

I suddenly wondered what they could do to half-breeds. Maybe they couldn't make them disappear like the regular fey; maybe a half-breed's human side prevented them from ceasing to exist. But what would draining their magic do to them? I looked at Thomas, standing forlornly in the center of the room, eyes empty of reason, and felt my skin crawl.

Leanansidhe must've been thinking the same thing. "This," she said, her voice cold and scary, "is unacceptable. Darlings…" She turned to us. "You need to go back, pets. Right now. Go back to the park and find what is doing this. I will not stand by while my exiles and half-breeds are killed right out in the open."

"Go back?" I frowned at her. "Why? There's nothing there. The park is completely dead of fey."

"Ethan darling." The Exile Queen regarded me with scary blue eyes. "You are not thinking, dove. The half-breed you found—" she glanced at Thomas, now sitting in a dazed lump on the carpet "—is not from New York. He was obviously taken and brought to Central Park. The park is empty, but so many half-breeds cannot simply vanish into thin air. And the normal fey are gone. Where did they all go, pet? They certainly didn't come to me, and as far as I know, no one has seen them in the mortal world."

I didn't know what she was getting at, but Kenzie spoke up, as if she'd just figured it out. "Something is there," she guessed. "Something is in the park."

Leanansidhe smiled at her. "I knew I liked you for a reason, darling."

"The glamour-eaters might have a lair in Central Park," Keirran added, nodding grimly. "That's why there are no fey there anymore. But where could they be? You'd think such a large population of exiles and half-breeds would notice a group of strange faeries wandering around."

"I don't know, darlings," Leanansidhe said, pulling her cigarette flute out of thin air. "But I think this is something you should find out. Sooner, rather than later."

"Why don't you come with us?" Keirran asked. "You haven't been banished from the mortal realm, Leanansidhe. You could see what's going on yourself."

Leanansidhe looked at him as if he'd just said the sky was green. "Me, darling? I would, but I'm afraid the Goblin Market rabble would make quite the mess while I'm gone. Sadly, I cannot go traipsing across the country whenever I please, pet—I have obligations here that make that impossible." She glanced at me and wrinkled her nose. "Ethan, darling, you're dripping blood all over my clean carpets. Someone should take care of that."

She snapped her fingers, and a pair of gnomes padded up, beckoning to me. I tensed, reminded of the piranha-palmed creatures, but I also knew many gnomes were healers among the fey. I let myself be taken to another room and, while the gnomes fussed over my arm, considered our next course of action.

Return to the park, Leanansidhe had said. Return to the place where a bunch of creepy, transparent, glamour-sucking faeries waited for us, maybe a whole nest of them. Kenzie was right; something was there, lurking in that park, unseen and unknown to fey and human alike. *The lady,* Thomas had mumbled. The lady and the big dark. What the heck did he mean by that?

The door creaked open, and Kenzie came into the room, dodging the gnome who padded out with a bloody rag. "Leanansidhe is keeping Thomas here for now," she said, perching on the stool beside mine. "She wants to see if he'll regain any of his memory, see if he can remember what happened to him. How's your arm?"

I held it up, drawing an annoyed reprimand from the gnome. They'd put some sort of smelly salve over the wound and wrapped it tightly with bandages so it no longer hurt; it was just numb. "I'll live."

"Yes, you will," muttered the gnome with a warning glower at me. "Though you're lucky it didn't get your hand—you might've lost a few fingers. Don't pick at the bandages, Mr. Chase." Gathering the supplies, it gave me a last glare and padded off with its partner, letting the door swing shut behind them.

Kenzie reached over and gently wrapped her hand around mine. I stared at our entwined fingers, dark thoughts bouncing around in my head. This was getting dangerous. No, forget that, this was already dangerous, more than ever. People were dying, vanishing from existence. A deadly new breed of fey was on the rise, killing their victims by draining their glamour, their very essence. Half-breeds were disappearing, right off the streets, from their homes and schools. And there was something else. Something dark and sinister, hidden somewhere in that park, waiting.

The big dark. The lady.

I felt lost, overwhelmed. As if I was a tiny speck of driftwood, bobbing in a huge ocean, waiting for something to swallow me whole. I wasn't ready for this. I didn't want to get pulled into this faery madness. What did they want from me? I wasn't my sister, half-fey and powerful, with the infamous Robin Goodfellow and the son of Mab at my side. I was only human, one human against a whole race of savage, dangerous faeries. And, as usual, I was going to put even more people in harm's way.

Kenzie ran her fingers over my skin, sending tingles up my arm. "I don't suppose there's any way I could convince you to stay behind," I murmured, already knowing the answer.

"Nope," said Kenzie with forced cheerfulness. I looked up, and she gave me a fierce smile. "Don't even think about it, Ethan. You'll need someone to watch your back. Make sure you don't get chomped by any more nasty faeries with sharp teeth. I didn't gain the Sight just to sit back and do nothing."

I sighed. "I know. But I don't have anything to protect you with anymore. Or *me*, for that matter." Gingerly, I clenched my fist, wincing at the needles of pain that shot up my arm. "If we're going to go look for this nest, I don't want a stick. It's not enough. I want my knife or something sharp between me and those faeries. I can't hold back with them any longer."

Cold dread suddenly gripped me. This wasn't a perverse game; me playing keep-away with a redcap motley in the library, or trying to avoid getting beaten up by Kingston's thugs. These fey, whatever they were, were savage and twisted killers. There would be no reasoning with them, no pleas for favors or bargains. It was kill or be torn to shreds myself.

I think I shivered, for Kenzie inched closer and leaned into me, resting her head on my shoulder. "We need a plan," she said calmly. "A strategy of some sort. I don't like the idea of rushing back with no clue of where to go. If we knew where this lair was..." She paused, as I closed my eyes and soaked in her warmth. "I wish I had a computer," she said. "Then I could at least research Central Park, try to figure out what this 'big dark' is. I don't suppose Leanansidhe has any laptops lying around?"

"Not a chance," I muttered. "And my phone is dead. I checked back in the real world."

"Me, too." She sighed and tapped her finger against my knee in thought. "Could we...maybe...go home?" she asked in a hesitant voice. "Not to stay," she added quickly. "I could check some things online, and you could grab your weapons or whatever it is you'll need. Our folks wouldn't have to know."

She snorted, and a bitter edge crept into her voice. "My dad might not even realize I've been gone."

I thought about it. "I don't know," I admitted at last. "I don't like the idea of going home and having those things follow me. Or waiting for me. And I don't want to drag your family into it, either."

"We're going to have to do something, Ethan." Kenzie's voice was soft, and her fingers very gently brushed the bandage on my wrist. "We're in way over our heads—we need all the help we can get."

"Yeah." Frustration rose up, and I resisted the urge to lash out, to snarl at something. Right now, the only someone around was Kenzie, and I wasn't going to take out my fear and anger on her. I wished there was someone I could go to, some grown-up who would understand. I'd never wanted to be the one everyone looked to for direction. Keirran wasn't here; this was my call. How had it all come to rest on me?

Wait. Maybe there *was* someone I could ask. I remembered his face in the locker room, the way he'd looked around as if he knew something was there. I remembered his words. *If you need help, Ethan, all you have to do is ask. If you're in trouble, you can come to me. For anything, no matter how small or crazy it might seem. Remember that.*

Guro. Guro might be the only one who would understand. He believed in the invisible things, the creatures you couldn't see with the naked eye. That's what he'd been trying to tell me in the locker room. His grandfather was a *Mang-Huhula,* a spiritual leader. Spirits to faeries wasn't that big of a leap, right?

Of course, I might be reading too much into it. He might think that I'd finally gone off the deep end and call the people in the white coats.

"What are you brooding over?" Kenzie murmured, her breath soft on my cheek.

I squeezed her hand and stood, pulling her up with me. "I think," I began, hoping the others would be okay with a detour, "that I'm going to have to ask Leanansidhe for one last favor."

She wasn't entirely happy with the idea of us running off to Louisiana again. "How will I know you won't just decide to go home, darlings?" the Dark Muse said, giving me a piercing stare. "You might see your old neighborhood, get homesick, return to your families, and leave me high and dry. That wouldn't work out for me, pets."

"I'm not running away," I said, crossing my arms. "I'm not going to lead those things right to my home. Besides, they might already be hanging around my neighborhood, looking for me. I'm coming back. I swear, I'm not backing out until this is finished, one way or another."

Leanansidhe raised a slender eyebrow, and I realized I'd just invoked one of the sacred vows of Faery. Damn. Well, I was in it for the long haul, now. Not that I couldn't have broken my promise if I wanted to; I was human and not bound by their complex word games, but making an oath like that, in front of a faery queen no less, meant I'd better carry it out or unpleasant things might happen. The fey took such vows seriously.

"Very well, darling." Leanansidhe sighed. "I still do not see the point of this ridiculous side quest, but do what you must. Since Grimalkin is no longer around, I will have to find someone else to take you home. When did you want to leave?"

"As soon as Keirran joins us."

"I'm here," came a quiet voice from the hallway, and the Iron prince came into the room. He looked tired, more solemn than usual, with shadows crouched under his eyes that hadn't been there before. Annwyl was not with him.

"Where are we going?" he asked, looking from me to Kenzie and back again. "Back to the park already?"

"Not yet." I held up my single rattan stick. "If we're going to be walking into this lady's lair or nest or whatever, I'm going to need a better weapon. I think I can convince my kali master to lend me one of his. He has a whole collection of knives and short swords."

And I want to talk to Guro one more time, let him know what's going on, that I didn't just drop out. I owe him that much, at least. And maybe he can tell my folks I'm all right. For now, anyway.

Keirran nodded. "Fair enough," he said.

"Where's Annwyl?" asked Kenzie. "Is she okay?"

"She's fine. The fight—the glamour-eaters—it took more out of her than we first realized. She's sleeping right now. Razor is with her—he'll come to me when she wakes up."

"Do you want to wait for her?" Kenzie asked. "We don't mind, if you wanted to let her sleep a bit."

"No." Keirran shook his head. "I'm ready. Let's go."

I watched him, the way he looked back nervously, as if he was afraid Annwyl could come through the door at any moment. "She doesn't know we're leaving," I guessed, narrowing my eyes. "You're taking off without her."

Keirran raked a guilty hand through his bangs. "You saw what they did to her," he said grimly. "Out of all of us, she's the one in the most danger. I can't take that risk again. She'll be safer here."

Kenzie shook her head. "So you're just leaving her behind? She's going to be *pissed*." Putting her hands on her hips, she glared at him, and he wouldn't meet her eyes. "I know I'd kick your ass if you pulled that stunt with me. Honestly, why do boys always think they know what's best for us? Why can't they just *talk*?"

"I've often wondered the same, darling," Leanansidhe

sighed. "It's one of the mysteries of the universe, trust me. But I need an answer, pets, so I know whether or not to call a guide. Are you three going to wait for the Summer girl, or are you going on without her?"

I looked at Keirran, questioning. He hesitated, looking back toward the door, eyes haunted. I saw the indecision on his face, before he shook his head and turned away. "No," he said, ignoring Kenzie's annoyed huff. "I want her to be safe. I'd rather have her angry at me than lose her to those monsters. Let's go."

It took most of the night. Leanansidhe's piskie guide knew of only one trod to my hometown; Guro's house was still clear across town where we came out, and we had to call a taxi to take us the rest of the way. During the half-hour cab ride, Kenzie dozed off against my shoulder, drawing a knowing smile from both Keirran and the driver. I didn't mind the journey, though I did find myself thinking that I wished Grimalkin was here—he would have found us a quicker, easier way to Guro's house—before I caught myself.

Whoa, when did you start relaying on the fey, Ethan? That can't happen, not now, not ever.

Careful not to disturb Kenzie, I crossed my arms and stared out the window, watching the streetlamps flash by. And I tried to convince myself that I still wanted nothing to do with Faery. As soon as this business with the glamour-eaters was done, so was I.

Somehow, I knew it wasn't going to be that simple.

The taxi finally pulled up to Guro's house in the early hours of the morning. I paid the driver with the last of my cash, then gazed up the driveway to the neat brick house sitting up top.

Hope Guro is an early riser.

I knocked on the front door, and immediately a dog started

barking from within, making me wince. Several seconds later, the door opened, and Guro's face stared at me through the screen. A big yellow lab peered out from behind his legs, wagging its tail.

"Ethan?"

"Hey, Guro." I gave an embarrassed smile. "Sorry it's so early. Hope I didn't wake you up."

Before I could even ask to come in, the screen door swung open and Guro beckoned us inside. "Come in," he said in a firm voice that set my heart racing. "Quickly, before anyone sees you."

We crowded through the door. The interior of his home looked pretty normal, though I don't know what I was expecting. Mats on the floor and knives on the walls, maybe? We followed him through the kitchen into the living room, where an older, scruffy-looking dog gave us a bored look from the sofa and didn't bother to get up.

"Sit, please." Guro turned to me, gesturing to the couch, and we all carefully perched on the edge. Kenzie sat next to the old dog and immediately started scratching his neck. Guro watched her a moment, then his dark gaze shifted back to me.

"Have you been home yet?"

"I…" Startled by his question, I shook my head. "No, Guro. How did you—"

"The news, Ethan. You've been on the news."

I jerked. Kenzie looked up at him with a small gasp.

Guro nodded grimly. "You, the girl and another boy," he went on, as a sick feeling settled in my stomach. "All vanished within a day of each other. The police have been searching for days. I don't know you—" he nodded at Keirran "—but I can only assume you're a part in this, whatever it is."

Keirran bowed his head respectfully. "I'm just a friend,"

he said. "I'm only here to help Ethan and Kenzie. Pay no attention to me."

Guro looked at him strangely. His eyes darkened, and for a second, I almost thought he could see through the glamour, through the Veil and Keirran's human disguise, to the faery beneath.

"Who was that at the door, dear?" A woman came into the room, dark-haired and dark-eyed, blinking at us in shock. A little girl of maybe six stared at us from her arms. "These…" She gasped, one hand going to her mouth. "Aren't these the children that were on TV? Shouldn't we call the police?"

I gave Guro a pleading, desperate look, and he sighed.

"Maria." He smiled and walked over to his wife. "I'm sorry. Would you be able to entertain our guests for a moment? I need to speak to my student alone." She looked at him sharply, and he took her hand. "I'll explain everything later."

The woman glanced from Guro to us and back again, before she nodded stiffly. "Of course," she said in a rigidly cheerful voice, as if she was trying to accept the whole bizarre situation. I felt bad for her; it wasn't every day three strange kids landed on your doorstep, two of whom were wanted by the police. But she smiled and held out a hand. "We can sit in the kitchen until your friend is done here."

Kenzie and Keirran looked at me. I nodded, and they rose, following the woman into the hall. I heard her asking if they wanted something to eat, if they'd had breakfast yet. Both dogs hopped up and trailed Kenzie as she left the room, and I was alone with my master.

Guro approached and sat on the chair across from me. He didn't ask questions. He didn't demand to know where I'd been, what I was doing. He just waited.

I took a deep breath. "I'm in trouble, Guro."

"That I figured," Guro said in a quiet, non-accusing voice. "What's happened? Start from the beginning."

"I'm…not even sure I can explain it." I ran my hands through my hair, trying to gather my thoughts. Why had I come here? Did I think Guro would believe me if I started talking about invisible faeries? "Do you remember what you said in the locker room that night? About not trusting what your eyes tell you?" I paused to see his reaction, but I didn't get much; he just nodded for me to go on. "Well…something was after me. Something that no one else can see. Invisible things."

"What type of invisible things?"

I hesitated, reluctant to use the word *faery,* knowing how crazy I already sounded. "Some people call them the Fair Folk. The Gentry. The Good Neighbors." No reaction from Guro, and I felt my heart sink. "I know it sounds insane, but I've always been able to see them, since I was a little kid. And *They* know I can see them, too. They've been after me all this time, and I don't think I can run from them any longer."

Guro was silent a moment. Then he said, very softly: "Does this have anything to do with what happened at the tournament?"

I looked up, a tiny spring of hope flaring in my chest. Guro didn't smile. "You were being chased, weren't you?" he asked solemnly. "I saw you. You and the girl both. I saw you run out the back door, and I saw something strike you just as you went outside."

"How—"

"Your blood was on the door frame." Guro's voice was grave, and I heard the worry behind it. "That, if anything, told me what I saw was real. I followed you out, but by the time I reached the back lot, you were both gone."

I held my breath.

"My grandfather, the *Mang-Huhula* who trained me, he

would often tell me stories of spirits, creatures invisible to the naked eye. He said there is a whole unknown world that exists around us, side by side, and no one knows it is there. Except for a few. A very rare few, who can see what no one else can. And the spirits of this world can be helpful or harmful, friendly or wicked, but above all, those who see the invisible world are constantly trapped by it. They will always walk between two lives, and they will have to find a way to balance them both."

"Do they ever succeed?" I asked bitterly.

"Sometimes." Guro's voice didn't change. "But they often have help. If they can accept it."

I chewed my lip, trying to put my thoughts into words. "I don't know what to do, Guro," I said at last. "I've been trying to stay away from all this—I didn't want to get involved. But they're threatening my friends and family now. I'm going to have to fight them, or they'll never leave me alone. I'm just… I'm scared of what they'll do to my family if I don't do something."

Guro didn't say anything for a moment. Then he stood and left the room for several minutes, while I sat on the couch and wondered if he was calling the police. If my story was still too crazy for him to accept, despite his apparent belief in "the invisible world." I was wondering if I should get Kenzie and Keirran and just leave, when he reappeared holding a flat wooden box. Setting it reverently on the coffee table between us, he looked at me with a serious expression.

"Remember when I told you I do not teach kali for violence?" he asked. I nodded.

"What *do* I teach it for?"

"Self-defense," I recited. Guro nodded at me to go on. "To…pass on the culture. To make sure the skills don't fade

away." Guro still waited. My answers were correct, but I still
wasn't saying what he wanted.

"And?"

I racked my brain for a few seconds, before I had it. "To
protect your family," I said quietly. "To defend the ones you
care about."

Guro smiled. Bending forward, he flipped the latches on
the case and pulled back the top.

I drew in a slow breath. The swords lay there on the green
felt, nestled in their leather sheaths. The same blades I had
used in the tournament.

Guro's gaze flickered to me. "These are yours," he explained. "I had them made a few years after you joined the
class. I had a feeling you might need them someday." He
smiled at my astonishment. "They have no history, not yet.
That will be up to you. And someday, hopefully, you can pass
them down to your son."

I unstrapped the swords and picked them up in a daze. I
could feel the balance, the lethal sharpness of the edges, and I
gripped the hilts tightly. Rising, I gave them a practice twirl,
hearing the faint hum of the blades cutting through the air.
They were still perfectly balanced, fitting into my hands like
they'd been waiting for me all along. I couldn't help but smile,
seeing my reflection in the polished surface of the weapons.

Okay, *now* I was ready to face whatever those glamour-
sucking bastards could throw at me.

"One more thing." Guro reached into the box and pulled
out a small metal disk hanging from a leather thong. A tri-
angle was etched into the center of the disk, and between the
lines was a strange symbol I didn't recognize.

"For protection," Guro said, holding it up. "This kept my
grandfather safe, and his father before him. It will protect you
now, as well."

Guro draped the charm around my neck. It was surprisingly heavy, the metal clinking against my iron cross as I tucked it into my shirt. "Thank you," I murmured.

"Whatever you have to face, Ethan, you don't have to do it alone."

Embarrassed now, I looked down. Guro seemed to pick up on my unease, for he turned away, toward the hall. "Come. Let's see what your friends have gotten themselves into."

Keirran was in the kitchen, sitting at the counter with his elbows resting on the granite surface, a mug of something hot near his elbow. The little girl sat next to him, scrawling on a sheet of paper with a crayon, and the half-faery—the prince of the Iron Realm—seemed wholly intrigued by it.

"A...lamia?" he asked as I came up behind him, peering over his shoulder. A squat, four-legged thing with two heads stood amid a plethora of crayon drawings, looking distinctly unrecognizable.

The kid frowned at him. "A pony, silly."

"Oh, of course. Silly me. What else can you draw?"

"Hey," I muttered, as the little girl huffed and started scribbling again. "Where's Kenzie?"

"In the office," Keirran replied, glancing up at me. "She asked if she could use the computer for a little while. I think she's researching the park. You should go check on her."

I smirked. "You gonna be okay out here?"

"There!" announced the girl, straightening triumphantly. "What's that?"

Keirran smiled and waved me off. I left the kitchen, nodding politely to Guro's wife as I wandered down the hall, hearing Keirran's hopeless guesses of dragons and manticores fade behind me.

I found Kenzie in a small office, sitting at a desk in the

corner, the two dogs curled around her chair. The younger lab raised his blocky head and thumped his tail, but Kenzie and the older dog didn't move. Her eyes were glued to the computer screen, one hand on the mouse as it glided over the desk. Releasing it, she typed something quickly, slender fingers flying over the keys, before hitting Enter. The current screen vanished and another took its place. The lab sat up and put his big head on her knee, looking up at her hopefully. Her gaze didn't stray from the computer screen, but she paused to scratch his ears. He groaned and panted against her leg.

I eased into the room. Reaching into my shirt, I withdrew Guro's amulet, pulling it over my head. Stepping up behind Kenzie, I draped it gently around her neck. She jerked, startled.

"Ethan? Jeez, I didn't hear you come in. Make some noise next time." She glanced at the strange charm hanging in front of her. "What's this?"

"A protection amulet. Guro gave it to me, but I want you to have it."

"Are you sure?"

"Yeah." I felt the weight of the swords at my waist. "I already have what I need." Looking past her to the computer screen, I leaned forward, bracing myself on the desk and chair. "What are you looking up?"

She turned back to the screen. "Well, I wanted to see if there was a place in Central Park that might be the nest or something. Thomas said something about a 'big dark,' so I wondered if maybe he meant the underground or something like that. I did some digging—" she scrolled the mouse over a link and clicked "—and I found something very interesting. Look at this."

I peered at the screen. "There's a cave? In Central Park?"

"Somewhere in the section called the Ramble." Kenzie scrolled down the site. "Not many people know about it, and it was sealed off a long time ago, but yeah…there's a cave in Central Park."

Suddenly, both dogs raised their heads and growled, long and low. Kenzie and I tensed, but neither of them were looking at us. At once, they bolted out of the room, barking madly, claws scrabbling over the floor. In the kitchen, the little girl screamed.

We rushed into the room. Keirran was on his feet, standing in front of the girl, while Guro's wife shouted something over the racket of the barking dogs. Both animals were in front of the refrigerator, going nuts. The younger lab was bouncing off the door as it barked and howled, trying to reach something on top.

A pair of electric green eyes glared down from the top of the freezer, and a spindly black form hissed at the two dogs below.

"No! Bad dogs! Bad! Go away!" it buzzed, and Keirran rushed forward.

"Razor! What are you doing here?"

"Master!" the gremlin howled, waving his long arms hopelessly. "Master help!"

I cringed. This was the last thing I'd wanted—to pull Guro and his family into this craziness. We had to get out of here before it went any further.

Grabbing Keirran's arm, I yanked him toward the door. "We're leaving," I snapped as he turned on me in surprise. "Right now! Tell your gremlin to follow us. Guro," I said as my instructor appeared in the door, frowning at the racket, "I have to go. Thank you for everything, but we can't stay here any longer."

"Ethan!" Guro called as I pushed Keirran toward the exit. I looked back warily, hoping he wouldn't insist that we stay. "Go home soon, do you hear me?" Guro said in a firm voice.

"I won't alert the authorities, not yet. But at least let your parents know that you're all right."

"I will," I promised and hurried outside with the others.

We rushed across the street, ducked between two houses, and came out in an abandoned lot choked with weeds. A huge oak tree, its hanging branches draped in moss, loomed out of the fog, and we stopped beneath the ragged curtains.

"Where's Razor?" Kenzie asked, just as the gremlin scurried up and leaped onto Keirran, jabbering frantically. The Iron prince winced as Razor scrabbled all over him, buzzing and yanking at his shirt.

"Ouch! Razor!" Keirran pried the gremlin away and held him at arm's length. "What's going on? I thought I told you to stay with Annwyl."

"Razor did!" the gremlin cried, pulling at his ears. "Razor stayed! Pretty elf girl didn't! Pretty elf girl left, wanted to find Master!"

"Annwyl?" Abruptly, Keirran let him go. Razor blipped out of sight and appeared in the nearby tree, still chattering but making no sense now. "She left? Where—?" The gremlin buzzed frantically, flailing his arms, and Keirran frowned. "Razor, slow down. I can't understand you. Where is she now?"

"She is with the lady, little boy."

We spun. A section of mist seemed to break off from the rest, gliding toward us, becoming substantial. The cat-thing with the old woman's face slid out of the fog, wrinkled lips pulled into an evil smile. Behind her, two more faeries appeared, the thin, bug-eyed things that had chased Kenzie and me into the Nevernever. The screech of weapons being drawn shivered across the misty air.

The cat-thing hissed, baring yellow teeth. "Strike me down, and the Summer girl will die," she warned. "The Iron monster speaks the truth. We watched as she entered the real world again, looking for you. We watched, and when she was away from the Between, we took her. She is with the lady now. And if I perish, the Summer faery will become a snack for the rest of my kin. It's up to you."

Keirran went pale and lowered his weapon. The faery smiled. "That's right, boy. Remember me? I watched you, after you killed my sister with your foul poison glamour. I saw you and your precious Summer girl lead the humans to the Exile Queen." She curled a withered lip. "Pah! Exile Queen. She is no more a true queen than that bloated slug Titania, sitting on her throne, feeding on her ill-gotten fame. Our lady will destroy these silly notions of Summer and Winter courts."

"I don't care about Titania," Keirran said, stepping forward. "Where's Annwyl? What have you done with her?"

The cat-faery smiled again. "For now, she is safe. When we took her, our lady gave specific orders that she was not to be harmed. How long she remains that way depends on you."

I saw Keirran's shoulders rise as he took a deep, steadying breath. "What do you want from us?" he asked.

"From the mortals? Nothing." The cat-thing barely glanced and me and Kenzie, giving a disdainful sniff. "They are human. The boy may have the Sight, but our lady is not interested in humans. They are of no use to her. She wants you, bright one. She sensed your strange glamour while you were in the park, the magic of Summer, Winter and Iron. She has never felt anything like it before." The faery bared her yellow fangs in a menacing smile. "Come with us to meet the lady, and the Summer girl will live. Otherwise, we will feed on her glamour, suck out her essence, and drain her memories until there is nothing left."

Keirran's arms shook as he clenched his fists. "Do you

promise?" he said firmly. "Do you promise not to harm her, if I come with you to see this lady?"

"Keirran!" I snapped, stepping toward him. "Don't! What are you doing?"

He turned on me, a bright, desperate look in his eyes.

"I have to," he whispered. "I have to do this, Ethan. You'd do the same if it was Kenzie."

Dammit, I would, too. And Keirran would do anything for Annwyl—he'd proven that already. But I couldn't let him march happily off to his destruction. Even if he was part fey, he was still family.

"You're going to get yourself killed," I argued. "We don't even know if they really took her. They could be lying to get you to come with them."

"Lying?" The cat-thing growled, sounding indignant and outraged. "We are fey. Mankind has forgotten us, the courts have abandoned us, but we are still as much a part of Faery as Summer and Winter. We do not lie. And your Summer girl will not survive the night if you do not come back with us, now. *That* is a promise. So, what will it be, boy?"

"All right," Keirran said, spinning back. "Yes. You have a deal. I'll come with you, if you swear not to harm my friends when we leave. Promise me that, at least."

The cat-faery sniffed. "As you wish."

"Keirran—"

He didn't look at me. "It's up to you, now," he whispered, and sheathed his blade. "Find us. Save everyone."

Razor buzzed frantically and leaped from the tree, landing on Keirran's shoulder. "No!" he howled, tugging on his collar, as if he could drag him away. "No leave, Master! No!"

"Razor, stay with Kenzie," Keirran murmured, and the gremlin shook his head, huge ears flapping, garbling nonsense. Keirran's voice hardened. "Go," he ordered, and Razor cringed back from the steely tone. "Now!"

With a soft wail, the gremlin vanished. Reappearing on Kenzie's shoulder, he buried his face in her hair and howled. Keirran ignored him. Straightening his shoulders, he walked steadily toward the trio of glamour-eaters, until he was just a few feet away. I noticed that the two thin faeries drifted a space away from him as he approached, as if afraid they would accidentally catch his deadly Iron glamour. "Let's go," I heard him say. "I'm sure the lady is waiting."

Do something, I urged myself. *Don't just stand there and watch him leave.* I thought of rushing the glamour-eaters and slicing them all to nothingness, but if Annwyl died because of it, Keirran would never forgive me. Clenching my fists, I could only watch as the fey drew back, one of the thin faeries turning to slash the very mist behind them. It parted like a curtain, revealing darkness beyond the hole. Darkness, and nothing else.

"Do not follow us, humans," the cat-faery hissed, and padded through the hole in the fog, tail twitching behind her. The thin fey jerked their claws at Keirran, and he stepped through the hole without looking back, fading into the darkness. The two fey pointed at us silently, threateningly, then swiftly vanished after him. The mist drew forward again, the tear in realities closed, and we were alone in the fog.

CHAPTER TWENTY
THE FORGOTTEN

Great. Now what?

I heard Kenzie trying to calm Razor down as I stared at the spot from which the glamour-eaters and the Iron prince had vanished a moment before. How were they able to create a trod right here? As I understood it, only the rulers of Faery—Oberon, Mab, Titania—or someone of equal power could create the paths into and out of the Nevernever. Even the fey couldn't just slip back and forth between worlds wherever they liked; they had to find a trod.

Unless someone of extreme power created that trod for them, knowing we'd be here.

Unless whatever lurked in Central Park could rival Oberon or Mab.

That was a scary thought.

Kenzie finally managed to get Razor to stop wailing. He sat on her shoulder, ears drooping, looking miserable. She sighed and turned to me. "Where to now? How do we get to Central Park from here?"

"I don't know," I said, fighting down my frustration. "We have to find a trod, but I don't know where any would be located. I never kept track of the paths into Faery. And even if we find one, humans can't open it by themselves."

Razor suddenly sniffed, raising his head. "Razor knows," he chirped, blinking huge green eyes. "Razor find trod, open trod. Trod to scary Muse lady. Razor knows."

"Where?" Kenzie asked, pulling the gremlin off her shoulder, holding him in both hands. "Razor, where?" He buzzed and squirmed in her grip.

"Park," he said, and she frowned. He pointed back at me. "Park near funny boy's house. Leads to scary lady's home."

"What?" I glared at him. "Why is there a trod to Leanansidhe's so close to my house? Was she sending her minions to spy on me, too?"

He yanked on his ears. "Master asked!" he wailed, flashing his teeth. "Master asked scary lady to make trod."

I stared at him, my anger fading. Keirran. Keirran had had Leanansidhe create a trod close to where I lived. Why?

Maybe he was curious. Maybe he wanted to see the other side of his family, the human side. Maybe he was hoping to meet us one day, but was afraid to reveal himself. I'd never seen him hanging around, but maybe he had been there, hidden and silent, watching us. Abruptly, I wondered if it had been lonely in the Iron Court, if he ever felt out of place, a half-human prince surrounded by fey.

Another thought came to me, the memory of a gremlin peering in my bedroom window. Could it have been Razor all along? Had Keirran been sending his pet to spy on me, since he couldn't come himself?

I'd have to ask him about that, if we rescued him from the lady. *When* we rescued him. I wouldn't let myself think that we might not.

"I know that park," I told Kenzie, as Razor scrambled to her shoulder again. "Let's go."

Another cab ride—Kenzie paid for it this time, since I was out of cash—and we were soon standing in a familiar neighborhood at the edge of the little park where I'd spoken to the dryad. It seemed like such a long time ago now. The sun had burned away the last of the mist, and people were beginning to stir inside their homes. I gazed toward the end of the street. Just a few blocks away stood my house, where Mom would be getting ready for work and Dad would still be asleep. So close. Were they thinking of me now? Did they worry?

"Ethan." Kenzie touched my elbow. "You okay?"

"Yeah," I muttered, turning away from the direction of my house. I couldn't think of home, not yet. "Sorry, I'm fine. Tell your gremlin to show us the trod."

Razor buzzed indignantly but hopped off Kenzie's shoulder and scampered to the old playground slide. Leaping to the railing, he jabbered and pointed frantically to the space beneath the steps. "Trod here!" he squeaked, looking at Kenzie for approval. "Trod to scary lady's house here! Razor did good?"

As Kenzie assured him that he did fine, I shook my head, still amazed that a trod to the infamous Exile Queen had been this close. But we couldn't waste any time. Todd, Annwyl and now Keirran were out there, with the lady, and every second was costly.

Taking Kenzie's hand, we ducked beneath the slide and into the Between once more.

The trod didn't dump us into Leanansidhe's basement this time. Rather, as we left the cold whiteness between worlds, we appeared in a closet that led to an empty bedroom. I felt a moment of dizziness as we stepped through the frame, and wondered if all this frequent trod jumping was hazardous to our health.

The room we entered was simple: a rumpled bed, a night-stand, a desk in the corner. All in shades of white or gray. The only thing of color in the room was a vase of wildflowers on the corner of the desk, Annwyl's handiwork, probably. Razor buzzed sadly as we came in, and his ears wilted.

"Master's room," he sniffled. Kenzie reached up and patted his head.

Voices and music drifted down the hallway as I opened the door. Not singing; just soft notes played at random, barely muffling a conversation. As we ventured down the corridor, the voices and notes grew stronger, until we came to a pair of double doors leading to a red-carpeted music room. An enormous piano sat in the center of the room, surrounded by various instruments on the walls and floor, many vibrating softly. A harp sat in a corner, the strings humming, though there was no one to play it. A lute plinked a quiet tune on the far wall, and a tambourine answered it, jingling softly. For a moment, it made me think that the instruments were talking to each other, as if they were sentient and alive, which was more than a little disturbing.

Then Leanansidhe glanced up from a sofa, and Grimalkin turned to stare at us with big golden eyes.

"Ethan, darling, there you are!" The Exile Queen rose in a fluttering of fabric and blue smoke, beckoning us into the room with her cigarette flute. "You've arrived just in time, pet. Grimalkin and I were just talking about you." She blinked as Kenzie and I stepped through the door, then looked down the empty hallway. "Um, where is the prince, darlings?"

"They have him," I said, and Leanansidhe's lips thinned dangerously. "They met us outside Guro's house and wanted Keirran to come back with them to see the lady."

"And you didn't *stop* him, pet?"

"I couldn't. The glamour-eaters kidnapped Annwyl and threatened to kill her if Keirran didn't do what they said."

"I see." Leanansidhe sighed, and a smoke hound went loping away over our heads. "I knew taking in that girl was a mistake. Well, this puts a rather large damper on our plans, doesn't it, darling? How do you intend to fix this little mess? I suggest you get started soon, before the Iron Queen hears that her darling son has gone missing. That wouldn't bode well for either of us, would it, dove?"

"I'll find him," I said, clenching my fist around a sword hilt. "We know where they are now."

"Oh?" The Exile Queen raised an eyebrow. "Do share, darling."

"The glamour-eaters said something about the Between." I watched as Leanansidhe's other eyebrow arched in surprise. "Maybe you aren't the only one who knows how to build a lair in the space between Faery and the mortal realm. If you can do it, others should be able to as well, right?"

"Technically, yes, darling." Leanansidhe's voice was stiff; obviously she didn't like the idea that she wasn't the only one to think of it. "But the Between is a very thin plane of existence, a curtain overlapping both realms you might say. For anything to survive here, it must have an anchor in the real world. Otherwise, a person could wander the Between forever."

"There's a cave in Central Park," Kenzie broke in, stepping up beside me. "It's a small cave, and it's been sealed off for years, but I bet that isn't a problem for faeries, right? If it exists in the real world, it could be an entrance to the Between."

"Well done, pet. That could very well be your entrance." The Exile Queen gave Kenzie an approving smile. "Of course, space isn't a problem here, as you might have noticed. That 'small cave' in the real world could be a huge cavern in the Between, or a tunnel system that runs for miles."

A huge hidden world, right under Central Park. Talk about eerie. "That's where we're going, then," I said. "Keirran, Annwyl and Todd must be down there somewhere." I turned to the girl. "Kenzie, let's go. The longer we stand around here, the harder it will be to find them."

On the piano bench, Grimalkin yawned and sat up. "Before you go rushing off into the unknown," he mused, regarding us lazily, "perhaps you would like to know what you are up against."

"I know what we're up against, cat."

"Oh? The intelligent strategist always learns as much as he can about his opposition." Grimalkin sniffed and examined a paw, giving it a lick. "But of course, if you wish to go charging off without a plan, send my regards to the Iron prince when you are inevitably discovered."

"Grimalkin and I have been discussing where these glamour-eaters could have come from," Leanansidhe said as I glared at the cat. He scratched behind an ear and ignored me. "They are not Iron fey, for they still have our deathly allergies to iron and technology. So it stands to reason that, at one point, they were just like us. Yet I have not been able to recognize a one of them, have you, darling?"

"No," I said. "I've never seen them before."

"Precisely." Grimalkin stood, and leaped from the bench to the sofa, regarding us coolly. He blinked once, then sat down, curling his tail around his feet as he got comfortable. After a moment, he spoke, his voice low and solemn.

"Do you know what happens to fey whom no one remembers anymore, human?"

Fey whom no one remembers anymore? I shook my head. "No. Should I?"

"They disappear," Grimalkin continued, ignoring my question. "One would say, they 'fade' from existence, much as the exiles do when banished to the mortal realm. Not just individual fey, however. Entire races can disappear and vanish into oblivion, because no one tells their stories, no one remembers their names, or what they looked like. There are rumors of a place, in the darkest reaches of the Nevernever, where these fey go to die, gradually slipping from existence, until they are simply not there anymore. Faded. Unremembered. Forgotten."

A chill slithered up my back. *"We are forgotten,"* the creepy faery had hissed to me, so long ago it seemed. *"No one remembers our names, that we ever existed."*

"Okay, great. We know what they are," I said. "That doesn't really explain why they're sucking the glamour from normal fey and half-breeds."

Grimalkin yawned.

"Of course it does, human," he stated, as if it were obvious. "Because they have none of their own. Glamour—the dreams and imagination of mortals—is what keeps us alive. Even half-breeds have a bit of magic inside them. But these creatures have been forgotten for so long, the only way for them to exist in the real world is to steal it from others. But it is only temporary. To truly exist, to live without fear, they need to be remembered again. Otherwise they are in danger of fading away once more."

"But…" Kenzie frowned, while Razor mumbled a half-hearted "bad kitty" from her shoulder, "how can they be re-membered, when no one knows what they are?"

"That," Grimalkin said, as I tried to wrap my brain around all of this, "is a very good question."

"It doesn't matter." I shook myself and turned to Leanansidhe, who raised an eyebrow and puffed her cigarette flute. "I'm going back for Keirran, Todd and the others, no matter what these things are. We need the trod to Central Park right now." Her eyes narrowed at my demanding tone, but I didn't back down. "We have to hurry. Keirran might not have a lot of time."

Grimalkin slid from the sofa, sauntering past us with his tail in the air. "This way, humans," he mused, ignoring Razor, who hissed and spat at him from Kenzie's shoulder. "I will take you to Central Park. Again."

"Are you coming with us this time?" Kenzie asked, and the cat snorted.

"I am not a tour guide, human," he said, peering over his shoulder. "I shall be returning to the Nevernever shortly, and the trod you wish to use happens to be on my way. I will not be tromping about Central Park with a legion of creatures bent on sucking away glamour. You will have to do your floundering without me."

"Yeah, that just breaks my heart," I returned.

Grimalkin pretended not to hear. With a flick of his tail, he turned and trotted out of the room with his head held high. Leanansidhe gave me an amused look.

"Bit of advice, darling," she said as we started to leave. "Unless you want to find yourselves in a dragon's lair or on the wrong end of a witch's bargain, it's never a good idea to annoy the cat."

"Right," I muttered. "I'll try to remember that when we're not fighting for our lives."

"Bad kitty," Razor agreed, as we hurried to catch up with Grimalkin.

CHAPTER TWENTY-ONE

THE BIG DARK

One more time, we stepped through the trod into Central Park, feeling the familiar tingle as we passed through the barrier. It was night now, and the streetlamps glimmered along the paths, though it wasn't very dark. The lights from the surrounding city lit up the sky, glowing with an artificial haze and making it impossible to see the stars.

I looked at Kenzie. "Where to now?"

"Um." She looked around, narrowing her eyes. "The Ramble is south of Belvedere Castle, where we found Thomas, so...this way, I think."

We started off, passing familiar trails and landmarks, though everything looked strange at night. We passed Belvedere Castle and continued walking, until the land around us grew heavily wooded, with only small, winding trails taking us through the trees.

"Where is this cave?" I asked, keeping my eyes trained on the forest, looking for ghostly shimmers of things moving through the darkness.

"I couldn't find any pictures, but I did find an article that said it's near a small inlet on the west side of the lake," was the answer. "Really, it's just a very small cave. More of a grotto, actually."

"Best lead we've got right now," I replied. "And you heard what Leanansidhe said. If these Forgotten things have a lair in the Between, size doesn't matter. They just need an entrance in from the real world."

Kenzie was silent a few minutes, before murmuring, "Do you think Keirran is okay?"

Man, I hope so. What would Meghan do if something happened to him? *What would* Ash *do?* That was a scary thought. "I'm sure he'll be fine," I told Kenzie, willing myself to believe it. "They can't drain his glamour without poisoning themselves, and they wouldn't have gone through all the trouble of kidnapping Annwyl if they wanted him dead."

"Maybe they want him as a hostage," Kenzie went on, her brow furrowed thoughtfully. "To get the Iron Queen to do what they want. Or to do nothing when they finally make their move."

Dammit, I hadn't thought of that. "We'll find him," I growled, clenching my fists. "All of them." I wasn't going to allow any more people to be dragged into this mess. I was not going to have my entire family manipulated by these things. If I had to look under every rock and bush in the entire park, I wasn't leaving without Keirran, Annwyl or Todd. This was going to end tonight.

The paths through the Ramble woods became even more twisted. The trees grew closer together, shutting out the light, until we were walking through shadow and near darkness. It was very quiet in this section of the park, the sounds of the city muffled by the trees, until you could almost imagine you were lost in this huge, sprawling forest hundreds of miles from everything.

"Ethan?" Kenzie murmured after a few minutes of silent walking.

"Yeah?"

"Don't you ever get scared?"

I glanced at her to see if she was serious. "Are you kidding?" I asked, as her solemn brown eyes met mine. "You don't think I'm scared right now? That marching into a nest of blood-thirsty faeries isn't freaking me out just a little?"

She snorted, giving me a wry look. "You could've fooled me, tough guy."

All right, I'd give her that. I'd done the whole "prickly bas-tard" thing for so long, I didn't know what was real anymore. "Truthfully?" I sighed, looking ahead into the trees. "I've been scared nearly my whole life. But one of the first rules I learned was that you never show it. Otherwise, They'll just torment you more." With a bitter chuckle, I dropped my head. "Sorry, you're probably sick of hearing me whine about the fey."

Kenzie didn't answer, but a moment later her hand slipped into mine. I curled my fingers around hers, squeezing gently, as we ventured farther into the tangled darkness of the Ram-ble.

Razor suddenly let out a hiss on Kenzie's shoulder. "Bad faeries coming," he buzzed, flattening his huge ears. Kenzie and I exchanged a worried glance, and my pulse started rac-ing under my skin. This was it. The lair was close.

"How many?" Kenzie whispered, and Razor hissed again. "Many. Coming quickly!"

I tugged her off the path. "Hide!"

We ducked behind a tree just as a horde of Forgotten sidled out of the woods, making no sound as they floated over a hill. They were pointed, thin faeries, the ones that had threatened me and Kenzie, the ones that had given me the scar on my shoulder. They flowed around the trees like wraiths and con-tinued on into the park, perhaps on the hunt for their nor-mal kin.

Kenzie and I huddled close to the tree trunk as the Forgotten drifted past us like ghosts, unseeing. I hugged her close, and her heart pounded against my chest, but none of the faeries looked our way. Maybe they didn't really notice us, maybe two humans in the park at night wasn't cause for attention. They were out hunting exiles and half-breeds, after all. We were just another human couple, for all they knew. I kept my head down and my body pressed close to Kenzie, like we were making out, as the faeries drifted by without a second glance.

Then Razor hissed at a Forgotten that passed uncomfortably close.

The thing stopped. Turned. I felt its cold eyes settle on me.

"Ethan Chase," it whispered. "I see you there."

Damn. Well, here we go.

I leaped away from Kenzie and drew my swords as the Forgotten gave a piercing shriek and lunged, slashing at me with long, needlelike talons.

I met the blow with an upward strike, and the razor edge of my weapon cut through the fragile limb as if was a twig, shearing it off. The Forgotten howled as its arm dissolved into mist and lurched back, flailing wildly with the other. I dodged the frantic blows, stepped close, and ripped my blade through the spindly body, cutting it in half. The faery split apart, fraying into strands of fog and disappeared.

Oh, yeah. Definitely better than wooden sticks.

A wailing sound jerked me to attention. The horde of Forgotten were coming back, black insect eyes blazing with fury, slit mouths open in alarm. Howling in their eerie voices, they glided through the trees, talons raised to tear me to shreds. I gripped my swords and whirled to face them.

"Kenzie, stay back!" I called, as the first faery reached me, ripping its claws at my face. I smacked its arm away with one sword and slashed down with the other, cutting through the spindly neck. Two more came right through the dissolving faery, grabbing at me, and I dodged aside, letting them pass while whipping the sword at the back of their heads. Turning, I lashed out with the second blade, catching another rushing me from behind. Then the rest of the horde closed in and everything melted into chaos—screaming, slashing claws, whirling blades—until I was aware of nothing except my next opponent and the blades in my hands. Claws scored me, tearing through clothes, raking my skin, but I barely registered the pain. I didn't know how many Forgotten I destroyed; I just reacted, and the air grew hazy with mist.

"Enough!"

The new voice rasped through the ranks of Forgotten, and the faeries drew back, staring at me with blackest hate. I stood there, panting, blood trickling down my arms from countless shallow cuts. The old woman with the cat's body stood a few yards away, flanked by more spindly Forgotten, observing the carnage with cold, slitted eyes.

"You again?" she spat at me, baring jagged yellow fangs. "You are not supposed to be here, Ethan Chase. We told you to stay out of our affairs. How did you find this place?"

I pointed my sword at her. "I'm here for my friends. Keirran, Annwyl and Todd. Let them go, right now."

She hissed a laugh. "You are in no position to give orders, boy. You are just one human—there are far more of us than you think. No, the lady will decide what to do with you. With the son and brother of the Iron Queen, the courts will not dare strike against us."

My hands were shaking, but I gripped the handle of my swords and stepped closer, causing several Forgotten to skitter back. "I'm not leaving without my friends. If I have to carve a path through each and every one of you to the lady herself, I'm taking them out of here." Twirling my blades, I gave the cat-faery an evil smirk. "I wonder how resistant your lady is to iron weapons."

But the ancient Forgotten simply smiled. "I would worry more about your own friends, boy."

A scream jerked my attention around. There was a short scuffle, and two Forgotten dragged Kenzie out from behind a tree. She snarled and kicked at them, but the spindly fey hissed and sank their claws into her arms, drawing blood. Gasping, she flinched, and one of them grabbed her hair, wrenching her head back.

I started forward, but the cat-lady bounded between us with a growl. "Not another step, little human!" she warned as I raised my weapons. "Or we will slit her open from ear to ear." One of the spindly fey raised a thin, pointed finger to Kenzie's throat, and I froze.

Razor suddenly landed on the cat-faery's head, hissing and baring his teeth. "Bad kitty!" he screeched, and the Forgotten howled. "Bad kitty! Not hurt pretty girl!"

He beat the faery's head with his fists, and the cat-thing roared. Reaching up, she yanked the gremlin from her neck and slammed him to the ground, crushing his small body between her bony fingers. Razor cried out, a shrill, painful wail, and the Forgotten's hand started to smoke.

With a screech, the cat-faery flung the gremlin away like he was on fire, shaking her fingers as if burned. "Wretched, wretched Iron fey!" she gasped, as I stared at the place Razor had fallen. I could see his tiny body, crumbled beneath a bush, eyes glowing weakly.

Before they flickered out.

No! I turned on the cat-faery, but she hissed an order, and the two Forgotten holding Kenzie forced her to her knees with a gasp. "I will give you one chance to surrender, human," the cat-thing growled, as the rest of the horde closed in, surrounding us. "Throw away your horrid iron weapons now, or this girl's blood will be on your hands. The lady will decide what to do with you both."

I slumped, desperation and failure making my arms heavy. *Dammit, I couldn't save anyone. Keirran, Todd, even Razor. I'm sorry, everyone.*

The cat-faery waited a moment longer, watching me with hateful eyes, before turning to the Forgotten holding Kenzie. "Kill her," she ordered, and my heart lurched. "Slit her throat."

"No! You win, okay?" Shifting my blades to both hands, I hurled them away, into the trees. They glinted for a brief second, catching the moonlight, before they fell into shadow and were lost from view.

"A wise move," the cat-thing purred, and nodded to the faeries holding the girl. They dragged her upright and shoved her forward, as the rest of the Forgotten closed in. She stumbled, and I caught her before she could fall. Her heart was racing, and I held her tight, feeling her tremble against me.

"You all right?" I whispered.

"Yeah," she replied, as the Forgotten made a tight circle around us, hemming us in. "I'm fine. But if they touch me again, I'm going to snap one of their stupid pointed legs off and stab them with it."

Jokes again. Kenzie being brave because she was terrified. As if I couldn't see the too-bright gleam in her eyes, the way she looked back at the place where Razor had fallen, crumpled and motionless. *I'm sorry,* I wanted to tell her. *This is my fault. I never should have brought you here.*

The circle of Forgotten began to drift forward, poking us with bony talons, forcing us to move. I looked back once, at the shadows that held the limp body of the gremlin, before being herded into the trees.

★ ★ ★

The Forgotten escorted us through the woods, down a winding path that looked much like every other trail in the Ramble, and deeper into the forest. We didn't walk far. The narrow cement path led us through a dense gully of boulders and shrubs, until we came to a strange stone arch nestled between two high outcroppings. The wall was made of rough stone blocks and was a good twenty or more feet high. The narrow arch set in the middle was only five or six feet across, barely wide enough for two people to pass through side-by-side.

It was also guarded by another Forgotten, a tall, skeletal creature that looked like a cross between a human and a vulture. It squatted atop the wall, bristling with black feathers, and its head was a giant bird skull with blazing green eye sockets. Long talons were clasped to its chest, like a huge bird of prey's, and even hunched over it was nearly ten feet tall. Kenzie shrank back with a gasp, and the cat-thing sneered at her.

"Don't worry, girl," she said as we approached the arch without the giant bird creature noticing us. "He doesn't bother humans. Only fey. He can see the location of a single faery miles away. Now that the park is virtually empty, we're going to have to hunt farther afield again. The lady is growing stronger, but she still requires glamour. We must accede to her wishes."

"You don't think the courts will catch on to what's happening?" I demanded, glaring at the Forgotten who poked me in the back when I stopped to stare at the huge creature. "You don't think they might notice the disappearance of so many fey?"

The cat-faery laughed. "They haven't so far," she cackled as we continued down the path, toward the arch and its monstrous guardian. "The Summer and Winter courts don't care about the exiles on this side of the Veil. And a few scraggly half-breeds are certainly below their notice. As long as we don't bother the fey in the Nevernever, they have no idea what is happening in the real world. The only unknown factor is the new Iron Court and its half-human queen." She smiled at me, showing yellow teeth. "But now, we have the bright one. And *you*."

We'd come to the opening in the wall, directly below the huge bird-creature perched overhead. Beyond the arch, I could see the path winding away, continuing between several large boulders and out of sight. But as the first of the Forgotten went through the arch, the air around them shimmered, and they disappeared.

I stopped, causing a couple of Forgotten to hiss impatiently and prod me in the back, but I didn't move. "Where does this go?" I asked, though I sort of knew the answer.

The cat-faery gestured, and the Forgotten crowded close, making sure we couldn't back away. "Your Dark Muse isn't the only one who can move through the Between, little boy. Our lady knew about the spaces between the Nevernever and the real world long before Leanansidhe ever thought to take over the courts. The cave here in the park is only the anchor—it exists in the same place, but we have fashioned it to our liking. This isn't the only entrance, either. We have dozens of tunnels running throughout the park, so we can appear anywhere, at any time. The silly faeries that lived here didn't even know what was going on until it was too late. But enough talking. The lady is waiting. Move."

She gestured, and the fey behind us dug a long talon into my ribs. I grunted in pain and went through the arch with Kenzie behind me.

As the blackness cleared and my eyes adjusted to the darkness, I looked around in astonishment. We were in a huge cavern, the ceiling spiraling up until I could just make out a tiny hazy circle directly overhead. That was the real world, way up there, beyond our reach. Down here, it looked like an enormous ant or termite nest, with tunnels snaking off in every direction, ledges running along walls, and bridges spanning the gulfs between. The walls and floor of the cave were spotted with thousands of glowing crystals, and they cast a pale, eerie luminance over the hundreds of Forgotten that roamed the cavern. Except for the thin faeries and the dwarves with killer hands, I didn't recognize any of these fey.

The Forgotten escorted us across the chamber, down a long, winding tunnel with fossils and bones poking out of the walls. More passageways and corridors wound off in every direction, bleached skeletons staring at us from the stone: lizards, birds, giant insects. I saw the fossil of what looked like a winged snake, coiled around a huge column, and wondered how much of the cave was real and how much was in the Between.

We walked through a long, narrow tunnel, under the rib cage of some giant beast, and entered another cavern. Here, the floor was dotted with large holes, and above us, the ceiling glittered with thousands of tiny crystals, looking like the night sky. A burly fey with an extra arm growing right out of his chest stood guard at the entrance, and eyed us critically as we approached.

"Eh? We're bringing humans down here now?" He peered at me with beady black eyes and curled a lip. "This one has the Sight, but no more glamour than the rocks on the ground. And the rest of the lot are all used up. What do we need 'em for?"

"That is not your concern," snapped the cat-faery, lashing her tail against her flanks. "You are not here to ask questions or attempt to be intelligent. Just make sure they do not escape."

The burly fey snorted. Turning away, it used its extra hand

to snatch a long wooden ladder leaning against the wall, then dropped it down into a pit.

"Get down there, mortal." A jab to the ribs prodded me forward. I walked to the edge and peered down. The ladder dropped away into black, and the sides of the hole were steep and smooth. I stared hard into the darkness, but I couldn't see the bottom.

Afraid that if I stood there much longer I'd get forcibly shoved into the black pit, I started down the ladder. My footsteps echoed dully against the wood, and with every step, the darkness grew thicker, until I could barely see the rungs in front of me.

I hope there's not something nasty down here, I thought, then immediately wished I hadn't.

My shoes finally hit a sandy floor, and I backed carefully away from the ladder, as Kenzie was coming down, as well. As soon as she hit the bottom, the ladder zipped up the wall and vanished through the opening, leaving us in near blackness.

I gazed around, waiting for my eyes to adjust. We stood in the center of a large chamber, the walls made of smooth, seamless stone. No handholds, no cracks or ledges, just flat, even rock. Above us, I could barely make out the hazy gray circles that were the holes in the floor above. The ground was covered in pale sand, with bits of garbage scattered here and there; the wrapper of a granola bar or a chewed apple core. Something had been down here recently, by the looks of it.

And then, a shuffle in the corner of the room made my heart skip a beat. My earlier thoughts were correct. Something *was* still down here with us. *Lots* of things. And they were getting closer.

KENZIE'S CONFESSION

Grabbing Kenzie, I pulled her behind me, backing away as several bodies shuffled forward into the beam of hazy light.

Humans. All of them. Young and old, male and female. The youngest was probably no more than thirteen, and the oldest had a gray beard down to his chest. There were about two dozen of them, all ragged and filthy-looking, like they hadn't bathed or eaten in a while.

Staring at them, my nerves prickled. There was something about this group that was just...wrong. Sure, they were ragged and filthy and had probably been captives of the Forgotten for a while now, but no one came forward to greet us or demand who we were. Their faces were blank, their features slack, and they gazed back with no emotion in their eyes, no spark of anger or fear or anything. It was like staring into a herd of curious, passive sheep.

Still, there were a lot of them, and I tensed, ready to fight if they attacked us. But the humans, after a somewhat disappointed glance, like they were expecting us to be food, turned away and shuffled back into the darkness.

I took a step forward. "Hey, wait!" I called, the echo bouncing around the pit. The humans didn't respond, and I raised my voice. "Just a second! Hold up!"

A few of them turned, regarding me without expression, but at least it was something. "I'm looking for a friend of mine," I went on, gazing past their ragged forms, trying to peer into the shadows. "His name is Todd Wyndham. Is there anyone by that name down here? He's about my age, blond hair, short."

The humans stared mutely, and I sighed, frustration and hopelessness threatening to smother me. End of the road, it seemed. We were stuck here, trapped by the Forgotten and surrounded by crazy humans, with no hope of rescuing Keirran or Annwyl. And Todd was still nowhere to be found.

There was a shuffle then, somewhere in the darkness, and a moment later a human pushed his way to the front of the crowd. He was about my age, small and thin, with scruffy blond hair and…

A jolt of shock zipped up my spine.

It was Todd. But he was *human*. The furry ears were gone, as were the claws and canines and piercing orange eyes. It was still Todd Wynham, there was no question about that; he still wore the same clothes as when I saw him last, though they were filthy and ragged now. But the change was so drastic it took me a few seconds to accept that this was the same person. I could only stare in disbelief. Except for the grime and the strange, empty look on his face, Todd seemed completely mortal, with no trace of the faery blood that ran through him a week ago.

"Todd?" Kenzie eased forward, holding out her hand. Todd watched her with blank hazel eyes and didn't move. "It is you! You're all right! Oh, thank goodness. They didn't hurt you, did they?"

I clenched my fists. She didn't know. She couldn't realize what had happened. Kenzie had only seen Todd as a human before; she didn't know anything was wrong.

But I knew. And a slow flame of rage began to smolder inside. *Well, you wanted to know what happened to half-breeds when their glamour was drained away, Ethan. There's your answer. All these humans were half-fey once, before the Forgotten took their magic.* Todd blinked slowly. "Who are you?" he asked in a monotone, and I shivered. Even his voice sounded wrong. Flat and hollow, like everything he was had been stripped away, leaving no emotion behind. I remembered the eager, defiant half-breed from before; comparing him to this hopeless stranger made me sick.

"You know me," Kenzie said, walking toward him. "Kenzie. Mackenzie, from school. Ethan is here, too. We've been looking everywhere for you."

"I don't know you," Todd stated in that same empty, chilling voice. "I don't remember *him,* or school or anything. I don't remember anything but this hole. But..." He looked away, into the darkness, his brow furrowing. "But...it feels like I should remember something. Something important. I think...I think I lost something." An agonized expression crossed his face, just for a moment, before it smoothed out again. "Or, maybe not," he continued with a shrug. "I can't remember. It must not have been very important."

I was shaking with fury, and took a deep breath to calm myself. *Bastards,* I thought, filled with a sudden, fiery hatred. *Killing faeries is one thing. But this?* I looked at Todd, at the slack face, the hollow eyes, and resisted the urge to punch the wall. *This is worse than killing. You stripped away everything that made him who he was, took something that he can't ever get back and left him...like this. To keep yourselves alive. I won't let you get away with that.*

"What about your parents?" Kenzie continued, still trying to cajole an answer out of the once half-faery. "Don't you remember them? Or any of your teachers?"

"No," was the flat reply, and Todd backed away, his eyes

clouding over, into the darkness. "I don't know you," he whispered. "Go away."

"Todd—" Kenzie tried again, but the human turned away from her, huddling down against the wall, burying his face in his knees.

"Leave me alone."

She tried coaxing him to talk again, asking him questions about home, school, how he came to be there, telling him about our own adventures. But she was met with a wall of silence. Todd didn't even look up from his knees. He seemed determined to pretend we didn't exist, and after a few minutes of watching this and getting nothing, I walked away, needing to move before I started shaking him. Kenzie's stubbornly cheerful voice followed me as I stalked into the shadows, and I left her to it; if anyone could persuade him to talk, she could.

Weaving through hunched forms of indifferent humans, I wandered the perimeter, halfheartedly searching for anything we might've missed. Anything that might allow us to escape. Nothing. Just steep, smooth walls and sand. We were well and truly stuck down here.

Putting my back against the wall, I slid to the floor, feeling cold sand through my jeans. I wondered what my parents were doing right now. I wondered how long the Forgotten would keep us down here. Weeks? Months? If they finally let us go, would we return to the mortal realm to find we'd been missing for twenty years, and everyone had given us up for dead?

Or, would they simply kill us and leave our bones to rot in this hole, gnawed on by a bunch of former half-breeds?

Kenzie joined me, looking tired and pale. Purple marks streaked her arms from where the Forgotten had grabbed her, and her eyes were dull with exhaustion. Anger flared, but it was damped by the feeling of hopelessness that clung to everything in this place. She gave me a brave smile as she came up, but I could see her mask crumbling, falling to pieces around her.

"Anything?" I asked, and she shook her head.

"No. I'll try again in a little while, when he's had a chance to think about it. I think poking him further will just make him retreat more." She slid down next to me, gazing out into the darkness. I felt the heat of her small body against mine, and an almost painful urge to reach out for her, to draw her close. But my own fear held me back. I had failed. Again. Not only Kenzie, but Todd, Keirran, Annwyl, everyone. I wished I had been stronger. That I could've kept everyone around me safe.

But most of all, I wished Kenzie didn't have to be here. That I'd never shown her my world. I'd give anything to get her out of this.

"How long do you think they'll keep us here?" Kenzie whispered after a few beats of silence.

"I don't know," I murmured, feeling the weight in my chest get bigger. Kenzie rubbed her arms, running her fingers over the bruises on her skin, making my stomach churn.

"We...we're gonna make it home, right?"

"Yeah." I half turned, forcing a smile. "Yeah, don't worry, we'll get out of here, and you'll be home before you know it. Your sister will be waiting for you, and your Dad will probably yell that you've been gone so long, but they'll both be relieved that you're back. And you can call my house and keep me updated on everything that happens at school, because my parents will probably ground me until I'm forty."

It was a kind lie, and we both knew it, but I couldn't tell her the truth. That I didn't know if we would make it home, that no one knew where we were, that right above our heads waited a legion of savage, desperate fey and their mysterious lady. Keirran was gone, Annwyl was missing, and the person we'd come to find was a hollow shell of himself. I'd hit rock bottom and had dragged her down with me, but I couldn't tell her that all hope was gone. Even though I had none of it myself.

So I lied. I told her we would make it home, and Kenzie returned the small smile, as if she really believed it. But then she shivered, and the mask crumpled. Bringing both knees to her chest, she wrapped her arms around them and closed her eyes.

"I'm scared," she admitted in a whisper. And I couldn't hold myself back any longer.

Reaching out, I pulled her into my lap and wrapped her in my arms. She clung to me, fists clenched in my shirt, and I folded her against my chest, feeling our hearts race together.

"I'm sorry," I whispered into her hair. "I wanted to protect you from all of this."

"I know," she whispered back. "And I know you're thinking this is your fault somehow, but it isn't." Her hand slipped up to my face, pressing softly against my cheek, and I closed my eyes. "Ethan, you're a sweet, infuriating, incredible guy, and I think I…might be falling for you. But there are things in my life you just can't protect me from."

My breath caught. I felt my heartbeat stutter, then pick up, a little faster than before. Kenzie hunched her shoulders, burying her face in my shirt, suddenly embarrassed. I wanted to tell her she had nothing to be afraid of; that I couldn't stay away from her if I tried, that she had somehow gotten past all my bullshit—the walls, the anger, the constant fear, guilt and self-loathing—and despite everything I'd done to drive her away and make her hate me, I couldn't imagine my life without her.

I wished I knew how to tell her as much. Instead, I held her and smoothed her hair, listening to our breaths mingle together. She was quiet for a long time, one hand around my neck, the other tracing patterns in my shirt.

"Ethan," she murmured, still not looking at me. "If—
when—we get home, what will happen, to *us?*"

"I don't know," I said honestly. "I guess…that will mostly
depend on you."

"Me?"

I nodded. "You've seen my life. You've seen how screwed
up it is. How dangerous it can be. I wouldn't force that on
anyone, but…" I trailed off, closing my eyes, pressing my forehead to hers. "But I can't stay away from you anymore. I'm
not even going to try. If you want me around, I'll be there."

"For how long?" Her words were the faintest whisper. If
we hadn't been so close, I wouldn't have caught them. Hurt,
I stared at her, and she peered up at me, her eyes going wide
at the look on my face.

"Oh, no! I'm sorry, Ethan. That wasn't for you. I just…" She
sighed, hanging her head again, clenching a fist in my shirt.
"All right," she whispered. "Enough of this, Kenzie. Before
this goes any further." She nodded to herself and looked up,
facing me fully. "I guess it's time you knew."

I waited, holding my breath. *Whatever secrets you have,* I
wanted to say, *whatever you've been hiding, it doesn't matter. Not
to me.* My whole life was one big lie, and I had more secrets
than one person should have in a lifetime. Nothing she said
could scare or shock me away from her.

But there was still that tiny sense of unease, that dark, ominous thing Kenzie had been keeping from me since we'd met.
I knew some secrets weren't meant to be shared, that knowing them could change your perspective of a person forever. I
suspected this might be one of those times. So I waited, as the
silence stretched between us, as Kenzie gathered her thoughts.
Finally, she pushed her hair back, still not looking at me, and
took a deep breath.

"Remember…when you asked why I would trade a piece

of my life away to Leanansidhe?" she began in a halting voice. "When I made that bargain to get the Sight. Do you remember what I said?"

I nodded, though she still wasn't looking at me. "That no one lives forever."

Kenzie shivered. "My mom died three years ago," she said, folding her arms protectively to her chest. "It was a car accident—there was nothing anyone could do. But I remember when I was little, she would always talk about traveling the world. She said when I got older, we would go see the pyramids together, or the Great Wall or the Eiffel Tower. She used to show me travel magazines and brochures, and we would plan out our trip. Sometimes by boat, or train or even by hot air balloon. And I believed her. Every summer, I asked if *this* was the year we would go." She sniffed, and a bitter note crept into her voice. "It never was, but dad swore that when he wasn't so busy, when work slowed down a bit, we would all take that trip together.

"But then she died," Kenzie went on softly, and swiped a hand across her eyes. "She died, and she never got the chance to see Egypt, or Paris or any of the places she wanted to see. And I always thought it was so sad, that it was such a waste. All those dreams, all those plans we had, she would never get to do any of them."

"I'm sorry, Kenzie."

She paused, taking a breath to compose herself, her voice growing stronger when she spoke again. "Afterward, I thought maybe Dad and I could...take that trip together, in her honor, you know? He was so devastated when he found out. I thought that if we could go someplace, just the two of us, he'd remember all the good times. And I wanted to remind him that he still had me, even though Mom was gone."

I remembered the way Kenzie had spoken about her father before, the anger and bitterness she'd shown, and my gut twisted. Somehow, I knew that hadn't happened.

"But, my dad…" Kenzie shook her head, her eyes dark. "When Mom died, he sort of…forgot about me. He never talked to me if he could help it, and just…threw himself into his job. He started working more and more at the office, just so he didn't have to come home. At first, I thought it was because he missed Mom so much, but that wasn't it. It was me. He didn't want to see me." At my furious look, she shrugged. "Maybe I reminded him too much of Mom. Or maybe he was just distancing himself, in case he lost me, too. I would try talking to him—I really missed her sometimes—but he'd just give me a wad of cash and then lock himself in his office to drink." Her eyes glimmered. "I didn't want money. I wanted someone to talk to me, to listen to me. I wanted him to be a dad."

Anger burned. And guilt. I thought of my family, of how we had lost Meghan all those years ago, and how my parents clung to me even more tightly, for fear of that same thing. I couldn't imagine them ignoring me, forgetting I existed, in case they woke up one day and found me gone. They were paranoid and overprotective, but that was infinitely better than the alternative. What was wrong with Kenzie's father? How could he ignore his only daughter, especially after she'd just lost her mom?

"That's insane," I muttered. "I'm sorry, Kenzie. Your dad sounds like a complete tool. You shouldn't have had to go through that alone." She didn't say anything, and I rubbed her arms, trying to get her to look at me, keeping my voice gentle. "So, you do all these crazy things because you don't want to end up like your mom?"

"No." Kenzie hunched her shoulders, looking off into the distance, and her eyes glimmered. "Well, that's part of it,

but..." She paused again and went on, even softer than before. "When Dad remarried, things got a little better. I had a
stepsister, Alexandria, so at least I wasn't stuck in a big empty
house all day, alone. But Dad still worked all the time, and
the nights he *was* home, he was so busy with his new wife
and Alex, he didn't pay much attention to me." She shrugged,
as if she'd gotten over it and didn't need any sympathy, but I
still seethed at her father.

"Then, about a year ago," Kenzie went on, "I started getting sick. Nausea, sudden dizzy spells, things like that. Dad
didn't notice, of course. No one really did...until I passed out
in the middle of class one afternoon. In history. I remember,
because I begged the school nurse not to call my dad. I knew
he'd be angry if he had to come pick me up in the middle of
the workday." Kenzie snorted, her eyes and voice bitter as she
stared at the ground. "I collapsed just picking up my books,
and the freaking *school nurse* had to tell him to take me to a
doctor. And he was still pissed about it. Like I got sick on purpose, like he thinks all the tests and treatments and doctor ap-
pointments are just a way of getting attention."

Something cold settled in my stomach, as many small
things clicked into place. The bruises. The protectiveness of
her friends at school. Her fearlessness and burning desire to see
all that she could. The dark thing hovered between us now,
turning my blood to ice as I finally figured it out. "You're sick
now, aren't you?" I whispered. "The serious kind."

"Yeah." She looked down, fiddling with my shirt, and took
a shaky breath. "Ethan I...I have leukemia." The words trailed
off into a whisper at the end, and she paused, but when she
continued her voice was calm and matter-of-fact. "The doctors won't tell me much, but I did some research, and the survival rate for the type I have, with treatment and chemo and

everything, is about forty percent. And that's if I even make
it through the first five years."

It felt as if someone had punched a hole in my stomach,
grabbed my insides and pulled them out again. I stared at Kenzie in horror, unable to catch my breath. Leukemia. Cancer.
Kenzie was…

"So, now you know the real reason I wanted the Sight.
Why I wanted to see the fey." She finally looked at me, one
corner of her lip turned up in a bitter smile. "That month I
traded to Leanansidhe? That's nothing. I probably won't live
to see thirty."

I wanted to do something, anything. I wanted to jump up
and punch the walls, scream out my frustration and the un-
fairness of it all. Why her? Why did it have to be Kenzie, who
was brave and kind and stubborn and absolutely perfect? It
wasn't right. "You should've gone back," I finally choked out.
"You shouldn't be here with me, not when you could be…" I
couldn't even get the word past my lips. The sudden thought
that this dark pit could be the last place she would ever see
nearly made me sick. "Kenzie, you should be with your family," I moaned in despair. "Why did you stay with me? You
should've gone home."

Kenzie's eyes gleamed. "To what?" she snapped, making a
sharp gesture. "Back to my dad, who can't even look at me?
Back to that empty house, where everyone tiptoes around and
whispers things they don't think I can hear? To the doctors
who won't tell me anything, who treat me like I have no idea
what's going on? Haven't you been listening, Ethan? What do
I have to go back to?"

"You would be safe—"

"Safe," she scoffed. "I don't have time to be safe. I want to
live. I want to travel the world. See things no one else has. Go
bungee jumping and skydiving and all those crazy things. If

I'm living on borrowed time, I want to make the most of it. And you showed me this whole other world, with dragons and magic and queens and talking cats. How could I pass that up?"

I couldn't answer, mostly because my own throat felt suspiciously tight. Kenzie reached out with both arms and laced her hands behind my head, gazing up at me. Her eyes were tender as she leaned in. "Ethan, this sickness, this thing inside me…I've made my peace with it. Whatever happens, I can't stop it. But there are things I want to do before I die, a whole list that I know I probably won't get to, but I'm sure as hell going to try. 'Seeing the fey' wasn't on the list, but 'go someplace no one has ever seen before' was. So is 'have my first kiss.'" She ducked her head, as if she was blushing. "Of course, there's never been a boy that I've wanted to kiss me," she whispered, biting her lip, "until I met you."

I was still reeling from her last words, so that admittance sent another jolt through my stomach, turning it inside out. That this strange, stubborn, defiantly cheerful girl—this girl who fought lindwurms and bargained with faery queens and faced her own mortality every single day, who followed me into Faery and didn't leave my side, even when she was offered a way home—this brave, selfless, incredible girl wanted me to kiss her.

Damn. I was in deep, wasn't I?

Yeah, and I don't care.

Kenzie was still staring at the ground, and I realized I hadn't answered her, still recovering from being blindsided by my own emotions. "But I understand if you don't want to," she went on in a forced, cheerful voice, dropping her arms. "It's not fair to you, to get involved with someone like me. It was stupid of me to say anything." She spoke quickly, trying to convince herself, and I shook myself out of my trance. "I don't know how long I'll have, and who wants to go through that?

It'll just end up breaking both our hearts. So, if you don't want to start anything, that's fine, I understand. I just—"

I kissed her, stopping any more arguments. She made a tiny noise of surprise before she relaxed into me with a sigh. Her arms laced around my neck; mine slid into her hair and down to the small of her back, holding us together. No more illusions, no more hiding from myself. I needed this girl; I needed her laughter and fearlessness, the way she kept pushing me, refusing to be intimidated. I'd kept people at arm's length for so long, scared of what the fey would do to them if I got close, but I couldn't do that anymore. Not to her.

It seemed a long time before we finally pulled back. The shuffle of the former half-breeds echoed around us, the pit was still dark and cold and unscalable, but I was no longer content just to sit here and accept our fate. Everything was different. I had something to fight for, a real reason to get home.

Kenzie didn't say anything immediately after. She blinked and looked a little dazed as I drew back. I couldn't help but smirk.

"Oh, wow," I teased quietly. "Did I actually render Mackenzie St. James speechless?"

She snorted. "Hardly, but you're welcome to try again."

Smiling, I pulled her to me for another kiss. She shifted so that her knees were straddling my waist and buried her hands in my hair, holding my head still. I wrapped my arms around the small of her back and let the feel of her lips take me away.

This time, Kenzie was the one who pulled back, all traces of amusement gone as she stared at me, my reflection peering back from her eyes. "Promise you won't disappear when we get home, tough guy," she whispered, and, though her tone was light, her gaze was solemn. "I like this Ethan. I don't want him to turn into the one I met at the tournament once we're safe."

"I can't promise that you won't ever see him again," I told

her. "The fey will still hang around me, no matter what I do. But I'm not going anywhere." Reaching up, I brushed the hair from her eyes, smiling ruefully. "I'm still not sure how this will work when we get home, but I want to be with you. And if you want me to be your boyfriend and go to parties and hang out with your meathead friends…I'll try. I'm not the best at being normal, but I'll give it a shot."

"Really?" She smiled, and her eyes glimmered. "You… you're not just saying that because you feel sorry for me, are you? I don't want to guilt you into doing anything, just because I'm sick."

No, Mackenzie. I fell for you long before then, I just didn't know it. "I'll prove it to you, then," I told her, running my hands up her back, drawing her closer. "Once we get out of here, I'll show you nothing has changed." *And everything's changed.* "Deal?"

She nodded, and a tear finally spilled over, running down her cheek. I brushed it away with my thumb. "Deal," she whispered, as I reached up to kiss her once more. "But, um… Ethan?"

"Yeah?"

"I think something is watching us."

CHAPTER TWENTY-THREE
THE ESCAPE

Warily, I looked up, just as something bright fell from the ceiling, flashing briefly as it struck the ground a few yards away.

Puzzled, I released Kenzie and stood, squinting as I walked up to it. When I could see it clearly in the darkness, my heart stood still.

My swords. Or one of them, anyway. Standing up point first in the sand. Incredulous, I picked it up, wondering how it got here.

There was a familiar buzz on the wall overhead. Heart leaping, I looked up to see a pair of smug, glowing green eyes. Razor grinned down at me, his teeth a blue-white crescent in the darkness. One spindly arm still clutched my second blade.

"Found you!" he buzzed.

Kenzie gasped, and the gremlin cackled, tossing the sword down. It soared through the air in a graceful arc and landed hilt up at my feet. Scuttling along the wall, the gremlin launched himself at Kenzie, landing in her arms with a gleeful cry. "Found you!" he exclaimed again, as she quickly shushed him. He beamed but dropped his voice to a staticky whisper. "Found you! Razor help! See, see? Razor brought swords silly boy dropped."

"Razor, are you all right?" Kenzie asked, holding him at

arm's length to look at him closely. One of his ears was torn, hanging limply at an angle, but other than that, he seemed okay. "That Forgotten threw you pretty hard," she mused, touching the wounded ear. "Are you hurt?"

"Bad kitty!" growled Razor, shaking his head as if he was shooing off a fly. "Evil, sneaky, nasty kitty! Boy should cut its nose off, yes. Tie rock to tail and throw kitty in lake. Watch kitty sink, ha!"

"Seems like he's fine," I said, sheathing my second blade. Relief and hope spread through me. Now that I was armed again, the future looked a lot less bleak. We might actually make it out of here. "Razor, did you happen to see Keirran anywhere? Or Annwyl?"

Before he could answer, a shuffle of movement up top silenced us, and we pressed back into the wall, staring up at the lip. A moment later, the old woman's voice floated down into the hole.

"Ethan Chase. The lady will see you now."

Kenzie shivered and pressed close, gripping my hand, as the gleam of the cat-faery's eyes appeared over the mouth of the pit. "Did you hear me, humans?" she called, sounding impatient. "When we lower the rungs, only the Chase boy is to come up. He will be escorted to the lady. Anyone who follows will be tossed back into the hole, without a ladder. So don't try anything."

Her wrinkled face split into an evil grin, and she disappeared. I turned to Kenzie.

"When I get up there," I whispered, "can you and Razor give me a distraction?" I glanced at Razor, hiding in her long black hair, then back to the girl. "I only need a few seconds. Think you can do that?"

She looked pale but determined. "Sure," she whispered. "No problem. Distractions are our specialty, right, Razor?"

The gremlin peeked out from the curtain of her hair and gave a quiet buzz. I brushed a strand from her eyes, trying to sound calm. "Wait until I'm almost at the very top," I told her, untucking my shirt, pulling the hem over the sword hilts. "Then, do whatever you have to do. Nothing dangerous, just make sure they're not looking at me when I come up. Also, here." I pulled out a sword, sheath and all, and handed it to her. "In case this doesn't go as planned. This will give you a fighting chance."

"Ethan."

I took her hand, fighting the urge to pull her close. "We're getting out of here, right now."

With a scraping sound, the ladder dropped into the pit. I squeezed Kenzie's arm and stepped forward, walking across the sand to the opposite wall. I saw Todd huddled in the corner, his head buried in his knees, not even looking at the ladder, and clenched my fists. *Dammit, what they did to you was unforgivable. Even if I can't fix that, I'll get you home, I swear. I'll get all of us home.*

My footsteps clunked loudly against the rungs as I started up, echoing my pounding heart.

Six steps from the top, I could see the hulking, three-armed Forgotten, yawning as it stared off into the distance.

Four steps from the top, I could see the old cat-faery and a pair of insect fey, one holding a coil of rope in its long talons. Another two guarded the entrance, floating a few inches above the ground.

Two steps from the top, Razor abruptly dropped onto the three-armed faery's head.

"*BAD KITTY!*" he screeched at the top of his lungs, making everything in the room jump in shock. The three-armed Forgotten gave a bellow and slapped at the thing on his head, but Razor leaped off just in time, and the huge fey smacked its own skull with enough force to knock it back a step.

I drew my sword and leaped out of the pit, blade flashing. I cut through one spindly body, dodged the second as it slashed at me, and sliced through its neck. Both dissolved into mist, and I went for the old cat-faery, intending to cut that evil grin from her withered face. She hissed and leaped away, landing behind the two guards at the mouth of the tunnel.

"Stop him!" she spat, and the Forgotten closed in on me, including the huge three-armed faery, a club clutched in his third hand. I dodged the first swing, parried the vicious claw swipes, and was forced back. "You cannot escape, Ethan Chase!" the cat-fey called triumphantly, as I fought to avoid being surrounded. The club swished over my head and smashed into the wall, showering me with rock. "Give up, and we will take you to the lady. Your death might be a painless one if you surrender no—aaaaaagh!"

Her warning melted into a yowl of pain as Razor dropped behind her, grabbed her skinny tail, and chomped down hard. The cat-faery spun, clawing at him, and I lost them both as the three fey crowded in. Battling Forgotten, I saw Kenzie pull herself out of the pit, sword in hand. Her eyes gleamed as she stepped up behind the hulking faery and swung a vicious blow at the back of its knees. Bellowing in pain, the Forgotten stumbled, lurched backward, and toppled over. Kenzie dodged aside as the big faery dropped into the pit with a howl.

Slicing through the last two guards, I lunged to where the cat-thing was twisting and clawing the air behind her, trying to reach the gremlin doggedly clinging to her tail. She looked up as I came in, made one last attempt to flee, but my sword flashed down across her neck and she erupted into mist.

Panting, I lowered my sword, stumbling back as Razor blinked, grinning as what had been the cat-faery rippled over the ground and evaporated. "Bad kitty," he buzzed, sounding smug as he looked up at me. "No more bad kitty. Ha!"

I smiled, turning to Kenzie, but then my heart seized up and I started to shout a warning.

The hulking Forgotten she had dropped into the pit had somehow clawed its way out again, looming behind her with its club raised. At the look on my face, she realized what was happening and started to turn, throwing up her arms, but the club swept down and I knew I would get there far too late.

And then...I don't know what happened. A dark, feature-less shadow sprang up, seemingly out of nowhere, between Kenzie and the huge Forgotten. A sword flashed, and the blow that probably would've crushed her skull hit her shoulder in-stead. The impact was still enough to knock her aside, and she crumpled against the wall, gasping in pain, as the shadow vanished as suddenly as it appeared.

Rage blinded me. Rushing forward, I leaped at the For-gotten with a scream, cutting at it viciously. It bellowed and swiped its club at my head, but I met the blow with my sword, severing the arm from its chest. Howling in pain, the faery resorted to pounding at me with its huge fists. I dodged back, snatching the fallen sword from the ground, and stepped up to meet the raging Forgotten. Ducking wild swings, I lunged past its guard and sank both blades into its chest with a snarl.

The Forgotten melted into fog, still bellowing curses. With-out a second glance, I rushed through its dissolving form to the body on the far side of the wall. Kenzie was struggling upright, grimacing, one hand cradling her arm. Razor hopped up and down nearby, buzzing with alarm.

"Kenzie!" Reaching her, I took her arm and very gen-tly felt along the limb, checking for lumps or broken bones. Miraculously everything seemed intact, despite the massive green bruise already starting to creep down her shoulder. *Badge of courage,* Guro would've called it. He would've been proud.

"Nothing's broken," I muttered in relief, and looked up at her. "Are you all right?"

She winced. "Well, considering today I have been stabbed, poked, pummeled and threatened with having my throat cut open, I guess I can't complain." Her brow furrowed, and she glanced around the cave. "Also, I thought there was... Did you see...?"

I nodded, remembering the shadow that had appeared, deflected the killing blow, and vanished just as suddenly. It had happened so fast; if Kenzie hadn't mentioned it, too, I might've thought I was seeing things.

"Oh, good. I thought I was having some weird near-death hallucination or something." Kenzie looked at the place the huge Forgotten had died and shuddered. "Any idea what just happened there?"

"No clue," I muttered. "But it probably saved your life. That's all I care about."

"Maybe for you," Kenzie said, wrinkling her nose. "But if I'm going to have some sort of shadowy guardian angel hanging around me, I kind of want to know why. In case I'm in the shower or something."

"Kenzie?" A faint, familiar voice drifted from the darkness before I could answer. We both jumped and gazed around wildly. "Ethan? Are you up there?"

"Annwyl?" Kenzie looked around, as Razor hopped to her shoulder. "Where are you?"

"Here," came the weak reply, as if muffled through the walls. I peered along the edge of the cave and saw a wooden door at the far corner of the room, nearly hidden in shadow. A thick wooden beam barred it shut. Hurrying over, we pushed the heavy beam out of the way and pulled on the door. It opened reluctantly, creaking in protest, and we stepped through.

Kenzie gasped. The room beyond was full of cages—bronze

or copper by the looks of them—hanging from the ceiling by thick chains. They groaned as they swung back and forth, narrow, cylindrical cells that barely gave enough room to turn around. All of them were empty, save one.

Annwyl huddled down in one of the cages, her knees drawn to her chest and her arms wrapped around them. In the darkness of the room, lit only by a single flickering torch on the far wall, she looked pale and sick and miserable as she raised her head, her eyes going wide.

"Ethan," she whispered in a trembling voice. "Kenzie. You're here. How...how did you find me?"

"We'll tell you later," Kenzie said, looking furious as she gripped the bars separating them. Razor buzzed furiously and leaped to the top of the cage, rattling the frame. "Right now, we're getting out of here. Where are the keys?"

Annwyl nodded to a post where a ring of bronze keys hung from a wooden peg. After unlocking the cage, we helped Annwyl climb down. The Summer girl stumbled weakly as she left the cage, leaning on me for support. The Forgotten had probably drained most of her glamour; she felt as thin and brittle as a bundle of twigs.

"Are there others?" I asked as she took several deep breaths, as if breathing clean air once again. Annwyl shuddered violently and shook her head.

"No," she whispered. "Just me." She turned and nodded to the empty cages, swinging from their chains. "When I was first brought here, there were a few other captives. Exiled fey like me. A satyr and a couple wood nymphs. One goblin. But...but then they were taken away by the guards. And they never came back. I was sure it was just a matter of time... before I was brought to her, as well."

"The lady," I muttered darkly. Annwyl shivered again.

"She...she *eats* them," she whispered, closing her eyes. "She

drains their glamour, sucks it into herself, just like her followers, until there's nothing left. That's why so many exiles
are gone. She needs a constant supply of magic to get strong
again, at least that's what her followers told me. So they go
out every night, capture exiles and half-breeds, and drag them
back here for her."

"Where's Keirran?" I asked, holding her at arm's length.
"Have you seen him?"

She shook her head frantically. "He's...with *her*," she said, on
the verge of tears. "I'm so worried...what if she's done something to him?" She covered her face with one hand. "What
will I do if he's gone?"

"Master!" Perched on Kenzie's shoulder again, Razor
echoed her misery, pulling on his ears. "Master gone!"

I sighed, trying to think over the gremlin's wailing. "All
right," I muttered, and turned to Kenzie. "We have to get
Todd and the others out of here. Do you remember the way
they brought us in?"

She winced, trying to shush the tiny Iron fey. "Barely. But
the cave is crawling with Forgotten. We'd have to fight our
way out."

Annwyl straightened then, taking a deep breath. "Wait," she
said, seeming to compose herself, her voice growing stronger.
"There is another way. I can sense where the trods are in this
place, and one empties under a bridge in the mortal world. It
isn't far from here."

"Can you lead everyone there? Open it?"

"Yes." Annwyl nodded, and her eyes glittered. "But I'm
not leaving without Keirran."

"I know. Come on." I led her out of the room, back to the
chamber that held the giant pit. Dragging the ladder from the
wall, I dropped it down into the hole.

"All right," I mumbled, peering into the darkness. Mutters

and shuffling footsteps drifted out of the pit, and I winced. "Wait here," I told Kenzie and Annwyl. "I'll be right back, hopefully with a bunch of crazy people."

"Wait," Kenzie said, stopping me. "I should go," she said, and held up a hand as I protested. "Ethan, if something comes into this room, I won't be able to stop it. You're the one with the mad sword skills. Besides, you're not the most comforting presence to lead a bunch of scared, crazy people to safety. If they start crying, you can't just crack your knuckles and threaten them to get them to move."

I frowned. "I wouldn't use my fists. A sword is much more threatening."

She rolled her eyes and handed me the gremlin, who scurried to my shoulder. "Just stand guard. I'll start sending them up."

A few minutes later, a crowd of ragged, dazed-looking humans clustered together in the tunnel, muttering and whispering to themselves. Todd was among them. He gazed around the cavern with a blank expression that made my skin crawl. I hoped that when we got him out of here he would go back to normal. No one looked at Annwyl or Razor, or seemed to notice them. They stood like sheep, passive and dull-witted, waiting for something to happen. Annwyl gazed at them all and shivered.

"How awful," she whispered, rubbing her arms. "They feel so...empty."

"Empty," Razor buzzed. "Empty, empty, empty."

"Is this everyone?" I asked Kenzie as she crawled back up the ladder. She nodded as Razor bounced back to her. "All right, everyone stay together. This is going to be interesting."

Drawing my weapons, I walked to the edge of the tunnel, where it split in two directions, and peered out. No Forgotten, not yet.

"Ethan." Kenzie and Annwyl joined me at the edge, the group following silently. Annwyl gripped my arm. "I'm not leaving. Not without him."

"I know. Don't worry." I shook off her fingers, then turned and handed a sword to Kenzie. "Get them out of here," I told her. "Take Annwyl, get to the exit, and don't look back. If anything tries to stop you, do whatever you can not to get caught again."

"What about you?"

I sighed, glancing down the tunnel. "I'm going back for Keirran."

She blinked. "Alone? You don't even know where he is."

"Yes, I do." Raking a hand through my hair, I faced the darkness, determined not to be afraid. "He'll be with the lady. Wherever *she* is, I'll find him, too."

"Master?" Razor perked up, eyes flaring with hope. "Razor come? Find Master?"

"No, you stay, Razor. Protect Kenzie."

The gremlin buzzed sadly but nodded.

Dark murmurs echoed behind us. The group of former half-breeds were shifting fretfully, muttering "the lady," over and over again, like a chant. It made my stomach turn with nerves.

"Here, then." Kenzie handed back the sword. "Take it. I won't need it this time."

"But—"

"Ethan, trust me, if something finds us, we won't be fighting—we'll be running. If you're going back, you're going to need it more than me."

"I'll come with you," Annwyl said.

"No." My voice came out sharp. "Kenzie needs you to open the trod when you get there. It won't work for humans. Besides, if something happens to you, if you get caught or threatened in any way, Keirran won't try to escape. He'll only come with me if he knows you're safe."

"I want to help. I won't abandon him—"

"Dammit, if you love him, the best thing you can do is leave!" I snapped, whirling on her. She blinked and drew back. "Keirran is here because of you! That's what got us into this mess in the first place." I glared at her, and the faery dropped her gaze. Sighing, I lowered my voice. "Annwyl, you have to trust me. I won't come back without him, I promise."

She struggled a moment longer, then nodded. "I'll hold you to that promise, human," she murmured at last.

Kenzie suddenly took my arm. "I will, too," she whispered as I looked into her eyes. She smiled faintly, trying to hide her fear, and squeezed my hand. "So you'd better come back, tough guy. You have a promise to keep, remember?"

The urge to kiss her then was almost overpowering. Gently, I cupped her cheek, trying to convey my promise, what I felt, without words. Kenzie put her hand over mine and closed her eyes. "Be careful," she whispered. I nodded.

"You, too."

Opening her eyes, she released me and stepped back. "We'll be at Belvedere Castle," she stated, her eyes suspiciously bright. "So meet us there when you find Keirran. We'll be waiting for you both."

Todd spoke up then, his voice echoing flatly over the rest. "If you're looking for the lady, she'll be on the very last floor," he stated. "That's where the screams used to come from."

A chill went through me. Giving Kenzie and the others one last look, I turned, gripping my weapons and disappeared into the tunnel.

CHAPTER TWENTY-FOUR
THE LADY

I made my way through the darkness of the Forgotten hive, keeping to the shadows, pressed flat against rocks or behind boulders. In a real cave, with no artificial light, it would be impossible to see your hand in front of your face. Here, in the Between, the cave glowed with luminescent crystals and mushrooms, scattered on the walls and along the ceiling. Colorful moss and ferns grew around a clear green pool in the center of the main cavern, where a small waterfall trickled in from the darkness above.

Forgotten drifted through the tunnels, pale and shimmery against the gloom, though there weren't as many as I'd first feared. Maybe most of them were out hunting exiles, since they had to feed on the glamour of the regular fey to live. Some were just transparent shadows, while others seemed much more solid, even gaining some color back. I noticed the less "real" the faery was, the more it tended to wander around in a daze, as if it couldn't remember what it was doing. I nearly ran right into a snakelike creature with multiple arms coming out of a tunnel, and dove behind a stalactite to avoid it, making a lot of noise as I did. The faery stared at my hiding spot for a few seconds, blinking, then appeared to lose interest and slithered off down another corridor. Breathing a sigh of relief, I continued.

Hugging the walls, I slowly made my way through the caverns and tunnels, searching for Keirran and the lady. I hoped Kenzie and Annwyl had gotten the others out, and I hoped they were safe. I couldn't worry about them now. If this lady was as powerful as I feared—the queen of the Forgotten, I suspected—then I had more than enough to worry about for myself.

Past another glittering pool, a stone archway rose out of the wall and floor, blue torches burning on either side. It looked pretty official, like the entrance to a queen's chamber, perhaps.

Gripping my weapons, I took a deep breath and walked beneath the arch.

The tunnel past the doorway was winding but short, and soon a faint glow hovered at the end. I crept forward, staying to the shadows, and peeked into the throne room of the Lady.

The cavern through the arch wasn't huge, though it glittered with thousands of blue, green and yellow crystals, some tiny, some as big as me, jutting out of the walls and floor. Several massive stone columns, twined with the skeletons of dragons and other monsters, lined the way to a crystal throne near the back of the room.

Sitting on that throne, flanked by motionless knights in bone armor, was a woman.

My breath caught. The Lady of the Forgotten wasn't monstrous, or cruel-looking or some terrible, crazy queen wailing insanities.

She was beautiful.

For a few seconds, I couldn't stop staring, couldn't even tear my eyes away. Like the rest of the Forgotten, the Lady was pale, but a bit of color tinged her cheeks and full lips, and her eyes were a striking crystal blue, though they shifted col-

ors in the dim light—from blue to green to amber and back
again. Her long hair was colorless, writhing away to mist at
the ends, as if she still wasn't quite solid. She wore billowing
robes with a high collar, and the face within was young, perfect and achingly sad.

For one crazy moment, my brain shut off, and I wondered
if we had this all wrong. Maybe the Lady was a prisoner of the
Forgotten, as well, maybe she had nothing to do with the disappearances and killings and horrible fate of the half-breeds.

But then I saw the wings, or rather, the shattered bones of
what had been wings, rising from her shoulders to frame the
chair. Like the other Forgotten. Her eyes shifted from green
to pure black, and I saw her reach a slender white hand out to
a figure standing at the foot of the throne.

"Keirran," I whispered. The Iron prince looked none the
worse for wear, unbound and free, as he took the offered hand
and stepped closer to the Lady. She ran long fingers through
his silver hair, and he didn't move, standing there with his
head bowed. I saw her lips move, and he might've said something back, but their voices were too soft to hear.

Anger flared, and I clenched my fists around my swords.
Keirran was still armed; I could see the sword across his back,
but he wouldn't do anything that would endanger Annwyl.
How strong was the Lady? If I burst in now, could we fight
our way out? I counted four guards surrounding the throne,
eyes glowing green beneath their bony helmets. They looked
pretty tough, but we might be able to take them down together. If I could only get his attention...

A second later, however, it didn't matter.

The Lady suddenly stopped talking to Keirran. Raising her
head, she looked right at me, still hidden in the shadows. I saw
her eyebrows lift in surprise, and then she smiled.

"Hello, Ethan Chase." Her voice was clear and soft, and her smile was heartbreaking "Welcome to my kingdom."

Dammit. I burst from my hiding spot, as Keirran whirled around, eyes widening in shock. "Ethan," he exclaimed as I walked forward, my blades held at my side. The guards started forward, but the Lady raised a hand, and they stopped. "What are you doing here?"

"What do you think I'm doing here?" I snapped. "I'm here to get you out. You can relax—Annwyl is safe." I met the Lady's gaze. "So are Todd and all the other half-breeds you kidnapped. And you won't hurt anyone else, I swear."

I wasn't expecting an answer. I expected Keirran to spin around, draw his sword, and all hell to break loose as we beat a hasty retreat for the exit. But Keirran didn't move, and the next words spoken weren't his. "What do you mean, Ethan Chase?" The Lady's voice surprised me, genuinely confused and shocked, trying to understand. "Tell me, how have I hurt your friends?"

"You're kidding, right?" I halted a few yards from the foot of the throne, glaring up at her. Keirran, rigid beside her, looked on warily. I wondered when he was going to step down, in case we had to fight our way out. Those bony knights at each corner of the throne looked pretty tough.

"Let me give you a rundown, then," I told the Forgotten queen, who cocked her head at me. "You kidnapped my friend Todd from his home and dragged him here. You kidnapped Annwyl to force Keirran to come to you. You've killed who knows how many exiles, and, oh, yeah....you turned all those half-breeds mortal by sucking out their glamour. How's that for harm, then?"

"The half-breeds were not to be harmed," the Lady said in a calm, reasonable voice. "We do not kill if there is no need. Eventually, they would have been returned to their homes. As for losing their 'fey-ness,' now that they are mortal, the Hidden World will never bother them again. They can live happier, safer lives now that they are normal. Wouldn't you agree that is the better option, Ethan Chase? You, who have been tormented by the fey all your life? Surely you understand."

"I... That's...that's not an excuse."

"Isn't it?" The Lady gave me a gentle smile. "They are happier now, or they will be, once they go home. No more nightmares about the fey. No more fear of what the 'pure-bloods' might do to them." She tilted her head again, sympathetic. "Don't *you* wish you could be normal?"

"What about the exiles?" I shot back, determined not to give her the upper hand in this bizarre debate. *Dammit, I shouldn't even have to argue about this. Keirran, what the hell are you doing?* "There's no question of what you did to them," I continued. "You can't tell me that they're happier being dead."

"No." The Lady closed her eyes briefly. "Sadly, I cannot. There is no excuse for it, and it breaks my heart, what we must do to our former brethren to survive."

A tiny motion from Keirran, just the slightest tightening of his jaw. *Well, at least that's something. I still don't know what you think you're doing, Prince. Unless she's got a debt or a glamour on you.* Somehow, I doubted it. The Iron prince looked fine when I first came in. He was still acting of his own free will.

"But," the Lady continued, "our survival is at stake here. I do what I must to ensure my people do not fade away again. If there was another way to live, to exist, I would gladly take it. As such, we feed only on exiles, those who have been banished to the mortal realm. That they will fade away eventually is small comfort to what we must do, but we must take our comfort where we can."

I finally looked at Keirran. "And you. You're okay with all this?"

Keirran bowed his head and didn't meet my gaze. The Lady reached out and touched the back of his neck.

"Keirran understands our plight," she whispered as I stared at him, disbelieving. "He knows I must protect my people from nonexistence. Mankind has been cruel and has forgotten us, as have the courts of Faery. We have just returned to the world again. How can we go back to nothing?"

I shook my head, incredulous. "I hate to break it to you, but I promised someone I wouldn't leave without the Iron prince, there." I stabbed a sword at Keirran, who raised his head and finally looked at me. I glared back. "And I'm going to keep my promise, even if I have to break both his legs and carry him out myself."

"Then, I am sorry, Ethan Chase." The Lady sat back, watching me sadly. "I wish we could have come to an agreement. But I cannot allow you to return to the Iron Queen with our location. Please understand—I do this only to protect my people."

The Lady lifted her hand, and the bone knights suddenly lunged forward, drawing their swords as they did. Their weapons were pure white and jagged on one end, like a giant razor tooth. I met the first warrior bearing down on me, knocking aside his sword and instantly whipping my second blade at his head. It happened in the space of a blink, but the faery dodged back, the sword missing him by inches.

Damn, they're fast. Another cut at me from the side, and I barely twisted away, feeling the jagged edge of the sword catch my shirt. Parrying yet another swing, I immediately had to dodge as the others closed in, not giving me any time to counter. They backed me toward a corner, desperately fending off blindingly quick stabs and thrusts. Too many. There were too many of them, and they were *good.* "Keirran!" I yelled, ducking behind a column. "A little help?"

The knights slowly followed me around the pillar, and through the short lull, I saw the Iron prince still standing beside the throne, watching. His face was blank; no emotion showed on his face or in his eyes as the knights closed on me again. Fear gripped my heart with icy talons. Even after everything, I still believed he would back me up when I needed it. "Keirran!" I yelled again, ducking as the knight's sword smashed into the column, spraying me with grit. "Dammit, what are you doing? Annwyl is safe—help me!"

He didn't move, though a tortured expression briefly crossed his face. Stunned and abruptly furious, I whirled, stepped inside a knight's guard as it cut at me, and lunged deep. My blade finally pierced the armored chest, lancing between the rib slits and sinking deep. The warrior convulsed, staggered away, and turned into mist.

But my reckless move had left my back open, and I wasn't able to dodge fast enough as another sword swept down, glancing off my leg. For just a second, it didn't hurt. But as I backed away, blood blossomed over my jeans, and then the pain hit in a crippling flood. I stumbled, gritting my teeth. The remaining three knights followed relentlessly, swords raised. All the while, Keirran stood beside the throne, not moving, as the Lady's remote blue eyes followed me over his head.

I can't believe he's going to stand there and watch me die. Panting, I desperately fended off another assault from all three knights, but a blade got through and hit my arm, causing me to drop one of my swords. I lashed out and scored a hit along the knight's jaw, and it reeled away in pain, but then another swung viciously at my head, and I knew I wouldn't be able to completely avoid this one.

I raised my sword, and the knight's blade smashed into it and my arm, knocking me to the side. My hurt leg crumpled beneath me, and I fell, the blade ripped from my hands, skidding across the floor. Dazed, I looked up to see the knights looming over me, sword raised for the killing blow.

That's it, then. I'm sorry, Kenzie. I wanted to be with you, but at least you're safe now. That's all that matters.

The blade flashed down. I closed my eyes.

The screech of weapons rang directly overhead, making my hair stand up. For a second, I held my breath, wondering when the pain would hit, wondering if I was already dead. When nothing happened, I opened my eyes.

Keirran knelt in front of me, arm raised, blocking the knight's sword with his own. The look on his face was one of grim determination. Standing, he threw off the knight and glared at the others, who eased back a step but didn't lower their weapons. Without looking in my direction but still keeping himself between me and the knights, he turned back to the throne.

"This isn't the way, my lady," he called. Cursing him mentally, I struggled to sit up, fighting the pain clawing at my arms, legs, shoulders, everywhere really. Keirran gave me a brief glance, as if making sure I was all right, still alive, and faced the Forgotten Queen again. "I sympathize with your plight, I do. But I can't allow you to harm my family. Killing the brother of the Iron Queen would only hurt your cause, and bring the wrath of all the courts down upon you and your followers. Please, let him go. Let us both go."

The Lady regarded him blankly, then raised her hand again. Instantly, the bone knights backed off, sheathing their weapons and returning to her side. Keirran still didn't look at me as he sheathed his own blade and gave a slight bow. "We'll be taking our leave, now," he stated, and though his voice was polite, it wasn't a question or a request. "I will think on what you said, but I ask that you do not try to stop us."

The Lady didn't reply, and Keirran finally bent down, putting my arm around his shoulders. I was half tempted to shove him off, but I didn't know if my leg would hold. Besides, the room seemed to be spinning.

"Nice of you to finally step in," I growled, as he lifted us both to our feet. Pain flared, and I grit my teeth, glaring at him. "Was that a change of heart at the end, or were you just waiting for the last dramatic moment?"

"I'm sorry," Keirran murmured, steadying us as I stumbled. "I was hoping…it wouldn't come to this." He sighed and gave me an earnest look. "Annwyl. Is she all right? Is she safe?"

"I already told you she was." My leg throbbed, making my temper flare. "No thanks to you! What the hell is wrong with you, Keirran? I thought you cared for Annwyl, or don't you care that they left her in a *cage,* all alone, while you were out here having tea with the Lady or whatever the hell you were doing?"

Keirran paled. "Annwyl," he whispered, closing his eyes. "I'm sorry. Forgive me, I didn't know…." Opening his eyes, he gave me a pleading look. "They wouldn't let me see her. I didn't know where she was. They told me she would be killed if I didn't cooperate."

"Well, you were certainly doing that," I shot back, and pushed him toward one of my fallen weapons. "Don't leave my swords. I want them in case your wonderful Lady decides to double-cross us."

"She wouldn't do that," Keirran said, dragging me over and kneeling to pick up my blade. "She's more honorable than you think. You just have to understand what's happened to her, what she's trying to accomplish—"

I snatched the weapon from him and glared. "Whose side are you on, anyway?"

That tortured look crossed his face again. "Ethan, please…"

"Never mind," I muttered, wincing as my leg started to throb. "Let's just get out of here, while I can still walk out."

We started across the floor again, but hadn't gone very far when the Lady's voice rang out again. "Prince Keirran," she called. "Wait, please. One more thing."

Keirran paused, but he didn't look back.

"The killings can stop," the Lady went on in a quiet but earnest voice. "No more exiles will be sacrificed to keep us alive, and no more half-breeds will be taken. I can order my people to do this, if that is what you want."

"Yes," Keirran said immediately, still not looking back. "It is."

"However," the Lady went on, "if I do this, you must come and speak with me again. One day soon I will call for you, and you must come to me, of your own free will. Not as a prisoner, but as a guest. An equal. Will you give me that much, at least?"

"Keirran," I muttered as he paused, "don't listen to her. She just wants you under her thumb again because you're the son of the Iron Queen. You *know* faery bargains never turn out right."

He didn't answer, staring straight ahead, at nothing.

"Iron Prince?" The Lady's voice was low, soothing. "What is your answer?"

"Keirran…" I warned.

His eyes hardened. "Agreed," he called back. "You have my word."

I wanted to punch him.

"Dammit, what is wrong with you?" I seethed as we left the queen's chamber. "Have you forgotten what she's done? Did you happen to see all the half-breeds she's kidnapped? Did you see what they did to them, drained all their magic so they're just shells of what they were? Have you forgotten all the exiles they've killed, just to keep themselves alive?" He didn't answer, and I narrowed my eyes. "Annwyl could've been one of them, or are you so enamored with your new lady friend that you forgot about her, too?"

The last was a low blow, but I wanted to make him angry, get him to argue with me. Or at least to confirm that he hadn't forgotten the atrocities committed here or what we'd come to do. But his blue eyes only got colder, though his voice remained calm.

"I wouldn't expect a human to understand."

"Then explain it to me," I said through gritted teeth, though hearing him say that sent a chill up my spine.

"I don't agree with her methods," Keirran said as two piranha-palm gnomes stepped aside for us, bowing to Keirran. "But she's only trying to achieve what every good ruler wants—the survival of her people. You don't know how horrible it is for exiles, for all of them, to face nothingness. Losing pieces of yourself every day, until you cease to exist."

"And the harm she's caused so that her people can survive?"

"That was wrong," Keirran agreed, furrowing his brow. "Others shouldn't have had to die. But the Forgotten are only trying to live and not fade away, just like the exiles. Just like everyone in Faery." He sighed and turned down a side tunnel filled with crystals and bone fragments. But the farther we walked, the more the gems and skeletons faded away, until the ground was just normal rock under our feet. Ahead, I could see the end of the tunnel and a small paved path that cut through the trees. The shadows of the cavern fell away. "There has to be a way for them to survive without hurting anyone else," Keirran muttered at last. I looked at him and frowned.

"And if there isn't?"

"Then we're all going to have to choose a side."

★ ★ ★

We left the cave of the Forgotten and stepped into the real world from beneath a stone bridge, emerging in Central Park again. I didn't know how long we had been in the Between, but the sky overhead blazed with stars, though the air held a stillness that said it was close to dawn. Keirran dragged me to a green bench on the side of the trail, and I collapsed on top of it with a groan.

The prince hovered anxiously on the edge of the path. "How's the leg?" he asked, sounding faintly guilty. *Not guilty enough,* I thought sourly. I prodded the gash and winced.

"Hurts like hell," I muttered, "but at least the bleeding's slowed down." Removing my belt, I wrapped it several times around my leg to make a rough bandage, clenching my jaw as I cinched it tight. The gash on my arm was still oozing sluggishly, but I'd have to take care of it later.

"Where to now?" Keirran asked.

"Belvedere Castle," I replied, desperately hoping Kenzie and the others were already there, waiting for us. "We agreed to meet there, when this was all over."

Keirran looked around the dense woods and sighed. "Any idea what direction it might be?"

"Not really," I gritted out and glared at him. "You're the one with faery blood. Aren't you supposed to have some innate sense of direction?"

"I'm not a compass," Keirran said mildly, still gazing around the forest. Finally, he shrugged. "Well, I guess we'll pick a trail and hope for the best. Can you walk?"

Despite my anger, I felt a tiny twinge of relief. He was starting to sound like his old self again. Maybe all that madness down in the Lady's throne room was because he'd been glamoured, after all.

"I'll be fine," I muttered, struggling to my feet. "But I'm

going to have to tell Kenzie that you're really not at all helpful on camping trips."

He chuckled, and it sounded relieved, too. "Be sure to break it to her gently," he said, and took my weight again.

Fifteen minutes later, we still had no idea where we were going. We were wandering up a twisty, narrow path, hoping it would take us someplace familiar, when Keirran suddenly stopped. A troubled look crossed his face, and I glanced around warily, wondering if I should pull my swords. Of course, it was going to be really awkward fighting while hopping around on one leg or leaning against Keirran. I had hoped our fighting was done for the night.

"What is it?" I asked. Keirran sighed.

"They're here."

"What? Who?"

"Master!"

A familiar wail rent the night, and Keirran grimaced, bracing himself, as Razor hurled himself at his chest. Scrabbling to his shoulders, the gremlin gibbered and bounced with joy. "Master, master! Master safe!"

"Hey, Razor." Keirran smiled, wincing helplessly as the gremlin continued to bounce on him. "Yeah, I'm happy to see you, too. Is the court far behind?"

I frowned at him. "Court?"

They emerged from the trees all around us, dozens of sidhe knights in gleaming armor, the symbol of a great iron tree on their breastplates. They slid out of the woods, amazingly silent for an army in plate mail, until they formed a glittering half circle around us. Leading them all was a pair of familiar faces: a dark faery dressed all in black with silver eyes, and a grinning redhead.

Keirran stiffened beside me.

"Well, well," Puck announced, smirking as he and Ash approached side-by-side. "Look who it is. See, ice-boy, I told you they'd be here."

Ash's glittering stare was leveled at Keirran, who quickly bowed his head but, to his credit, didn't cringe or back away. Which took guts, I had to admit, facing down that icy glare.

"Are you two all right?" From Ash's tone, I couldn't tell if he was relieved, secretly amused or completely furious. His gaze swept over me, quietly assessing, and his eyes narrowed. "Ethan, you're badly wounded. What happened?"

"I'm fine." A weak claim, I knew, as my shirt and half my pant leg were covered in blood. Beside me, Keirran was rigid, motionless. Razor gave a worried buzz from his neck. *What's the matter?* I thought. *Afraid I'm going to tell Daddy that you nearly let me be skewered to death?* "I got into a fight with a few guards." I shrugged, then grimaced as the motion tore the dried wound on my shoulder. "Turns out, fighting multiple opponents in armor isn't a very smart idea."

"You think?" Puck came forward, shooing Keirran away and pointing me to a nearby rock. "Sit down. Jeez, kid, do I look like a nurse? Why are you always bleeding whenever I see you? You're worse than ice-boy."

Ash ignored that comment as Puck briskly started tying bandages around my various cuts and gashes, being not particularly gentle. "Where are they?" the dark faery demanded.

I clenched my teeth as Puck yanked a strip of cloth around my arm. "There's a trod under a bridge that will take you to their lair," I said, pointing back down the path. "I'd be careful, though. There's a lot of them running around."

"Don't hurt them," Keirran burst out, and everyone, even Razor, glanced at him in surprise. "They're not dangerous," he pleaded, as I gave him an are-you-crazy look. He ignored me. "They're just…misguided."

Puck snorted, looking up from my shoulder. "Sorry, but are

we talking about the same creepy little faeries that tried to kill us atop the castle that night? Evil gnomes, toothy hands, tried to suck out everyone's glamour—this ringing any bells?" He stood, wiping off his hands, and I pushed myself to my feet, gingerly putting weight on my leg. It was just numb now, making me wonder what Puck had done to it. Magic, glamour or something else? Whatever it was, I wasn't complaining.

"The killings will stop," Keirran insisted. "The queen promised me they would stop."

"They have a queen?" Ash's voice had gone soft and lethal, and even Puck looked concerned. Keirran drew in a sharp breath, realizing his mistake.

"Huh, another queen," Puck mused, an evil grin crossing his face. "Maybe we should drop in and introduce ourselves, ice-boy. Do the whole, hey, we were just in the neighborhood, and we were just wondering if you had any plans to take over the Nevernever. Have a fruit basket."

"Father, please." Keirran met Ash's gaze. "Let them go. They're only trying to survive."

The dark faery stared Keirran down a few moments, then shook his head. "We didn't come here to start a war," he said, and Keirran relaxed. "We came here for you and Ethan. The courts will have to decide what to do with the emergence of another queen. Right now, let's get you both out of here. And, Keirran—" he glared at his son, who flinched under that icy gaze "—this isn't over. The queen will be waiting for you when we get home. I hope you have a good explanation."

Meghan, I thought as Keirran and Puck took my weight again, and we started hobbling down the path. Questions swirled, all centered on her and Keirran. I needed to talk to my sister, not just to ask about my nephew and the "other" side of my family, but to let her know that I understood. I knew why she left us so long ago. Or at least, I was beginning to.

I couldn't speak to her now, but I would, soon. Keirran was my way back to Faery, back to my sister, because now that we'd met, I was pretty sure not even the Iron Queen herself could keep him away.

"Ah." Puck sighed, shaking his head as we headed into the forest. "This brings back memories." He glanced over his shoulder and grinned. "Don't they remind you of a pair, ice-boy, from way back when?"

Ash snorted. "Don't remind me."

EPILOGUE

Belvedere Castle looked eerie and strange under the moonlight, with armored knights standing guard along the top and the banner of the Iron Queen flapping in the wind. It was as if we'd stepped through time into King Arthur's court or something. But the small group of humans clustered on the balcony sort of ruined that image, though it was obvious they couldn't see the unearthly knights milling around them. Occasionally one would break away from the group and walk toward the steps, though when they reached the edge they would turn and wander back, a dazed look on their face. So, a glamour barrier had been placed over the castle, preventing them from going anywhere. Probably a good idea; the former half-breeds didn't even know who they were and wouldn't survive for long, out there on their own. Still, it was faery magic, repressing the will of normal humans, keeping them trapped, and it made my skin crawl.

"What will happen to the half-breeds now that they're human?" I asked as we approached the first flight of stairs, knights bowing to us on either side.

Ash shook his head. "I don't know." Gazing up at the top of the steps, he narrowed his eyes. "Some of them are probably Leanansidhe's, so she might take them back, see if they regain their memories. Beyond that…" He shrugged. "Some of them may have been reported missing. We'll let the human authorities know they're here. Their own will have to take care of them now."

"One of them is a friend of ours," I said. "He's been missing for days. We need to take him back to Louisiana with us."

Ash nodded. "I'll make sure he gets home."

Keirran stopped at the foot of the stairs, his breath catching. I gritted my teeth as the abrupt halt jolted my leg, then followed his gaze up to where Annwyl stood at the top of the steps, waiting for him.

I sighed and pulled my arm from his shoulders. "Go on," I said, rolling my eyes, and he instantly leaped up the steps, taking them three at a time, until he reached the top. Uncaring of Ash, Puck or any of the surrounding knights, he pulled the Summer girl into his arms and kissed her deeply, while Razor jabbered with delight, beaming his manic smile at them both.

Puck shot a look at Ash, his green eyes solemn. "I told you, ice-boy. That kid of yours is trouble. And that's coming from *me*."

Ash scrubbed a hand over his face. "Leanansidhe," he muttered, and shook his head. "So that's where he's been disappearing to." He sighed, and his silver gaze narrowed. "The three of us are going to have to have a talk."

Where's Kenzie? I thought, gazing up the stairs. If Annwyl and the former half-breeds were safe, she had to be here, too. But I didn't see her near the top of the steps with Keirran and Annwyl, or in the cluster of humans wandering around the balcony. I felt a tiny prick of hurt, that she wasn't here to greet me and tried to ignore it. She must have her reasons.

Though you'd think me standing here bleeding all over the place would warrant some type of reaction.

"Sire." Glitch suddenly appeared from the trees, leading another squad of knights behind him. The lightning in his hair glowed purple as he bowed. "We found a second entrance to the strange faeries' lair," he said solemnly, and Ash nodded. "However, the cave was empty when we investigated. There was evidence of other trods, leading in from various points in the park, but nothing remained of the inhabitants themselves. They cleared out very recently."

I looked at Ash, frowning. "You had a second squad, coming from another direction," I guessed. He ignored me, giving Glitch a brief nod.

"Good work. Though if they've fled, there is nothing to do but wait for them to reemerge. Return to Mag Tuiredh and inform the queen. Tell her I will return shortly with Keirran."

"Yes, sire." Glitch bowed, took his knights, and vanished into the darkness.

"Guess that's our cue, as well," Puck said, stepping away from me. "Back to Arcadia, then?"

"Not yet." Ash turned to gaze into the forest, his eyes solemn. "I want to do one more sweep, one last search around the cave, just in case we missed anything." He glanced over his shoulder, smirking. "Care to join me, Goodfellow?"

"Oh, ice-boy. A moonlight stroll with you? Do you even have to ask?"

"Ethan," Ash said, as Puck gave me a friendly arm punch and sauntered into the trees, "we'll return in a few minutes. Tell Keirran that if he even *thinks* about moving from this spot, I will freeze his legs to the floor of his room." His eyes flashed silver, and I didn't doubt his threat. "Also..." He sighed, glancing over my shoulder. "Let him know that the Summer girl probably shouldn't be here when we get back. She's been through enough."

Surprised, I nodded. *Huh. Guess you're not a complete heartless bastard, after all,* I thought grudgingly, as the dark faery turned and melted into the woods with Puck. *I didn't think you'd be the type to look the other way.* Catching myself, I snorted. *I still don't like you, though. You can still drop dead anytime.*

"They won't find anything," Keirran stated, a few steps away, and I turned. The Iron prince stood behind Annwyl with his arms around her waist, gazing over her shoulder. His eyes were dark as he stared into the forest. "The Lady will have taken her followers and fled to another part of the Between. Maybe she'll never reemerge. Maybe we'll never see them again."

"I hope so." Annwyl sighed, and Razor hissed in agreement. But Keirran continued to stare into the trees, as if he hoped the Lady would step out of the shadows and call to him.

And, one day, she will.

"Where's Kenzie?" I asked, clutching the railing as I limped up the stairs, pushing dark thoughts out of my head for now. Keirran and Annwyl hurried down to help, but I waved away their offered hands. "I didn't see her with any of the humans," I continued, marching doggedly forward, up the stairs. "Is she okay?"

"She's talking to one of the half-breeds," Annwyl said. "Todd? The smaller human. I think he was starting to remember her, at least a little bit. He was crying when I saw them last."

I nodded and hurried toward the top, pushing myself to go faster, though my leg was beginning to throb again. As I persisted up the steps, I heard Annwyl's and Keirran's voices drift up behind me.

"I think I should go, too," Annwyl said. "While I still can, if Leanansidhe even takes me back." Her voice grew softer, frightened. "I don't know what will happen to us, Keirran. Everyone saw…"

"I don't care." Keirran's voice was stubbornly calm. "Let

them exile me if they want. I'm not backing down now. I'll beg Leanansidhe to take you back, if that's what it takes." A dark, determined note crept into his words. "I won't watch you fade away into nothing," he swore in a low voice. "There has to be a way. I'll *find* a way."

Leaving them embracing in the middle of the stairs, I reached the balcony where the group of humans still milled aimlessly about, looking as if they were sleepwalking. Pushing my way through the crowd, I spotted a pair of figures sitting by the wall, one hunched over with his head buried in his knees, the other crouched beside him, a slender hand on his shoulder.

Kenzie looked up, and her eyes widened when she saw me. Bending close to Todd, she whispered something in his ear, and he nodded without raising his head.

Standing, she walked across the balcony, dodged the humans that shuffled in front of her, and then we were face-to-face.

"Oh, Ethan." The whisper was half relief, half horror. Her eyes flickered to my face, the blood streaking my arm, splattered across my shirt and jeans. She looked as if she wanted to hug me close but was afraid of hurting me. I gave her a tired smile. "Are you all right?"

"Yeah." I took one step toward her, so that only a breath separated us. "I'm fine enough to do this." And I pulled her into my arms.

Her arms came around me instantly, hugging me back. Closing my eyes, I held her tight, feeling her slim body pressed against mine. She clung to me fiercely, as if daring something to take me away, and I relaxed into her, feeling nothing but relief. I was alive, Todd was safe, and everyone I cared for was all right. That was enough for now.

She finally pulled back, gazing up at me, tracing a shallow

cut on my cheek. "Hi, tough guy," she whispered. "Looks like you made it."

I smiled. Taking her hand, I led her over to the railing, where the wall dropped away and we could see the pond, the forest and most of the park stretched out before us.

I jerked my head toward the lump huddled in the opposite corner. "How is he?"

"Todd?" She sighed, shaking her head. "He still doesn't remember me. Or our school. Or any of his friends. But he said he does remember a woman, very vaguely. His mom, I hope. He started crying after that, so I couldn't get much more out of him." She leaned against the railing, resting her arms on the ledge. "I hope he can get back to normal."

"Me, too," I said, though I seriously doubted it. How could you be normal again when a huge piece of you had been stripped away? Was there even a cure, a remedy, something that could restore a creature's glamour, once it had been lost?

I suddenly realized the irony: here I was, wishing I could give someone back their magic, to return them to the world of Faery, when a few days ago I didn't want anything to do with the fey.

When did I change so much?

Kenzie sighed again, gazing out over the pond. The moonlight gleamed off her hair, outlining her slender body, casting a hazy light around her. And I knew. I knew exactly when I had changed.

It started the day I met you.

"It sure has been a crazy week," she murmured, resting her chin on the back of her hands. "Getting kidnapped, being chased around the Nevernever, faeries and Forgotten and talking cats. Things will seem very dull when we go home." She groaned, hiding her face in her arms. "God, we are going to be in *sooooooo* much trouble when we get back."

I stepped behind her, putting my hands on her waist. "Yeah," I agreed, making her groan again. "So let's not think about that right now." There would be plenty of time to worry about the trouble we were in, the Forgotten, the Lady, Kenzie's disease and Keirran's promise. Right now, I didn't want to think about them. The only thing on my mind was a promise of my own.

I wrapped my arms around Kenzie's waist and brought my lips close to her ear. "Remember what I promised you?" I murmured. "Down in the cave?"

She froze for a second, then turned slowly, her eyes wide and luminous in the moonlight. Smiling, I drew her close, slipping one arm around her waist, the other sliding up to her neck. I lowered my head as her eyes fluttered shut. And on that balcony under the stars, in front of everyone who might be watching, I kissed her.

And for the first time, I wasn't afraid.

★ ★ ★ ★ ★

ACKNOWLEDGMENTS

First and foremost, a huge shout out to my Guro, Ron. Thanks for answering all my crazy kali questions, for all the "badges of courage" I picked up in sparring, and for making Hit-People-With-Sticks class the best night of the week. I could not have written this book without you.

To Natashya Wilson, T. S. Ferguson, and all the awesome Harlequin TEEN people, you guys rock. Tashya, you especially deserve a standing ovation. I don't know how you juggle so much and still manage to make it look easy.

To my agent, Laurie McLean. This has been one crazy ride, and I'm so grateful to be taking it with you. Let's keep shooting for the stars.

And of course, to my husband, sparring partner, first editor, and best friend, Nick. To many more years of writing, laughs and giving each other "badges of courage" in kali. You keep me young (and deadly).

QUESTIONS FOR DISCUSSION

1. Ethan almost gets into a fight on his first day of school. What did you think about his response to Brian Kingston's bullying of Todd? What would you have done? What do you think is an effective way of responding to a bully?

2. When we first meet Todd, he seems to be the victim of bullies. Later we learn that perhaps the situation is not as simple as Ethan first believes. Todd even lets Ethan take the fall for his retaliation against Kingston. Why do you think Ethan still decides to look for Todd and help him? Did you agree with Ethan's actions, or would you have done something else?

3. Ethan is angry with his sister, Meghan, for what he sees as her desertion of their family. What do you think of the way he handles his feelings? What do you think Meghan would say if she knew how he felt? If someone left you and stayed away to protect you, how would that make you feel? What kinds of things do you do to protect people you care about?

4. Kenzie gives Leanansidhe a month of her life in exchange for gaining the Sight. What do you think of her decision? Are there any circumstances under which you would knowingly give up a month of your life?

5. Guro Javier believes Ethan when Ethan comes to him for help. What, if any, circumstances in your life require you to believe in something you can't see? What do you think would happen if Ethan did open up to kids at school?

6. Julie Kagawa's Iron Fey world began with the addition of the Iron faeries, who live with metal and technology that is poisonous to traditional faeries. Now she has added another type of faery to this world, the Forgotten. What do you think can make someone live on after death? What does immortality mean to you?

7. The Forgotten must steal the glamour of other faeries to survive. How do you feel about their circumstances? What would you do if you knew your life depended on stealing someone else's?

Turn the page for an exclusive excerpt from book 2
of Julie Kagawa's dark and riveting
BLOOD OF EDEN *series*
THE ETERNITY CURE

In a future world, vampires rule and humans are blood cattle.
New vampire Allison Sekemoto is on a quest to find and save her
creator, Kanin, from the sadistic vampire Sarren. Blood calls to
blood—but Allie's path has never been as simple as it seems....

Coming in May 2013

A "big white house" and a pointed finger was all I had to go on, but I found what the human was talking about easily enough. Almost due north from the tower, past a crumbling street lined with rusty cars and across another swampy lawn, a bristling fence rose out of the ground to scar the horizon. Twelve feet tall, made of black iron bars topped with coils of barbed wire, it was a familiar sight. I'd seen many walls in my travels across the country; concrete and wood, steel and stone. They were everywhere, surrounding every settlement, from tiny farms to entire cities. They all had one purpose: to keep rabids from slaughtering the population.

And there were a lot of rabids shambling about the perimeter, a pale, dead swarm. They prowled the walls, always searching, always hungry, looking for a way in. As I stopped in the shadow of a tree to watch, I noticed something weird. The rabids didn't rush the fence, clawing and biting, like they had the tower. They skulked around the edge, always a couple feet away, never touching the iron bars.

Looming above the gates, a squat white building crouched in the weeds. The entrance to the place was circular, lined with columns, and I could make out flickering lights through the windows.

Kanin, I thought. *Sarren. Where are you? I can feel you in there, somewhere.*

The breeze shifted, and the stench of the rabids hit me full force, making my nose wrinkle. They probably weren't going to let me saunter up and knock on the Prince's door, and I really didn't want another fight so soon after my last two. I was Hungry, and any more blood loss would drive me closer to the monster. Besides, there were a lot of rabids this time, a whole huge swarm, not just a few. Taking on this many would venture very close to suicide. Even I could be dragged under and torn apart by sheer numbers.

Frowning, I pondered my plan of attack. I needed to get inside, past the rabids, without being seen. The fence was only twelve feet tall; maybe I could vault over it?

One of the rabids snarled and shoved another that had jostled it, sending it stumbling toward the fence. Hissing, the other rabid put out a hand to catch itself and landed square on the iron bars.

There was a blinding flash and an explosion of sparks, and the rabid shrieked, convulsing on the metal. Its body jerked in spasms, sending the other rabids skittering back. Finally, the smoke pouring off its blackened skin erupted into flame and consumed the monster from the inside.

Okay, definitely not touching the fence.

I growled in frustration. Dawn wasn't far, and soon I would have to fall back to find shelter from the sun. Which meant abandoning any plans to get past the gate until tomorrow night. I was so close! I was right here, mere yards from my target, and the only thing keeping me from my goal was a rabid horde and a length of electrified metal.

Wait. Dawn was approaching. Which meant that the rabids would have to sleep soon. They couldn't face the light any better than a vampire; they would have to burrow into the ground to escape the burning rays of the sun.

Under normal circumstances, I would, as well.

But these weren't normal circumstances. And I wasn't your average vampire. Kanin had taught me better than that.

To keep up the appearance of being human, I'd trained myself to stay awake when the sun rose. Even though it was very, very difficult and something that went against my vampire instincts, I could remain awake and active if I had to. For a little while, at least. But the rabids were slaves to instinct and wouldn't even try to resist. They would vanish into the earth, and with the threat of rabids gone, the power that ran through the fence would probably be shut off. There'd be no need to keep it running in the daytime, especially with fuel or whatever powered the fence in short supply. If I could stay awake long enough, I'd have a clear shot to the house and whoever was inside it. I just had to deal with the sun.

It might not be smart, continuing my quest in the daylight. I would be slow, my reactions muted. But if Sarren was in that house, he would be slowed, as well. He might even be asleep, not expecting Kanin's vengeful daughter to come looking for him here. I could get the jump on him, if I could stay awake myself.

I scanned the grounds, marking where the shadows were thickest, where the trees grew close together. Smartly, the area surrounding the fence was clear of brush and trees, with no places a rabid could climb or hide from the sun. Indirect sunlight wouldn't harm us, but it could still cause a great deal of pain.

Finally, as the sky lightened and the sun grew close to breaking the horizon, the horde began to disappear. Breaking away from the fence, they skulked away to bury themselves in the soft mud, their pale bodies vanishing beneath water and earth until there wasn't a rabid to be seen.

I stayed up, leaning against the trunk of a thick oak, fighting the urge to follow the vicious creatures beneath the earth, to sleep and hide from the sun. It was madly difficult to stay awake. My thoughts grew sluggish, my body heavy and tired. I waited until the sun had risen nearly above the trees, to allow time for the fence to be shut down. It would be hilariously tragic if I avoided the rabids and the sun only to be fried to a crisp on a damn electric fence because I was too impatient. But my training to remain aboveground paid off. About twenty or so minutes after the horde disappeared, the faint hum coming from the metal barrier finally clicked off.

Now came the most dangerous part.

Pulling up my coat, I drew it over my head and tugged the sleeves down so they covered my hands. Direct sunlight on my skin would cause it to blacken, rupture and eventually burst into flame, but I could buy myself some time if it was covered.

Still, I was not looking forward to this.

All my vampire instincts were screaming at me to stop when I stepped out from under the branches, feeling even the weak rays of dawn beating down on me. Keeping my head down, I hurried across the grounds, moving from tree to tree and darting into shade whenever I could. The stretch closest to the fence was the most dangerous, with no trees, no cover, nothing but short grass and the sun heating the back of my coat. I clenched my teeth, hunched my shoulders and kept moving.

I scooped up a branch as I approached the black iron barrier, hurling it in front of me. It arced through the air and struck the bars with a faint clatter before dropping to the ground. No sparks, no flash of light, no smoke rising from the wood. I didn't know much about electric fences, but I took that as a good sign as I drew close enough to touch the bars.

Let's hope that fence is really off.

I leaped toward the top, feeling a brief stab of fear as my fingers curled around the bars. Thankfully, they remained cold and dead beneath my hands, and I scrambled over the fence in half a second, landing on the other side in a crouch.

In the brief moment it took me to leap over the iron barrier, my coat had slipped off my head, exposing it to the sun. My relief at being inside the fence without cooking myself was short-lived as a blinding flare of pain seared my face and hands. I gasped, frantically tugging my coat up while scrambling under the nearest tree. Crouching down, I examined my hands and winced. They were red and painful from just a few seconds of being hit by the sun.

I've got to get inside.

Keeping close to the ground, I hurried across the tangled, snowy lawn, feeling horribly exposed as I drew closer to the building. If someone pushed aside those heavy curtains that covered the huge windows, they would most definitely spot me. But the windows and grounds remained dark and empty as I reached the oval wall and darted beneath an archway, relieved to be out of the light.

Okay. Now what?

The faint tug, that subtle hint of knowing, was stronger than ever as I crept up the stairs and peeked through a curtained window. The strange, circular room beyond was dark and surprisingly intact. A table stood in the center, and several chairs sat around it, all thankfully deserted. Beyond that room was an empty hallway, and even more rooms beyond that.

I stifled a groan. Judging from the size of this place, finding one comatose vampire in such a huge house was going to be a challenge. But I couldn't give up. Kanin was in there somewhere. And so was Sarren.

The glass on the windows was shockingly unbroken, but

the window itself was unlocked. I slid through the frame and dropped silently onto the hardwood floor, glancing warily about. Humans lived here, I realized; a lot of them. I could smell them on the air, the lingering scent of warm bodies and blood. If Sarren was here, he'd likely painted the walls with it.

But I didn't run into any humans, alive or dead, as I made my way through the gigantic house, and that worried me. Especially since it was obvious this place was well taken care of. Nothing appeared broken. The walls and floor were clean and uncluttered, the furniture, though old, remarkably intact. The vampire Prince who lived here either had a lot of servants to keep the place up and running, or he was unbelievably dedicated to cleaning.

I kept expecting to run into someone, a human at the least and Sarren or the Prince at the worst. I continued to scan the shadows and the dozens of empty rooms, wary and alert, searching for movement. But the house remained dark and lifeless as I crept up a long flight of steps, down an equally long corridor and stopped outside a thick wooden door at the end.

This…this is it.

I could feel it, the pull that I'd followed over half the country to this spot, the sudden knowing that what I searched for was so close. Kanin was here. He was just on the other side. Or…I stopped myself from grasping the handle…would it be Sarren that I'd face, grinning manically as I opened the door? Would he be asleep, lying helpless on a bed? Or was he expecting me, as I'd begun to imagine from the silent, empty house? Something was wrong. Getting here had been way too easy. Whoever was on the other side of that door knew I was coming.

Carefully, I grasped my sword and eased it out, being sure the metal didn't scrape against the sheath. If Sarren was expecting me, I'd be ready, too. If Kanin was in there, I wasn't leaving until I got him out safe.

Grasping the door handle, I wrenched it to the side and flung the door open.

A figure stood at the back, waiting for me as I'd feared. He wore a black leather duster, and his thick dark hair tumbled to his broad shoulders. Leaning against the wall with his arms crossed, he didn't even raise an eyebrow as the door banged open. A pale, handsome face met mine over the room, lips curled into an evil smile. But it was the wrong face. I'd gotten everything wrong. I'd followed the wrong pull—and this vampire was supposed to be dead.

"Hello, sister," Jackal greeted, his gold eyes shining in the dim light. "It's about time you showed up."

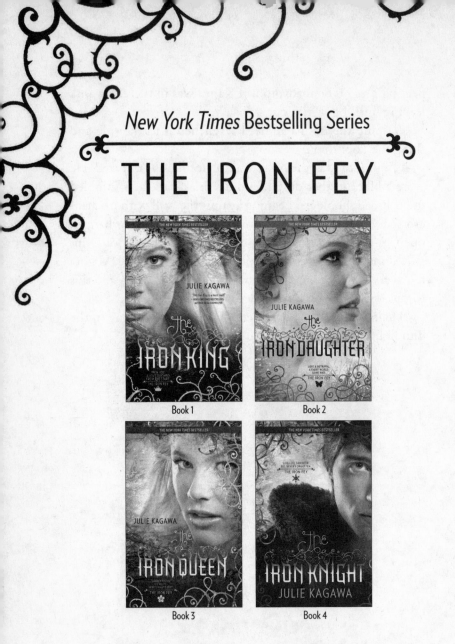
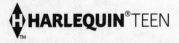

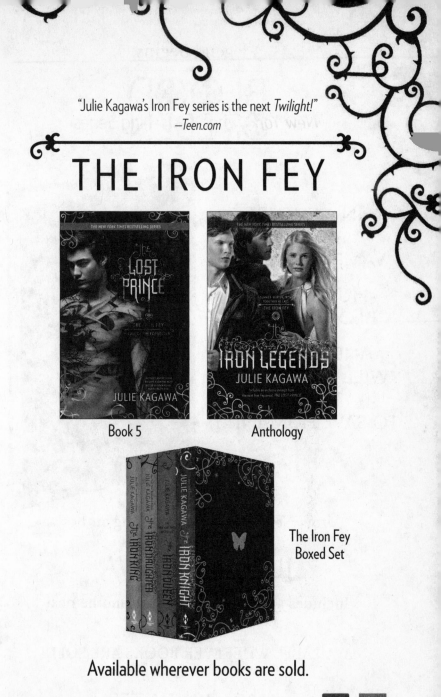

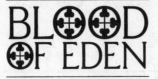
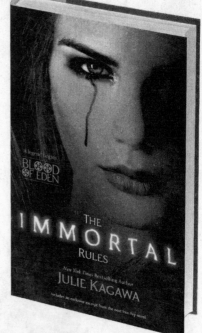
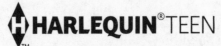

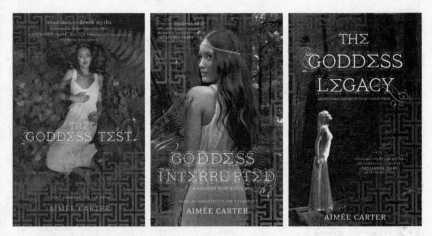
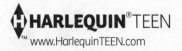

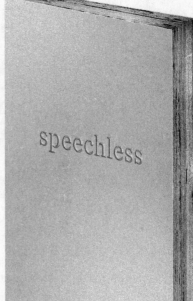
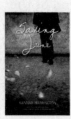
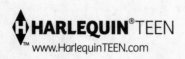